Gastroenterology For General Surgeons

Matthias W. Wichmann
Timothy K. McCullough
Ian C. Roberts-Thomson
Guy J. Maddern
Editors

Gastroenterology For General Surgeons

Springer

Editors
Matthias W. Wichmann
Department of Surgery
Mount Gambier Hospital
Mount Gambier
Australia

Timothy K. McCullough
Department of Surgery
Mount Gambier Hospital
Mount Gambier
Australia

Ian C. Roberts-Thomson
Adelaide Medical School
University of Adelaide
Adelaide
Australia

Guy J. Maddern
The Queen Elizabeth Hospital
University of Adelaide
Woodville South
Australia

ISBN 978-3-319-92767-1 ISBN 978-3-319-92768-8 (eBook)
https://doi.org/10.1007/978-3-319-92768-8

This Springer imprint is published by the registered company Springer Nature Switzerland AG.
The registered company address is: Gewerbestrasse 11, 6330 Cham, Switzerland

This book is dedicated to the memory of my surgical teacher, mentor and shining example Univ. Prof. Dr. med. Dr. h.c. Friedrich-Wilhelm Schildberg who passed away in September 2018 at the age of 84 years.
In gratitude, Matthias Wichmann.

Preface

Dear colleague, life is too short for bad books, but rest assured this is not one of them.

If you are working in an environment where support by a specialist gastroenterologist is limited,

if you are concerned that your knowledge about current gastroenterological problems and their management requires updating,

or if you are interested in a good book about the current nonsurgical treatment of diseases of the gastrointestinal tract,

then this book is for you.

This volume has been a challenge to edit and write for the general surgeons. We are therefore grateful to have secured the outstanding support and contributions of our coeditor Professor Ian C. Roberts-Thomson—an outstanding gastroenterologist. Without his never-ending enthusiasm, it would have been difficult to complete this work.

The book addresses nonsurgical conditions affecting the gastrointestinal tract. We sincerely hope it meets your expectations and will help to further improve your management of these diseases.

We are indebted to a large number of colleagues who offered their knowledge and time to contribute to this book. We are all aware it is difficult to find the time in our busy work schedule. We are most grateful to our contributing authors.

We would like to thank Springer-Verlag and their staff for the opportunity to publish our work with them.

Remarkable developments have occurred in gastroenterology and gastrointestinal surgery over the past 50 years. Some of us remember the introduction of flexible endoscopy. Larger numbers can recall the introduction of ultrasonography, computed tomography, and magnetic resonance imaging. Blood tests are now more accurate at differentiating inflammatory causes for pain from non-inflammatory conditions. Laparoscopic surgery was in its infancy in 1990 but is currently the procedure of choice for many gastrointestinal disorders.

There has also been a dramatic change in the incidence of various diseases with falls in the incidence of appendicitis and peptic ulcers and rises in the incidence of nonalcoholic fatty liver disease and inflammatory bowel disorders.

Fifty years ago, there were only minor areas of overlap between the interests of gastroenterologists and general surgeons, but boundaries have been blurred by the passage of time and then came the Internet and more knowledgeable and sometimes more demanding patients.

Aspects of medical care that have remained unchanged include the benefits of a careful evaluation of symptoms and clinical signs, the allocation of time for an adequate explanation for symptoms, and the development of a doctor-patient relationship that aids the management of chronic symptoms.

We hope that you enjoy reading this book and, more importantly, that the information contained in this book results in better outcomes for patients and greater satisfaction for surgeons.

Mount Gambier, SA, Australia
Woodville South, SA, Australia

The Editors

Contents

1 Functional Dyspepsia and the Irritable Bowel Syndrome

Ian C. Roberts-Thomson

1.1 Introduction

Intermittent gastrointestinal symptoms are a normal component of human life. Common examples include epigastric discomfort after larger meals, apparent intolerance of foods such as spices and coffee and a bowel habit that is somewhat irregular in response to variation in diet, alcohol use and stress. These symptoms are interpreted as a consequence of lifestyle factors by most people and only rarely as a reason to seek medical advice. However, some individuals have more prominent symptoms, either intermittently or persistently, which are perceived as abnormal and that impair the expectation of a "normal" quality of life. When investigations are unhelpful, these symptoms are often labelled as "functional" although this term sheds little light on the nature of pathogenic mechanisms. Symptoms that focus on the upper gastrointestinal tract are usually called either functional or non-ulcer dyspepsia. Symptoms that focus on the lower gastrointestinal tract are typically called the irritable bowel syndrome. Additional categories include functional biliary-type pain, discussed in Chapter 17, and chronic abdominal pain of unknown cause, often called the functional abdominal pain syndrome. While some patients readily fit into one of the above categories, many are more difficult to categorize because of symptoms that include both the upper and lower gastrointestinal tracts.

I. C. Roberts-Thomson (✉)
School of Medicine, University of Adelaide, Adelaide, SA, Australia
e-mail: ian.robertsthomson@adelaide.edu.au

M. W. Wichmann et al. (eds.), *Gastroenterology For General Surgeons*,
https://doi.org/10.1007/978-3-319-92768-8_1

1.2 Epidemiology

Intermittent dyspepsia is common, particularly in adults. The prevalence in Caucasian populations has been estimated at 5–15%, but this varies considerably depending on the survey method [questionnaire or interview], methods for the definition of symptoms and the length of the observation period. Even higher prevalence rates occur when symptoms are expanded to include those of esophageal reflux such as regurgitation and heartburn. Most studies indicate that the prevalence in women is modestly higher than that in men. Prevalence rates do not appear to be influenced by age as there is a similar number with new-onset symptoms to those whose symptoms resolve spontaneously.

The proportion of patients with dyspepsia who seek medical attention has been estimated at approximately 50%. This probably includes those with more severe symptoms of recent onset, but other factors can be relevant including fear of serious illness, serious illness in a friend or relative and anxiety or psychological stress. Other people with dyspepsia simply tolerate their symptoms, experiment with over-the-counter products or consult a variety of non-medical practitioners.

In contrast to dyspepsia, there is more reliable data on the prevalence of the irritable bowel syndrome. Using criteria agreed by an international panel [Rome I–IV criteria], the global prevalence of the irritable bowel syndrome is approximately 10%. Prevalence rates may be highest in South America and lowest in Africa. In Western populations, the prevalence in women is somewhat higher than that in men with the majority of patients in the age group 30–50 years. In Asia, the irritable bowel syndrome is more prevalent in younger age groups but is equally common among males and females.

Not all people with irritable bowel symptoms consult medical practitioners. In Western countries, women are more likely to seek help than men, perhaps because symptoms are more frequent and severe. Women are also less likely to attribute symptoms to anxiety and stress. In contrast, men are more likely to consult medical practitioners in some parts of Asia [e.g. India], perhaps because of cultural differences in the interpretation and response to symptoms.

The functional abdominal pain syndrome is much less common than functional dyspepsia or the irritable bowel syndrome with a population prevalence of approximately 1%. The majority of these patients are women who often exhibit chronic pain behaviour and significant psychological disturbance.

The financial burden of functional gastrointestinal disorders on personal and national health budgets is substantial. The National Health Insurance database in South Korea estimated that 6% of the population sought medical care for irritable bowel symptoms at least once per year. This generated outpatient visits, investigations and hospitalization that accounted for approximately 0.5% of the total medical budget. In many other countries without national insurance schemes, these costs are borne by the patient, sometimes by diverting funds from critical areas such as food and housing. In the USA, direct costs associated with functional bowel disorders have been estimated at $20 billion per year.

1.3 Symptoms of Functional Gastrointestinal Disorders

The term dyspepsia describes a variety of symptoms localised to the epigastric region. The major symptoms are those of postprandial fullness, early satiety, epigastric pain and epigastric burning. However, additional symptoms may be present such as nausea, prominent burping and abdominal bloating. The presence of esophageal symptoms is relatively common in clinical practice, but significant esophageal symptoms would place patients outside the relatively strict category of functional dyspepsia. This difficulty with terminology has led to the development of consensus views on definitions [Rome criteria] that have particular relevance for the development and interpretation of clinical studies. In the Rome III consensus, functional dyspepsia was subdivided into two groups: a postprandial distress syndrome that included postprandial fullness and early satiety and an epigastric pain syndrome characterized by epigastric pain or burning. This subdivision was supported by epidemiologic studies showing that there was no major overlap of symptoms between the two groups.

In the Rome consensus, postprandial fullness describes an unpleasant sensation of prolonged persistence of food in the stomach after meals. Early satiety is a sensation that the stomach is full or overfull soon after starting a meal with the result that the meal cannot be finished. Epigastric pain describes an intense and unpleasant sensation in the epigastrium which can lead to concern about the presence of significant disease. Epigastric burning describes an unpleasant sensation of heat or discomfort in the epigastrium, often but not always related to meals.

In contrast, the major symptoms of the irritable bowel syndrome are recurrent abdominal pain [often related to defecation], a change in the frequency of defecation and changes in the appearance of stools. These are often accompanied by abdominal bloating and sometimes by other gastrointestinal symptoms such as nausea. Again, patients have been subdivided according to bowel habit into those with diarrhea as a prominent symptom [IBS with diarrhea], constipation as a prominent symptom [IBS with constipation], alternating diarrhea and constipation [IBS with mixed symptoms] and unsubtyped IBS. These subtypes may improve the homogeneity of patients in clinical trials and assist with the study of pathophysiologic mechanisms and therapy. Rome IV criteria for the diagnosis of functional dyspepsia and irritable bowel syndrome are listed in Table 1.1.

Care needs to be taken in categorizing the presence of diarrhea and constipation in individual patients. For example, most patients appropriately describe diarrhea as the presence of loose stools, but diarrhea may be an alternative description for fecal incontinence. Other important historical features are the duration of symptoms, the presence or otherwise of fluctuating symptoms, stool characteristics, associated symptoms, diet and medication. Constipation can be even more difficult as assessment is complicated by issues such as hard stools, difficult defecation and laxative use. One definition of a normal bowel habit ranges from two stools per day to two stools per week, but this is more complex in individuals who "only have a bowel action with laxatives". The prevalence of self-perceived constipation in adult communities usually ranges from 10% to 20% and is more common in women than in men.

Table 1.1 Rome IV criteria for the diagnosis of functional dyspepsia and the irritable bowel syndrome

Functional dyspepsia – postprandial distress syndrome
• Bothersome postprandial fullness, occurring after ordinary-sized meals, at least several times per week
• Early satiation that prevents finishing a regular meal, at least several times per week
Supportive criteria include upper abdominal bloating, postprandial nausea and excessive belching. The epigastric pain syndrome may coexist
Functional dyspepsia – epigastric pain syndrome
• Pain or burning localized to the epigastrium, of at least moderate severity, at least once per week. Pain is intermittent, not generalized and not relieved by defecation and does not fulfil the criteria for biliary pain
Supportive criteria include pain induced or relieved by ingestion of a meal. The postprandial distress syndrome may coexist. A component of retrosternal pain excludes the strict definition of functional dyspepsia but is common in clinical practice. Many older studies have defined dyspepsia as predominant epigastric pain for at least 1 month, sometimes associated with epigastric fullness, nausea, vomiting or mild heartburn
Irritable bowel syndrome
• Recurrent abdominal pain on most days associated with at least two of the following three symptoms: pain related to defecation, changes in the frequency of stool and changes in the form [appearance] of stool
Supportive criteria include the absence of warning symptoms. For both functional dyspepsia and the irritable bowel syndrome, patients included in contemporary clinical trials have usually fulfilled criteria for 3 months and describe the onset of symptoms as >6 months

Whether patients with functional disorders are more likely than control subjects to have symptoms outside the gastrointestinal tract is still being debated. However, some authors highlight unexplained symptoms such as headaches, urinary symptoms and other pain syndromes as evidence for a more generalized pain disorder not restricted to the gastrointestinal tract. There is also the issue of psychiatric disorders that could be of primary importance or secondary to persistent gastrointestinal symptoms.

1.4 Pathogenesis

Several factors appear to influence susceptibility to functional disorders. These include genetic factors, psychosocial distress, psychiatric disorders, visceral hypersensitivity, activation of mucosal immunity, altered gastrointestinal motility, dietary influences and changes in the intestinal microbiome and intestinal permeability. Although mutations influencing intestinal fluid transport and carbohydrate metabolism have been identified, these mutations are rare and only account for symptoms in a small minority of patients.

A controversial area is the importance of psychiatric disorders and changes in the brain-gut axis. Patients with functional disorders have a higher than expected frequency of childhood abuse, anxiety and depression and frequently describe abdominal symptoms that are aggravated by stress. In addition, some show an exaggerated response to stress with higher circulating levels of corticotropin-releasing factor. These observations support the hypothesis of brain-to-gut pathways, but a primary role for the central nervous system seems likely in fewer than 50% of patients.

An interesting subgroup of patients develops an irritable bowel syndrome after an episode of gastroenteritis. Various infectious agents have been implicated including bacteria, viruses and protozoa, but bacterial infections with *Salmonella* and *Campylobacter* species have been most prominent in the UK. The frequency of persistent irritable bowel-type symptoms after an episode of gastroenteritis has been estimated at 10–20%. Many of these patients have histological features of persistent, low-grade inflammation with an increase in mucosal lymphocytes and mast cells in the small and large bowel. For functional dyspepsia, a consensus view is that gastric infection with *Helicobacter pylori* [*H. pylori*] causes or aggravates symptoms in a minority of patients. There is also some evidence for an increase in mucosal eosinophils in the upper gastrointestinal tract in the subgroup of patients with postprandial distress syndrome.

Some patients with functional disorders have changes in gastrointestinal motility. For example, approximately 25% of patients with functional dyspepsia have delayed gastric emptying. In the irritable bowel syndrome, transit time through the small and large bowel is often accelerated with diarrhea and delayed with constipation. Another area is the sensory function of the gastrointestinal tract that appears to be hypersensitive [visceral hypersensitivity] to stimuli such as balloons that inflate various parts of the bowel. In most patients, this is not associated with hypersensitivity to stimuli applied to the skin.

Other factors include diet, the intestinal microbiome and gastrointestinal permeability. Functional symptoms are aggravated by food in up to 50% of patients, particularly those with functional dyspepsia. Intolerance of specific foods is also common although blinded trials only show resolution of symptoms during withdrawal and reproduction of symptoms during rechallenge in a minority of patients. These non-immune mechanisms need to be distinguished from food allergy [e.g. peanuts, cows' milk and eggs] mediated by IgE. More recently a group of poorly absorbed, short-chain carbohydrates have been implicated in the pathogenesis of irritable bowel symptoms. These compounds described under the acronym FODMAPs include fructose, lactose, fructans, galacto-oligosaccharides and polyols. They may aggravate irritable bowel symptoms by osmotic activity in the small bowel and gas production with distension in the large bowel. The role of the intestinal microbiome in the pathogenesis of functional symptoms has not yet been clarified. Some patients appear to have mild bacterial overgrowth in the small bowel, while others have evidence of reduced microbial diversity in faeces but no characteristic microbial marker. There is also evidence of abnormal intestinal permeability in some patients, particularly those with diarrhea, but whether this is related to changes in the intestinal microbiome remains unclear. Greater intestinal permeability could explain mild bowel inflammation and changes in visceral sensitivity.

Functional gastrointestinal symptoms cannot be explained by a single algorithm. In some patients, it seems likely that the central nervous system is the primary mediator with secondary effects on the enteric nervous system. Whether these effects are related to overactivity of the hypothalamic-pituitary-adrenal axis, the autonomic nervous system or other pathways remain unclear. In other patients, the primary stimulus arises in the gut with a gut-to-brain axis. This applies to the postinfectious irritable bowel and diet-induced symptoms and may apply to changes in the intestinal microbiome with potential changes in intestinal permeability.

1.5 Towards a Positive Diagnosis of Functional Syndromes

Surveys suggest that up to 50% of patients seen by specialist physicians or surgeons because of unexplained abdominal symptoms have a functional disorder. The challenge for both the general practitioner and the specialist is to avoid missing important diagnoses and, at the same time, to avoid unhelpful and expensive investigations. At one end of the spectrum is the younger adult with long-standing symptoms who has had a number of negative investigations. At the other end is the older adult with symptoms of recent onset who may have had only limited or no investigation. Clearly, the probability of a non-functional disorder is higher in the latter group.

Guidance on the probability of non-functional disorders, particularly cancer, has resulted in the publication of alarm or "red flag" symptoms. For upper gastrointestinal symptoms, these include dysphagia, severe pain, protracted vomiting, unintentional weight loss, anaemia and a positive fecal occult blood test [guaiac test]. Unfortunately, the reality is that most cancers exhibiting one or more of these symptoms are relatively advanced and sometimes have a poor prognosis. For lower gastrointestinal symptoms, alarm features include age over 50 years with no previous colon cancer screening, a recent change in bowel habit, overt gastrointestinal bleeding, nocturnal pain or passage of stools, unintentional weight loss and a positive fecal occult blood test [usually an immunochemical test].

A short list of non-functional disorders that can cause upper gastrointestinal symptoms is provided in Table 1.2. Chronic duodenal or gastric ulcers are found at endoscopy in up to 10% of patients. A further 10% have endoscopic evidence of reflux esophagitis with at least some inflammation or mucosal ulceration in the lower esophagus. Gastric or esophageal cancers are diagnosed in fewer than 2% of patients.

In patients with lower gastrointestinal symptoms, the differential diagnosis is influenced by the nature of the presenting symptoms, particularly the presence of diarrhea or constipation. One difficulty is the role of diverticulosis in the pathogenesis of symptoms. Diverticula are uncommon below the age of 50 years but increase in frequency thereafter to affect up to 50% of adults by the age of 70 years. While the majority of affected individuals are asymptomatic, a minority with more extensive disease can have an irregular bowel habit, intermittent pain and changes in the appearance of stools. A short list of non-functional disorders presenting with either diarrhea or constipation is provided in Table 1.3.

Screening tests for the presence of non-functional disease have been recommended by several authors. For functional dyspepsia-type symptoms, these may include a full blood examination, ESR, urea, electrolytes and liver function tests.

Table 1.2 Non-functional disorders that can cause intermittent upper gastrointestinal symptoms[a]

• Reflux esophagitis
• Chronic duodenal ulcer
• Chronic gastric ulcer
• Gallstone disease
• Adverse effects from medication
• Diabetic gastroparesis
• Chronic pancreatitis
• Gastric cancer
• Pancreatic neoplasms
• Miscellaneous: hernias, mechanical disorders, angina and others

[a]In approximate order of frequency

Table 1.3 Non-functional disorders that can cause intermittent lower gastrointestinal symptoms[a]

• Severe diverticulosis
• Colorectal cancer [and larger polyps]
• Inflammatory bowel disease
• Microscopic [lymphocytic] colitis
• Adverse effects from medication
• Celiac disease
• Radiation colitis
• Rectal prolapse and solitary rectal ulcer syndrome
• Fecal impaction and incontinence
• Laxative abuse
• Ovarian cancer
• Miscellaneous: thyroid disease, bacterial overgrowth syndromes, neuroendocrine tumours of pancreas and others

[a]In approximate order of frequency

Other options include serological tests for *H. pylori* antibodies and celiac disease. A negative test for *H. pylori* largely excludes duodenal ulceration, but gastric ulceration may still occur in those who use non-steroidal, anti-inflammatory drugs. Patients with persistent symptoms often proceed to endoscopy, but abnormalities are unusual in younger adults.

For irritable bowel-type patients, screening tests will be influenced by the presence of constipation or diarrhea. A full blood examination, ESR and/or C-reactive protein and urea, electrolytes and liver function tests are appropriate in most individuals. In those with diarrhea, additional tests may include fecal occult blood, fecal calprotectin, fecal microscopy and culture, celiac serology and thyroid function tests. In older women, a pelvic ultrasound study may be appropriate in those with symptoms of short duration to exclude ovarian cancer. The majority of older patients, especially those with diarrhea, will proceed to colonoscopy to exclude colorectal cancer, inflammatory bowel disease and microscopic colitis. The role of bile acid malabsorption in the pathogenesis of chronic diarrhea remains uncertain, and testing is not readily available at present.

Unfortunately, there is no accurate diagnostic test for either functional dyspepsia or the irritable bowel syndrome. Nevertheless, these functional disorders should not be simply a diagnosis of exclusion. Evidence for the stability of functional diagnoses comes from several longitudinal studies indicating that the emergence of important new diagnoses in patients previously diagnosed with functional disorders is rare. Furthermore, another study showed that patients diagnosed with functional disorders on the basis of symptoms rarely had positive findings from more extensive investigation.

1.6 Research Investigations in Functional Disorders

Several techniques have been described in an attempt to define mechanisms of potential relevance to the pathogenesis of both functional dyspepsia and the irritable bowel syndrome. Some of these relate to motility and sensation in the gastrointestinal tract, while others have explored potential changes in the function of parts of the central nervous system. In functional dyspepsia, gastrointestinal investigations have included motility in the stomach and duodenum, rates of gastric emptying and accommodation and sensation, mostly in thc stomach. Similar studies have been performed in the colon and rectum in the irritable bowel syndrome.

The major methods for the assessment of gastric emptying have included scintigraphy of radiolabelled solid and liquid meals, breath tests using radiolabelled octanoic acid and specialized tests using ultrasound and magnetic resonance imaging. Although some patients have delayed gastric emptying [approximately 25%], a consensus view is that there is no clear relationship between delayed emptying and subtypes of functional dyspepsia. Similarly, research studies using a gastric balloon [barostat] have revealed gastric hypersensitivity and impaired accommodation in 30%–40% of patients but no or only weak correlations between test abnormalities and symptoms. Manometry of the stomach and duodenum is a highly specialized area but does not, as yet, appear to assist with the diagnosis of functional dyspepsia.

Similar studies have been performed in individuals with the irritable bowel syndrome. In the diarrhea-predominant group, several studies have shown that the majority have rapid transit through the colon and that some have rapid transit through the small bowel. In the constipation-predominant group, transit through the colon may be normal or slow. Visceral hypersensitivity is also a common feature with more prominent symptoms after balloon distension, gaseous distension or standard meals. Changes in motility have also been confirmed by manometric studies in the colon, but none have been specific for subtypes of the irritable bowel syndrome.

Yet another area of interest has been brain structure and function because of the likelihood of central influences on abdominal symptoms. Subtle changes have been noted on neuroimaging studies such as positron emission tomography and magnetic resonance imaging, but the significance of these changes remains unclear. A particular area of interest is the role of the autonomic nervous system which is linked to both the enteric nervous system and to states of arousal and emotion. However, activation of the autonomic nervous system is difficult to study, and it is possible that activation can be restricted to particular organs such as the gastrointestinal tract. Finally, it is difficult to ignore the association between functional syndromes and psychological issues that include personality profiles, family relationships, physical and sexual abuse, societal myths and cultural differences.

1.7 Treatment

As both functional dyspepsia and the irritable bowel syndrome are heterogeneous disorders, it comes as no surprise that there is no simple algorithm in relation to therapy. One important aspect is an effective doctor-patient relationship that provides reassurance, a positive diagnosis and at least a partial explanation for symptoms. Referral to a psychiatrist or psychologist is often resisted by patients although a meta-analysis showed some benefit from cognitive behavioural therapy and hypnotherapy. Regular exercise programmes, meditation and other stress-reduction methods also appear to be of some help. Another consideration in the interpretation of randomized trials of medication is improvement in symptoms in 30–40% of patients treated with placebo.

Recognition of the potential role of FODMAPs has led to renewed interest in the dietary management of functional disorders. In functional dyspepsia, this may include small regular meals and limits on the intake of coffee, alcohol, fatty foods and other foods identified as potential aggravating factors. For the irritable bowel syndrome, insoluble fibre in the form of bran may improve constipation but aggravate pain and bloating. These adverse effects do not appear to occur with soluble fibre in the form of psyllium husks. In randomized trials, the low-FODMAP diet was of similar or greater benefit for irritable bowel symptoms than conventional dietary recommendations. Additional data on these specialised diets is awaited with interest.

A wide range of prescription and over-the-counter medication is available for the treatment of functional disorders. These include agents with effects on gastrointestinal motility, gastric acid secretion and gut microbiota as well as agents with effects on anxiety and depression. Some of these drugs have been superior to placebo in randomized trials, but the degree of benefit is often small. As a result, it is common for patients to experiment with alternative therapies such as herbal preparations, probiotics and other products such as melatonin. Some of these preparations appear to be helpful in individual patients, but large randomized trials have not been reported.

In functional dyspepsia, it is common for patients to be treated with drugs that reduce gastric acid secretion such as histamine [H2] receptor antagonists or proton pump inhibitors. Currently, proton pump inhibitors are more widely used, but efficacy is modest and is largely restricted to those with heartburn and the subgroup with epigastric pain. In a typical study, improvement occurs in 50% of patients treated with anti-secretory drugs versus 30% of those treated with placebo. The number needed to treat [NNT] for one to have significant benefit over treatment with placebo has been estimated at six. Another option is a serological test for *H. pylori* followed by therapy in those with positive results. Although different results have emerged from different trials, a consensus view is that eradication of *H. pylori* is of benefit with a NNT of between 7 and 13. As functional dyspepsia is sometimes associated with delayed gastric emptying, there has been a continuing interest in drugs that enhance gastric motility. Potential agents include metoclopramide, cisapride, mosapride and domperidone, but the former three drugs are unsuitable for long-term use because of side-effects. Domperidone appears to be relatively safe, but there is a debate as to efficacy, and the drug has not been approved for use in the USA. In contrast, there is good evidence for benefit from tricyclic antidepressant drugs although improvement in symptoms is not necessarily accompanied by improvement in features such as delayed gastric emptying. Various drugs have been used in clinical trials including amitriptyline, nortriptyline, imipramine and desipramine with an NNT of approximately six. Reasons for benefit remain unclear but include a degree of sedation and improvement in sleep patterns. However, some patients are reluctant to take medication for "depression", while others have anticholinergic side-effects such as dry mouth, constipation and urinary retention. Interestingly, serotonin reuptake inhibitors do not appear to be helpful, perhaps because the medication sometimes results in nausea and dyspepsia.

Drug therapy for patients with the irritable bowel syndrome often needs to be individualized because of variation in symptoms, particularly in relation to bowel habit. In those with diarrhea as the major symptom, the intermittent or regular use of loperamide may suffice. When diarrhea is accompanied by significant pain, tricyclic antidepressants usually slow intestinal transit and often have beneficial effects on pain. Alternative agents for those with more difficult diarrhea include alosetron, a 5-hydroxytryptamine type 3 receptor agonist, and eluxadoline, a novel drug that acts on opioid receptors. Both drugs are expensive and have been associated with significant adverse events. Rifaximin, a poorly absorbed antibiotic, also appears to be helpful in patients with the irritable bowel syndrome who are not troubled by constipation. In randomized trials, the drug was superior to placebo for global symptoms and abdominal bloating.

For the irritable bowel syndrome with constipation, initial measures usually focus on the treatment of constipation. This may involve an increase in dietary fibre although this is sometimes accompanied by a temporary increase in abdominal pain and bloating. Alternative measures include the use of soluble fibre [psyllium husk], lactulose or polyethylene glycol. For patients with difficult constipation, options include the novel drugs, lubiprostone and linaclotide, that increase fluid secretion into the gastrointestinal tract. Both drugs usually improve constipation but are expensive and only have modest effects on pain and global symptoms. Antispasmodic drugs including peppermint oil appear to be helpful in some individuals but have rarely been exposed to randomized trials.

1.8 Conclusion

Functional gastrointestinal disorders are common throughout the world with significant effects on the quality of life of affected individuals. Furthermore, they generate a substantial economic burden because of costs associated with medical consultation, investigation, hospitalization and therapy. The major disorders are functional dyspepsia and the irritable bowel syndrome, but there is heterogeneity in relation to symptoms and overlap between the two disorders. Although functional disorders are broadly seen as disorders of the brain-gut axis, there is evidence that the primary event resides in the brain in some patients and the gut in others. The challenge for medical research is to define biological mechanisms in more detail and to integrate these pathways with factors such as genetic and epigenetic influences, gender, early life stressors and psychological and psychiatric disorders.

There is no simple algorithm for the management of functional disorders. Arguably, the most helpful measure is a good doctor-patient relationship with appropriate advice on diet and lifestyle. Medication is beneficial in up to 60% of patients, but this compares with placebo benefit in 30%. In functional dyspepsia, relatively inexpensive therapies of established benefit include acid suppression medication, eradication of *H. pylori* and tricyclic antidepressant drugs. For the irritable bowel syndrome, tricyclic antidepressants are helpful for diarrhea, and several other agents are useful in individual settings. The prospect of a highly effective therapy for functional syndromes seems remote at present unless visceral sensation can be modified without the emergence of major adverse events.

Recommended Reading

Chang L, Di Lorenzo C, Farrugia G, et al. Functional bowel disorders: a roadmap to guide the next generation of research. Gastroenterology. 2018;154:723–35.

Drossman DA, Hasler WL. Rome 1 V Functional GI disorders: disorders of gut-brain interaction. Gastroenterology. 2016;150:1257–61.

Ford AC, Lacy BE, Talley NJ. Irritable bowel syndrome. N Engl J Med. 2017;376:2566–78.

Gwee K-A, Ghoshal UC, Chen M. Irritable bowel syndrome in Asia: pathogenesis, natural history, epidemiology and management. J Gastroenterol Hepatol. 2018;33:99–110.

Moayyedi PM, Lacy BE, Andrews CN, Enns RA, Howden CW, Vakil N. ACG and CAG clinical guidelines: management of dyspepsia. Am J Gastroenterol. 2017;112:988–1013.

Sahoo S, Padhy SK. Cross-cultural and psychological issues in irritable bowel syndrome. J Gastroenterol Hepatol. 2017;32:1679–85.

Tack J, Talley NJ. Functional dyspepsia-symptoms, definitions and validity of the Rome 111 criteria. Nat Rev Gastroenterol Hepatol. 2013;10:134–41.

Talley NJ, Silverstein MD, Agreus L, Sonnenberg A, Holtmann G. AGA Technical review: evaluation of dyspepsia. Gastroenterology. 1998;114:582–95.

Vanheel H, Carbone F, Valvekens L, et al. Pathophysiological abnormalities in functional dyspepsia subgroups according to the Rome 111 criteria. Am J Gastroenterol. 2017;112:132–40.

Diverticular Disease 2

Matthias W. Wichmann

2.1 Epidemiology/Risk Factors/Pathogenesis

Diverticulosis of the large bowel is defined by the presence of multiple diverticula in the bowel wall (Fig. 2.1). A colonic diverticulum is a protrusion of the bowel wall at the position where the vasa recta penetrate the circular muscle layer of the colon. Since only the mucosa and submucosa herniate, the colonic diverticulum is a "false" or pulsion diverticulum. This defect of the bowel wall is only covered by serosa.

During recent years there has been a continuous increase of hospital admissions for both uncomplicated and complicated diverticular disease, with approximately 100 new cases per 100,000 population diagnosed annually. At age 60, 40–60% of the population have developed diverticula. Male and female patients are equally affected. Of interest, the distribution of diverticulosis within the colon varies by geography. Patients from western and industrialized nations have sigmoid diverticula in 95% of all cases. In Asia, diverticulosis is predominantly localized in the ascending colon.

Risk factors for the development of diverticulosis and subsequent progression to diverticular disease include environmental and lifestyle factors, but the connection between disease and exposure to potential risk factors is largely unclear. The role of *fiber* in the development of diverticulosis is unclear. While early studies suggested that a diet low in fiber would contribute to the development of diverticular disease, this has not been confirmed in more recent publications. A diet low in fiber and high in total *fat* or *red meat* however significantly increases the risk of diverticular disease. Lack of *physical activity* combined with low dietary fiber intake increases the risk of symptomatic diverticular disease. *Obesity* increases the risk of complicated diverticular disease (infection, bleeding). *Smoking* increases the risk for

M. W. Wichmann (✉)
Department of Surgery, Mount Gambier General Hospital, Mount Gambier, SA, Australia
e-mail: matthias.wichmann@sa.gov.au

M. W. Wichmann et al. (eds.), *Gastroenterology For General Surgeons*,
https://doi.org/10.1007/978-3-319-92768-8_2

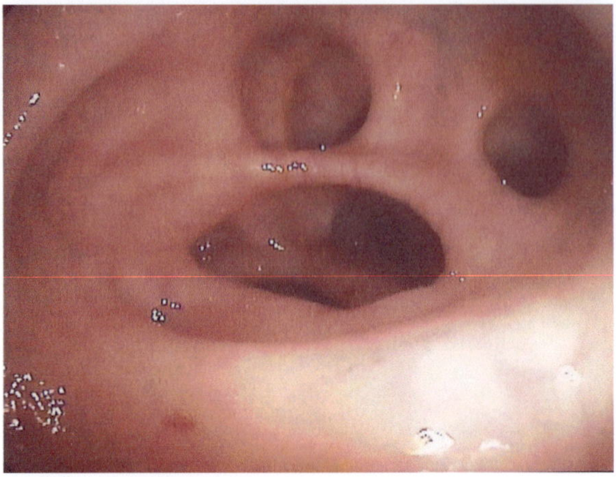

Fig. 2.1 Colonoscopic impression of uncomplicated diverticulosis

complicated diverticular disease (perforation, abscess). *Medications* associated with increased risks of diverticular disease (infection, bleeding) are nonsteroidal anti-inflammatory drugs, steroids, and opiates.

No increased risk for the development of diverticular disease has been associated with the following lifestyle choices: caffeine, alcohol, nuts, corn, and popcorn consumption.

No single risk factor will cause the development of diverticular disease, but the combination of several of the "classical" risk factors (lack of fiber, fat, red meat, lack of physical activity, obesity, smoking, NSAIDS, steroids, opiates) can be identified in most patients with symptomatic diverticular disease.

There is no effective *secondary prophylaxis* once diverticular disease has developed.

The *pathogenesis* for the development of diverticula is not completely clear. It appears that abnormal colonic motility with hypersegmentation of the large bowel (exaggerated segmentation contractions) and subsequently increased intraluminal pressure predispose to the development of diverticula. This hypothesis makes sense when looking at diverticular disease of the sigmoid colon (smallest diameter, high pressure zone at rectosigmoid junction). Higher intraluminal pressures in this segment of the bowel can be explained with Laplace's law according to which pressure is proportional to wall tension and inversely proportional to the radius. The "high pressure zone hypothesis" does not help to explain the higher prevalence of right-sided diverticular disease in the Asian population. The development of *complicated diverticular disease* with bleeding and/or infection/perforation is somewhat easier to explain. Bleeding occurs due to the close proximity of the vasa recta to the diverticulum. Structural changes of the artery and mechanical injury can lead to rupture and blood loss into the lumen. Infection results from a perforation of the diverticulum through erosion of the wall. Smaller infections are usually contained, but free perforations or fistulating processes can also occur.

2.2 Diagnosis/Differential Diagnosis

Acute diverticulitis is a clinical diagnosis based on lower abdominal pain (usually left lower quadrant), worsening pain on palpation, and inflammatory changes in blood testing (white blood cell count, C-reactive protein). The diagnosis should be confirmed by computed tomography (CT) of the abdomen and pelvis. The CT also identifies noncomplicated acute diverticulitis (Fig. 2.2) versus complicated (perforation, abscess, obstruction, fistula) (Figs. 2.3 and 2.4).

Differential diagnoses to be considered in patients presenting with suspected acute diverticulitis include:

- Irritable bowel syndrome
- Colon cancer
- Inflammatory bowel disease
- Urinary tract infection
- Infectious/neoplastic conditions of the ovaries/adnexa

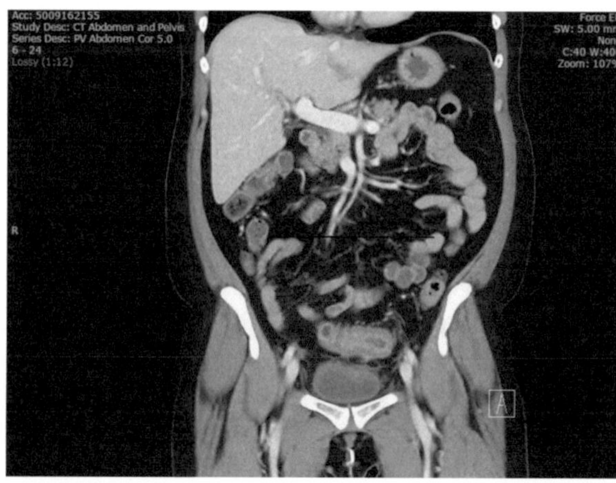

Fig. 2.2 CT scan of uncomplicated acute diverticulitis (patient TB—day 1)

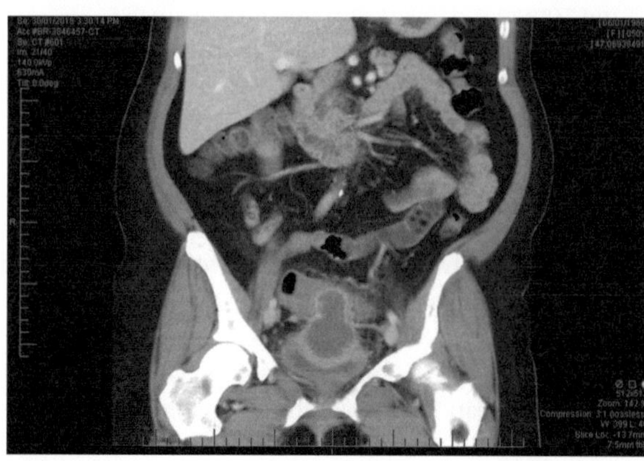

Fig. 2.3 CT scan of complicated acute diverticulitis (patient TB—day 3)

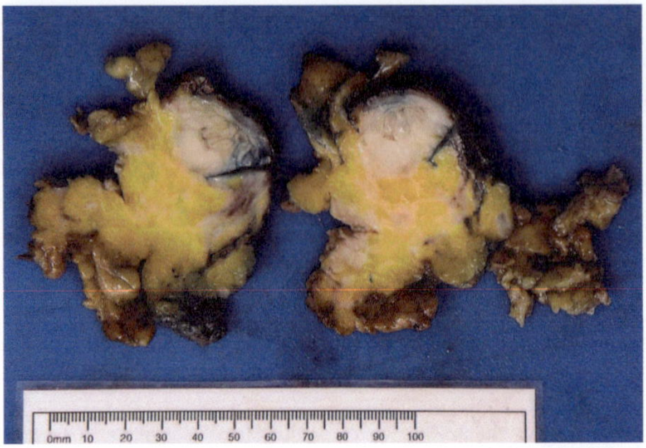

Fig. 2.4 Perforated diverticulum with impacted bone (postoperative diagnosis) causing obstruction

2.3 Nonsurgical Management

Acute diverticulitis can be managed with inpatient or outpatient treatment depending on the patient's presentation, the severity of disease, and other circumstances (remoteness, time of presentation, available support structures).

Acute uncomplicated diverticulitis can usually be treated conservatively. Conservative treatment may include one initial dose of IV antibiotics followed by oral antibiotics and subsequent outpatient reassessment (3 days after initial presentation, until complete resolution of symptoms). Alternatively, the patient may need to be admitted for IV antibiotics and clinical observation. Hospital admission for management of uncomplicated acute diverticulitis is necessary in patients with immunosuppression, fever, uncontrolled pain, advanced age, or significant comorbidities.

Successful conservative management of acute uncomplicated diverticulitis carries the risk of recurrent disease in approximately 2% of all patients per annum. Only patients with increased risks of complications or mortality should be discussed for elective surgery: organ transplant patient, immunosuppression, diabetes, and chronic organ dysfunction (lung, kidney, liver).

Acute noncomplicated diverticulitis requires oral antibiotic treatment for 7–10 days after diagnosis (Table 2.1). The treatment must cover the gastrointestinal flora of Gram-negative and anaerobe bacteria, especially *E. coli* and *B. fragilis*. There is no evidence to support dietary changes for patients selected for outpatient management.

Acute complicated diverticulitis requires inpatient treatment. Antibiotic treatment should be given intravenously (Table 2.2), and in addition to this complication-specific treatment as well as pain management is necessary:

- Frank perforation—emergency surgery (see below)
- Microperforation—no additional treatment needed

Table 2.1 Oral antibiotic treatment regimens suitable for outpatient treatment of acute uncomplicated diverticulitis

Medication	Dosage	Frequency	Duration
1. Amoxicillin + clavulanate	875 + 125 mg	12 hourly	5 days
2. Cephalexin	500 mg	6 hourly	5 days
+ Metronidazole	400 mg	12 hourly	5 days
3. Metronidazole	400 mg	12 hourly	5 days
+ Trimethoprim+ sulfamethoxazole	160 + 800 mg	12 hourly	5 days
(For patients with immediate penicillin hypersensitivity)			

Table 2.2 Intravenous antibiotic treatment regimens suitable for inpatient treatment of acute severe or complicated diverticulitis

Medication	Dosage	Frequency	Duration
1. Amoxicillin/ampicillin	1000 mg	6 hourly	3 days
+ Gentamicin	4–7 mg/kg for 1 dose		
(2nd/3rd dose depending on kidney function)			
+ Metronidazole	500 mg	12 hourly	3 days
(Change to regimen 2, 3, or 4 if clinical findings did not improve after 3 days)			
2. Piperacillin + tazobactam	4000 + 500 mg	8 hourly	@
3. Ticarcillin + clavulanate	3000 + 100 mg	6 hourly	@
Choose regimen 2 or 3 for patients with contraindication to gentamicin			
4. Metronidazole	500 mg	12 hourly	@
+ Ceftriaxone or cefotaxime	1000 mg	Daily	
Choose regimen 4 for patients hypersensitive to penicillin			

@Continue treatment until afebrile for 24–48 h

- Abscess—can be seen in up to 50% of patients with acute complicated diverticulitis. Small abscesses (<3 cm) can be treated without intervention; larger abscesses should be drained percutaneously (CT-guided drainage)
- Obstruction—urgent surgery (see below)
- Fistula formation—this can occur between the large bowel and the bladder, vagina, uterus, and other segments of the small/large bowel; (urgent) surgery (see below)

Complicated diverticular disease is best classified using the *Hinchey criteria*:

- Pericolic or mesenteric abscess
- Walled-off pelvic abscess
- Generalized purulent peritonitis
- Generalized fecal peritonitis

Successful nonsurgical treatment of acute uncomplicated as well as complicated diverticulitis requires a *colonoscopy* at approximately 6 weeks after initial presentation (once all symptoms have resolved) to exclude an underlying bowel cancer (unless complete colonoscopy was done within 1 year prior to presentation with acute diverticulitis). After successful treatment of acute complicated diverticulitis (percutaneous abscess drainage, conservative treatment of small abscess/microabscess), *elective surgery* needs to be planned to avoid the morbidity and mortality associated with a recurrent episode of diverticulitis (incidence up to 40%, mortality of elective vs. emergency surgery 0.3% vs. 4.6%).

Dietary intervention does not prevent recurrent disease after acute diverticulitis, and patients do not need to avoid seeds, corn, and nuts.

2.4 Surgical Management

Most patients presenting with complications of diverticular disease can be treated conservatively, but approximately 15% will require surgery.

Emergency surgery is required with free perforation and subsequent fecal peritonitis. This condition is associated with a mortality rate of up to 25%.

Urgent surgery (within the same admission) must be considered for patients presenting with failure of medical treatment, obstruction, abscess formation (Fig. 2.4) not responding to conservative treatment (CT-guided drainage, antibiotic medication), and fistula formation causing urosepsis/pyelonephritis.

Elective surgery should be performed on patients with fistula formation (if not considered for urgent surgery) and on patients with chronic smoldering diverticulitis (initial response to medical treatment followed by recurrent pain, change in bowel habits, and per rectal bleeding). Also patients after successful conservative management of complicated diverticulitis should be prepared for elective resection (preoperative colonoscopy and physiological optimization). Urgent and elective surgeries both have a mortality of up to 5%.

The decision whether or not to operate on a patient suffering from recurrent diverticulitis should be influenced by the following considerations:

- More than 40% of patients after successful nonoperative management of acute diverticulitis are at risk to develop recurrent diverticulitis
- Prior uncomplicated episodes of acute diverticulitis do not predict a higher incidence or higher severity of recurrent diverticulitis
- Complications and colostomy rates are not affected by the number of previous episodes of acute diverticulitis
- More episodes of diverticulitis are not associated with a higher rate of conversion from laparoscopic to open surgery
- The mortality rate of emergency surgery is significantly higher than the mortality rate of elective surgery (0.3% vs. 4.6%)
- Patients with persistent symptoms at 6–8 weeks after onset of symptoms may suffer from chronic smoldering diverticulitis and should be considered for surgery
- Availability of emergency services to patients in case of recurrent disease (travel plans, remote living)
- Immunocompromised patients often require emergency surgery when presenting with a second attack due to atypical and/or late presentation

2.4.1 Surgical Technique

The choice of surgical approach depends on patient factors as well as surgeon factors. The aim of surgery is to remove the affected segment of the bowel. This can be achieved with open as well as laparoscopic surgery. Depending on the patient's presentation, surgery can be performed in a single-stage (resection and primary anastomosis, no diverting stoma), two-stage (resection ± anastomosis, diverting stoma/end-colostomy), or even three-stage (drainage of abscess/peritonitis, resection + anastomosis, diverting stoma) approach.

Single-stage surgery should be limited to the few patients where the bowel is well-perfused and non-edematous and the anastomosis is tension-free. Most patients require a *two-stage* approach with or without (Hartmann's operation) primary anastomosis. When deciding to perform a Hartmann's procedure, it is important to consider that only half of these patients will have a colostomy closure after recovering from the initial surgery. *Three-stage* surgery may be necessary in patients with colonic perforation due to diverticular disease.

In *unstable patients* unfit for definite surgery, a damage control procedure with limited bowel resection and end-colostomy should be favored.

Laparoscopic surgery has several advantages including lower rates of wound infection, blood transfusion, postoperative ileus, hospital stay, and incisional hernia. More significant complications (leakage, stricture, bowel laceration, bowel obstruction, abscess formation) have been reported to be independent of surgical approach (laparoscopic or open surgery).

Surgery for diverticular disease can be expected to cure the patient; nonetheless up to 10% of patients require repeat surgery for recurrent complicated diverticular disease. Up to 25% of patients suffer from persistent pain similar to the symptoms reported prior to surgery.

2.5 When to Transfer

Nonoperative management of complicated diverticular disease may require CT-guided abscess drainage. If this cannot be offered, a transfer to a center with interventional radiology support must be offered. Emergency surgery may require postoperative care in high-dependency or intensive care units. If this cannot be provided and the patient can still be transferred, this should be considered prior to surgical intervention.

Recommended Reading

McDermott FD, et al. Minimally invasive and surgical management strategies tailored to the severity of acute diverticulitis. Br J Surg. 2014;101(1):e90–9.

Rezapour M, et al. Diverticular disease: an update on pathogenesis and management. Gut Liver. 2018;12(2):125–32. https://doi.org/10.5009/gnl16552.

Therapeutic Guidelines – Gastrointestinal Version 5 (2011).

Tursi A, et al. Current management of patients with diverticulosis and diverticular disease: a survey from the Second International Symposium on Diverticular Disease. J Clin Gastroenterol. 2016;50(Suppl 1):S97–100.
UpToDate®: Acute colonic diverticulitis: Medical Management.
UpToDate®: Acute colonic diverticulitis: Surgical Management.
UpToDate®: Colonic diverticulosis and diverticular disease: epidemiology, risk factors, and pathogenesis.

3 Gastroenteropancreatic Neuroendocrine Tumours

Florian Bösch, Christoph Auernhammer, Christine Spitzweg, and Martin Angele

3.1 Introduction

Gastroenteropancreatic neuroendocrine tumors (GEP-NETs) are rare neoplasms and represent a heterogeneous group of tumors. These tumors can arise from neuroendocrine cells throughout the body and were formerly referred to as gastrointestinal carcinoids (a term introduced by Oberndorfer more than 100 years ago) and islet cell tumors of the pancreas. Functional tumors produce peptides and hormones and cause characteristic symptoms (including diarrhea and/or flush in carcinoid syndrome, hypoglycaemia in insulinoma, gastrointestinal ulcers in Zollinger-Ellison syndrome). Non-functional tumors lack characteristic symptoms and become clinically apparent due to tumor mass effects (i.e. jaundice, abdominal pain).

Using criteria established by the WHO in 2010, neuroendocrine tumors are classified into well-differentiated neuroendocrine tumors (NET) and poorly differentiated neuroendocrine carcinomas (NEC). Grading (G1–G3) is defined on the basis of mitotic count and/or Ki67 staining. The classification system is well established and predicts the biological behaviour of the tumor with high probability (Fig. 3.1).

Due to their rarity, incidence data on GEP-NETs are difficult to obtain and are mainly based on national cancer registries and small retrospective analyses. Nonetheless incidence is rising, which might be due to improved understanding of the disease and superior imaging modalities. The incidence rate varies between

F. Bösch · C. Auernhammer · C. Spitzweg · M. Angele (✉)
Department of General, Visceral, and Transplant Surgery,
Ludwig-Maximilians-University Munich, Munich, Germany
e-mail: Florina.Boesch@med.uni-muenchen.de;
Christoph.Auernhammer@med.uni-muenchen.de;
christine.spitzweg@med.uni-muenchen.de;
martin.angele@med.uni-muenchen.de

M. W. Wichmann et al. (eds.), *Gastroenterology For General Surgeons*,
https://doi.org/10.1007/978-3-319-92768-8_3

Fig. 3.1 Grading classification according to the WHO (HPF mitotic counts per 10 high power fields)

Grading	Ki-67 index	Mitotic rate
G1	≤ 2 %	< 2 / 10 HPF
G2	3 – 20 %	2 - 20 / 10 HPF
G3	> 20 %	> 20 / 10 HPF

studies and is about 1.3–3.5/100,000 per year. The mean age at initial diagnosis is dependent on the primary tumor and peaks in the late 50s; however, appendiceal NETs may arise at the age of 40–50 years. Prognosis is determined by the presence of distant metastases and particularly by the proliferative activity/grading. NETs occurring in the small intestine are the most prevalent, with an annual incidence of 0.67–0.81/100,000 per year representing approximately 35% of all cases. The second most common GEP-NET arises from the appendix with a yearly incidence of 0.15–0.6/100,000 and is usually diagnosed incidentally during appendectomy. Pancreatic NETs are subdivided into functional and non-functional and have an incidence of 0.1–0.3/100,000 per year.

Due to the complexity of GEP-NETs, patients should be treated by an experienced multidisciplinary team. The only chance of cure is complete tumor resection. Nonetheless, even tumor debulking may be beneficial if >90% of the tumour burden can be removed. A surgical approach may also be recommended for relief of tumor-related symptoms in stage IV patients.

3.2 Diagnosis

3.2.1 Imaging Modalities

Cross-sectional imaging using CT or MRI is the cornerstone of initial staging to rule out locoregional or distant metastases. The modalities should follow modern protocols with contrast media, which is adapted to the investigated organ (i.e. MRI with liver-specific contrast agent and various sequences including DWI and T2 to detect liver metastases). GEP-NETs are best detected in the arterial phase of a triple-phase CT scan, and the hyperenhancement of the primary tumor as well as of liver metastases with intravenous contrast agent is characteristic for GEP-NETs.

Most GEP-NETs express somatostatin receptors on their surface, commonly type 2. As a consequence a PET/CT scan specifically targeting the somatostatin receptor (i.e. ^{68}Gallium-DOTA-TATE, ^{68}Gallium-DOTA-TOC) shows very high sensitivity. Detection of functional somatostatin receptor expression facilitates the therapeutic use of peptide receptor radionuclide treatment in NET G1/G2 tumours. In contrast, most poorly differentiated NECs lose somatostatin receptor expression; thus ^{18}fluorodeoxyglucose PET/CT is the preferred diagnostic imaging procedure. Somatostatin receptor-targeted radionuclide therapy is not feasible in NECs.

Thorough preoperative staging, with appropriate tumor-specific diagnostic modalities, is vital. A colonoscopy is mandatory: either to diagnose a small tumor in the terminal ileum or to rule out a secondary colonic malignancy. Carcinoid syndrome (see Sect. 2.3) may affect the heart, leading to fibrosis of the valvular endocardium and right ventricular insufficiency. In patients who show clinical signs of a carcinoid syndrome and/or elevated 5-HIAA in the urine, a transthoracic echocardiogram and cardiologic assessment are strongly recommended; NT-pro-BNP has been recommended as an additional screening parameter. Endoscopic ultrasound (EUS) is mandatory in the case of gastric and rectal NETs and should be done before commencement of treatment as the therapeutic strategy correlates with the extent of invasion of the intestinal wall and locoregional lymph nodes. Moreover, EUS combined with fine needle aspiration is useful to detect and diagnose pancreatic NETs. In the case of small or multiple pancreatic NETs, EUS is advantageous to localize the tumors and adjacent vessels. EUS is also helpful to determine the localization of the pancreatic NET with respect to the pancreatic duct to assess feasibility of tumor enucleation.

3.2.2 Endocrine Testing

No validated tumor markers for screening for GEP-NETs exist, as the sensitivity and specificity of plasma chromogranin A (CgA) is limited. However in patients with known GEP-NETs, plasma CgA is recommended as a general tumor marker and surrogate marker for follow-up. CgA should be assessed for every GEP-NET entity and may have prognostic value.

In patients with small intestine NETs, 24-hour urinary 5-hydroxyindoleacetic acid (5-HIAA) should be measured at initial diagnosis. 5-HIAA has a sensitivity of almost 100% and a specificity of 85–90% for carcinoid syndrome. However, it is important to be aware that 5-HIAA tests are easily influenced by certain medications and food.

Specific tests exist for diagnosing functional pancreatic NETs, such as a supervised 72-hour fast to confirm the presence of an insulinoma. Endogenous hyperinsulinemia with symptoms of hypoglycaemia, paired with inadequately elevated levels of insulin, C-peptide and/or proinsulin, can indicate an insulinoma.

Forty percent of gastrinomas are located in the pancreatic head inducing peptic ulcers and watery diarrhea. A gastrinoma can be diagnosed if gastrin is >1000 pg/mL and gastric pH is <2. In 60% of gastrinoma patients, gastrin levels are only mildly elevated (<1000 pg/mL), and a subsequent secretin test is necessary to support the diagnosis. Serum gastrin levels are influenced by multiple factors, in particular proton pump inhibitors which should be stopped 7–10 days prior to testing.

3.2.3 Carcinoid Syndrome

Carcinoid syndrome is uncommon (5–10%); however, symptoms are severe. Most commonly small intestine NETs with liver metastases cause carcinoid syndrome because serotonin bypasses the first pass effect of the liver. The main symptoms are flushing (60–85%), diarrhea (60–80%), intermittent bronchial wheezing (<10%) and right heart valve fibrosis (carcinoid heart syndrome; up to 20%).

Carcinoid crisis is a serious exacerbation of carcinoid syndrome and potentially fatal, with continuous flushing, severe abdominal pain, hypo- or hypertension, severe bronchospasm and cardiac arrhythmia. It can be induced by severe stress or intraoperatively by manipulating the tumor. Therefore, somatostatin analogues (SSA) have to be increased perioperatively to prevent carcinoid crisis. Intra- and postoperative continuous intravenous infusion of octreotide is recommended.

To reduce symptoms like flushing and diarrhea, biotherapy with SSAs is effective in approximately 70%. Long-acting SSAs bind to somatostatin receptors and are injected every 28 days. Moreover, two randomized prospective studies demonstrated that therapy with SSAs also results in significantly prolonged progression-free survival due to its antiproliferative effect.

3.3 Therapy

3.3.1 Pancreas

Pancreatic NETs (pNETs) are divided into functional (f-pNETs) and non-functional pNETs (nf-pNETs). nf-pNETs are more frequent (>60%) but are commonly diagnosed in the advanced stage as they are typically asymptomatic. f-pNETs such as insulinoma (1–32/1,000,000 per year) and gastrinoma (0.5–21.5/1,000,000 per year) are rare.

3.3.1.1 Insulinoma

Patients with insulinomas should undergo exploration and resection independent of a possible hereditary disorder (10% of patients will have a MEN1 mutation) with the main objective to control hypoglycaemia-associated symptoms. If multiple insulinomas (10% of patients) are suspected, the whole pancreas has to be exposed, bidigitally palpated, and an intraoperative ultrasound performed. Insulinomas are often small; thus enucleation is feasible. A laparoscopic approach is practicable for preoperatively anatomically located tumours, which are not closer than 3 mm to the main pancreatic duct. To prevent pancreatic fistula, a formal resection is necessary if the main duct is not definable.

MEN1 patients may suffer from insulinoma and nf-pNET simultaneously, which requires a diligent preoperative diagnostic strategy, including preoperative arterial calcium stimulation and venous sampling (ASVS), with measurement of insulin to functionally localize the insulinoma within the pancreas. If the insulinoma cannot be detected, a blind distal resection is not recommended.

The rate of malignancy in insulinoma is less than 10%; however these patients require a radical resection with an oncological lymphadenectomy.

3.3.1.2 Gastrinoma

Gastrinoma are classified as sporadic (70%) or hereditary (30%, MEN1), with the distinction prognostically and therapeutically relevant.

Sporadic gastrinomas are mostly solitary tumors in the duodenum (70%) or the pancreas (25%). These tumors should be treated by parenchyma-sparing resection (i.e. enucleation) and lymph node dissection in the gastrinoma triangle (hepatoduodenal ligament-ligament of Treitz-duodenal sweep). In certain cases, such as recurrent disease or if the tumor is close to the main pancreatic duct, a partial pancreatectomy is indicated. A blind resection is not mandatory due to efficacy of proton pump inhibitors; however a lymph node dissection in the gastrinoma triangle should be performed.

Patients with sporadic Zollinger-Ellison syndrome can be cured by surgery in 20–45% of cases, whereas MEN1-associated gastrinomas are not curable by surgery (0–1%). Gastrinomas <2 cm are generally not treated surgically, but these cases should be discussed by the multidisciplinary team. Patients with gastrinomas >2 cm should undergo oncological resection with lymph node dissection.

3.3.1.3 Rare Functional pNET

Other rare tumors (glucagonoma, SSoma, GRHoma, ACTHoma, VIPoma) cause symptoms depending on the secreted hormone (diabetes mellitus, acromegaly, Cushing's syndrome, Verner-Morrison syndrome). Such cases should be referred to specialized centres, if curative surgery is feasible.

3.3.1.4 Non-functional pNET

Improvements in diagnostic modalities have resulted in a higher incidence of nf-pNETs. The biological behaviour of these tumors is uncertain; hence proliferation index (Ki67) and tumour diameter are used for better characterization.

Nf-pNETs <2 cm are rarely malignant (6% of cases), and therefore the therapeutic strategy for surgical treatment has to be discussed by a multidisciplinary team. If a conservative approach is chosen, a continuous follow-up every 3 months should be performed within the first year. Thereafter a follow-up every 6 months for at least 3 years is recommended. However, data for conservative management are weak and need to be confirmed in larger series. If there is any doubt concerning malignancy, surgical management is indicated.

Surgical resection is crucial for patients with nf-pNETs >2 cm. A pancreaticoduodenectomy should be performed if the tumor is located in the pancreatic head, while a distal pancreatectomy with splenectomy is indicated for nf-pNETs in the tail of the pancreas. Any operation has to be combined with an oncological lymphadenectomy. Due to good prognosis, extended multivisceral surgery is an option for patients with extensive tumors. Liver resection for metastases is indicated if at least 90% of the hepatic tumour load can be removed. MEN1 patients often have multifocal tumors; thus complete tumor resection is not feasible. Parenchyma-sparing resections should be applied for tumors >2 cm in size. In exceptional cases, total pancreatectomy might be necessary.

3.3.2 Stomach

Gastric NETs (gNETs) have an incidence of approximately 0.2/100,000 per year, accounting for 23% of GEP-NETs. The type of the gNET influences the therapeutic strategy.

Type 1 gastric NETs are the most prevalent (70–80%), are often small (<2 cm), multifocal and most commonly show a low proliferative index. Described as ECLomas (enterochromaffin-like cell carcinoids), they are secondary to chronic hypergastrinaemia and associated with chronic atrophic gastritis. Since metastatic risk correlates with size, tumors >1 cm should be resected endoscopically, using either endoscopic mucosal resection (EMR) or endoscopic submucosal dissection (ESD). Active surveillance is appropriate for tumors <1 cm. Tumors >2 cm are rare and like node-positive gNETs, a domain of surgery. Overall survival is excellent for gNETs type 1 < 2 cm; however the recurrence rate is high as chronic atrophic gastritis, and concomitant hypergastrinaemia which act as growth stimulus remain present. Therefore, lifelong endoscopic follow-up at least every 1–2 years is recommended.

Type 2 gNETs are associated with Zollinger-Ellison syndrome (ZES) and rarely occur. Hypergastrinaemia due to a gastrinoma leads to these tumors, which have a higher metastatic potential (10–30%). These tumors are also often multiple, small (<2 cm) and mostly well differentiated. Endoscopic resection might be feasible, but treatment strategy is dictated by ZES and additional GEP-NETs in the duodenum or pancreas.

Type 3 gNETs are also rare, and therapy of these tumors is equivalent to gastric adenocarcinomas. Type 3 gNETs—in contrast to type 1 and type 2—are not associated with hypergastrinaemia. Mostly these are solitary, large tumors, which might be centrally exulcerated at diagnosis. These tumors are highly metastatic in over 50% of cases upon initial diagnosis. Therefore a total gastrectomy combined with a D2 lymphadenectomy is indicated.

3.3.3 Small Intestine

Neuroendocrine tumors of the small intestine (si-NETs) are commonly well differentiated (G1 or G2). Upon diagnosis si-NETs are mostly very small, but advanced disease is common. These tumors metastasize early into lymph nodes and are often associated with a desmoplastic reaction of the mesentery. The desmoplastic reaction subsequently results in bowel obstruction and impaired perfusion of the small intestinal segment causing abdominal pain or ileus (Fig. 3.2). Therefore, up to 50% of patients with si-NETs are diagnosed during emergency laparotomy due to an ileus.

si-NETs can secrete serotonin, causing carcinoid syndrome. Carcinoid syndrome is an indirect sign of liver metastases when the secreted serotonin bypasses the first pass effect of the liver. Transthoracic echocardiography should be done preoperatively in these patients to rule out fibrosis of the valvular endocardium. If a carcinoid

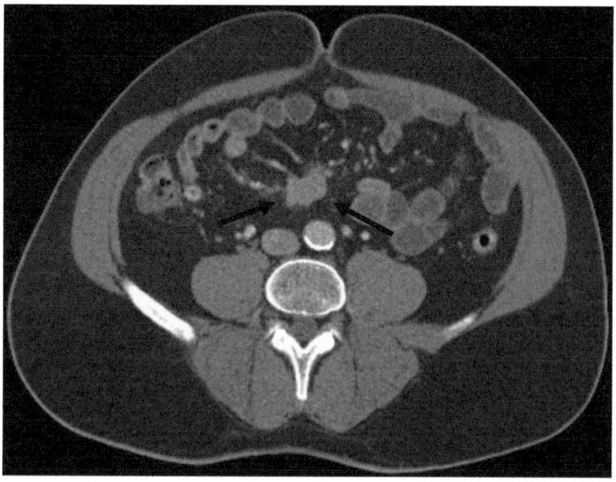

Fig. 3.2 CT scan of a patient with a si-NET forming a desmoplastic reaction (arrows)

syndrome is clinically apparent, perioperative treatment with somatostatin analogues is necessary to avoid a life-threatening carcinoid crisis.

The 5-year survival rate correlates with the tumor stage and is about 80–100% if metastases are not present. If lymph node metastases are evident, the 5-year survival rate decreases to 70–80% and to 35–70% if distant metastases occur.

3.3.3.1 Surgical Approach

Due to the high probability of lymph node metastases, even for small tumors, an oncological resection with wide lymph node dissection is mandatory. Approximately 30% of patients with tumors <1 cm will have lymph node metastases. This rate increases up to 80% in patients with tumors >2 cm. Since most si-NETs are located in the terminal ileum, a right-sided hemicolectomy has to be performed. Often the desmoplastic lymph nodes encase the superior mesenteric artery and its branches (Fig. 3.3). However infiltration of the mesenteric root is not common; thus primary tumor resection combined with high lymph node dissection is indicated.

Bimanual palpation of the entire small intestine is necessary to rule out multifocal si-NETs, which are present in 20% of cases. In the case of multifocality, surgical resection is beneficial and should follow oncological principles with open abdominal approach recommended. If laparoscopic surgery is performed, the same oncological standards have to be fulfilled. This can be achieved by a small incision to allow digital palpation of the entire small intestine. However, a laparoscopic approach is not suitable for multifocal tumours and large mesenteric metastases. After curative treatment, adjuvant therapy is not recommend. Surveillance should occur for at least 10 years.

Recurrences often originate from lymph nodes, which were not resected at initial operation. Therefore, reoperation is recommended if oncological standards were not followed. If the si-NET was incidentally detected, proper staging should be performed before reoperation.

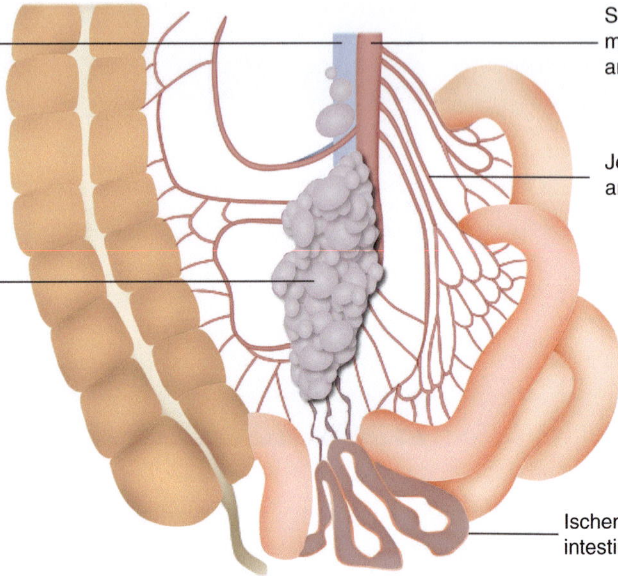

Fig. 3.3 The desmoplastic reaction is extensively involving the mesenteric root

Patients with metastatic disease are often seen and can be divided into different groups:

Patients with limited hepatic metastases, where a curative surgical approach is feasible, should undergo primary tumor resection and liver resection. Dependent on the extent of the hepatic tumor load, hepatic resection can be combined with the primary resection or two-staged after convalescence.

In case of distant metastases with extended mesenteric tumor mass leading to an ileus, the approach is palliative. The main goal is alleviation of symptoms. An intestinal bypass is not recommended as the mesenteric mass will increase in size, subsequently occluding the bypass. Therefore, the gold standard is a limited resection.

If curative liver surgery is not feasible, a primary tumor resection with wide lymph node dissection is recommended. Liver-directed therapy like transarterial chemoembolization (TACE) or selective internal radiation therapy (SIRT) may be suitable for these patients. Stage IV patients may benefit from primary tumor resection and tumor debulking. Overall survival can be improved, and tumor-related symptoms are relieved after tumor debulking. Nonetheless, patients with stage IV disease should be discussed by the multidisciplinary team and multimodal concepts adapted for every patient.

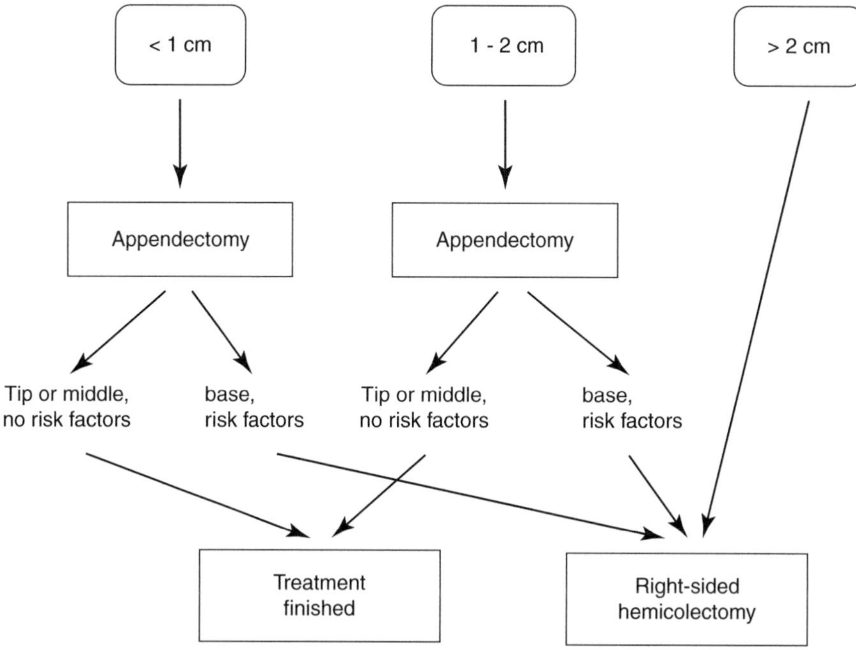

Fig. 3.4 Therapeutic algorithm for appendiceal NET

3.3.4 Appendix

Appendiceal NETs are most commonly diagnosed incidentally during appendectomy with the majority of tumors located in the tip of the appendix. The therapeutic strategy primarily depends on size and localization.

Three groups can be defined by reference to the size (<1 cm, 1–2 cm, >2 cm) of the tumor (Fig. 3.4).

Two thirds of patients have a tumor <1 cm located in the tip or mid of the appendix and are postoperatively classified as G1, L0, V0 and R0. Those can be cured by a simple appendectomy. Exceptions are only rare cases, which show risk factors defined in the second group. Almost 100% long-term survival rates are achieved. No follow-up is required.

The second group is the most challenging and accounts for 5–25% of appendiceal NETs. Tumors are 1–2 cm in size and might be treated sufficiently by appendectomy. But there are several risk factors defined which require a right-sided hemicolectomy with lymphadenectomy. These risk factors are G2 (Ki-67 $\geq$ 3%), lymphatic (L1) or vascular invasion (V1), an invasion depth of >3 mm into the mesoappendix, tumor location in the appendiceal base (instead of tip or mid of the appendix) or infiltration of the resection margin after appendectomy (R1). If patients are young and tumors are exceeding 1.5 cm, a right-sided hemicolectomy might individually be discussed even without risk factors because of the higher probability of positive lymph nodes. Regarding follow-up, no formal guidelines exist, but patients with risk factors should be followed up.

Approximately 10% of patients have appendiceal NETs >2 cm. Locoregional lymph node metastases occur in 40% of these patients; therefore a right-sided hemicolectomy is indicated. After curative surgery, a structured follow-up is recommended. Because of the inappropriate lymph node dissection, an ileocecal resection should not be performed.

Goblet cell carcinoids of the appendix are a rare subtype of mixed adenoneuroendocrine carcinomas (MANEC). The oncological therapy of these tumors should be performed in a multidisciplinary setting. Since these tumours have a disposition to early peritoneal metastases, a multimodal therapeutic approach is indicated. Therapy might include surgery with right-sided hemicolectomy, ovarectomy, peritonectomy, HIPEC (hyperthermic intraperitoneal chemotherapy) as well as adjuvant chemotherapy similar to colon carcinoma.

3.3.5 Colon and Rectum

Colorectal NETs account for 7–12% of all GEP-NETs and should be discussed separately.

Colonic NETs are commonly asymptomatic and diagnosed during a colonoscopy. At initial diagnosis up to 30% of patients have metastases. Minimal staging includes a complete colonoscopy and CT scan. Patients with tumours >2 cm should undergo a colonic resection, similar to adenocarcinomas of the same origin. If there are no metastases and the tumor is <2 cm, the patient can be treated endoscopically with ESD. Five-year survival rate for colonic NETs is 62% but reaches 100% for patients with a T1 tumour.

The therapeutic approach of rectal NETs is dependent on tumor size; subsequently there are three groups: tumors <1 cm, 1–2 cm and > 2 cm. Minimal staging of rectal NETs consists of a complete colonoscopy and assessment of local lymph nodes. For that purpose endosonography and/or MRI are recommended. If no metastases are evident, an endoscopic resection can be performed in tumors <1 cm. Therapeutic decisions for patients with tumors between 1 and 2 cm should be discussed in the multidisciplinary team meeting and findings discussed with the patient. In this group, lymph node metastases are reported in up to 42% of patients. If an endoscopic approach is chosen, a full-thickness resection via transanal endoscopic microsurgery should be performed. Patients with tumors >2 cm should undergo an oncological resection similar to adenocarcinomas of the rectum. Well-differentiated rectal NETs have the most favourable 5-year survival rate of all GEP-NETs, reaching 88%.

3.4 Follow-Up

Follow-up for GEP-NETs depends primarily on primary tumor localization, grading and classification. Patients should be referred to a specialized GEP-NET centre for further therapy and follow-up. Due to slow progression and the high percentage of late (>5 years) recurrence of GEP-NET following curative resection, follow-up should extend longer than 5 years (different guidelines recommend 10 years to lifelong), although in this respect, no prospective data exist.

Surveillance of patients with pancreatic NETs requires imaging every 3–9 months and measurement of biochemical markers. Sporadic insulinomas do not require further follow-up if there is no recurrence after 6 months.

Gastric NETs type 1 should undergo endoscopic follow-up after resection at least every 2 years. Type 3 gNETs should be followed up as for adenocarcinoma of the stomach.

Patients with si-NETs who had a curative resection should be screened every 6–12 months, or every 3–6 months if a non-curative resection was performed. Follow-up includes a triphasic CT or MRI scan and the measurement of CgA and 5-HIAA. If recurrence is suspected, a DOTA-TATE or DOTA-TOC PET/CT scan should be done. According to ENETS guidelines, lifelong follow-up is recommended for patients with si-NET.

Recommendations for follow-up for patients with appendiceal NETs are tripartite. Patients with a tumour <1 cm and no signs of malignancy or risk factors are cured by appendectomy and need no further examinations. Follow-up is recommended for patients with tumours >2 cm or with signs of malignancy or risk factors. These patients should be followed up either with CT or MRI scans. MRI may be beneficial since these patients are often young and fertile requiring long-time surveillance. No data exists on follow-up for patients with tumours between 1 and 2 cm. In cases without risk factors, follow-up seems unnecessary but should be done in the presence of additional risk factors.

Recommended Reading

Auernhammer CJ, Goke B. Therapeutic strategies for advanced neuroendocrine carcinomas of jejunum/ileum and pancreatic origin. Gut. 2011;60:1009–21.

Caplin ME, Pavel M, Cwikla JB, Phan AT, Raderer M, Sedlackova E, et al. Lanreotide in metastatic enteropancreatic neuroendocrine tumors. N Engl J Med. 2014;371:224–33.

Delle Fave G, O'Toole D, Sundin A, Taal B, Ferolla P, Ramage JK, et al. ENETS consensus guidelines update for Gastroduodenal neuroendocrine neoplasms. Neuroendocrinology. 2016;103:119–24.

Falconi M, Eriksson B, Kaltsas G, Bartsch DK, Capdevila J, Caplin M, et al. ENETS consensus guidelines update for the management of patients with functional pancreatic neuroendocrine tumors and non-functional pancreatic neuroendocrine tumors. Neuroendocrinology. 2016;103:153–71.

Fendrich V, Bartsch DK. Surgical therapy of sporadic pancreatic neuroendocrine Neoplasias G1/G2. Visc Med. 2017;33:344–50.

Garcia-Carbonero R, Sorbye H, Baudin E, Raymond E, Wiedenmann B, Niederle B, et al. ENETS consensus guidelines for high-grade gastroenteropancreatic neuroendocrine tumors and neuroendocrine carcinomas. Neuroendocrinology. 2016;103:186–94.

Giesel FL, Kratochwil C, Mehndiratta A, Wulfert S, Moltz JH, Zechmann CM, et al. Comparison of neuroendocrine tumor detection and characterization using DOTATOC-PET in correlation with contrast enhanced CT and delayed contrast enhanced MRI. Eur J Radiol. 2012;81:2820–5.

Haug AR, Cindea-Drimus R, Auernhammer CJ, Reincke M, Wangler B, Uebleis C, et al. The role of 68Ga-DOTATATE PET/CT in suspected neuroendocrine tumors. J Nucl Med. 2012;53:1686–92.

Khan MS, Luong TV, Watkins J, Toumpanakis C, Caplin ME, Meyer T. A comparison of Ki-67 and mitotic count as prognostic markers for metastatic pancreatic and midgut neuroendocrine neoplasms. Br J Cancer. 2013;108:1838–45.

Kim HH, Kim GH, Kim JH, Choi MG, Song GA, Kim SE. The efficacy of endoscopic submucosal dissection of type I gastric carcinoid tumors compared with conventional endoscopic mucosal resection. Gastroenterol Res Pract. 2014;2014:253860.

Kloppel G, Couvelard A, Perren A, Komminoth P, McNicol AM, Nilsson O, et al. ENETS consensus guidelines for the standards of care in neuroendocrine tumors: towards a standardized approach to the diagnosis of gastroenteropancreatic neuroendocrine tumors and their prognostic stratification. Neuroendocrinology. 2009;90:162–6.

Landry CS, Lin HY, Phan A, Charnsangavej C, Abdalla EK, Aloia T, et al. Resection of at-risk mesenteric lymph nodes is associated with improved survival in patients with small bowel neuroendocrine tumors. World J Surg. 2013;37:1695–700.

Maasberg S, Jurgensen C, Scheerer F, Pschowski R, Felder S, Begum N, et al. Endoscopic therapy for gastroduodenal neuroendocrine neoplasms. Chirurg. 2016;87:271–9.

Niederle B, Pape UF, Costa F, Gross D, Kelestimur F, Knigge U, et al. ENETS consensus guidelines update for neuroendocrine neoplasms of the jejunum and ileum. Neuroendocrinology. 2016;103:125–38.

Oberg K, Couvelard A, Delle Fave G, Gross D, Grossman A, Jensen RT, et al. ENETS consensus guidelines for standard of care in neuroendocrine tumours: biochemical markers. Neuroendocrinology. 2017;105:201–11.

Pape UF, Niederle B, Costa F, Gross D, Kelestimur F, Kianmanesh R, et al. ENETS consensus guidelines for neuroendocrine neoplasms of the appendix (excluding goblet cell carcinomas). Neuroendocrinology. 2016;103:144–52.

Pape UF, Perren A, Niederle B, Gross D, Gress T, Costa F, et al. ENETS consensus guidelines for the management of patients with neuroendocrine neoplasms from the jejuno-ileum and the appendix including goblet cell carcinomas. Neuroendocrinology. 2012;95:135–56.

Pavel M, Baudin E, Couvelard A, Krenning E, Oberg K, Steinmuller T, et al. ENETS consensus guidelines for the management of patients with liver and other distant metastases from neuroendocrine neoplasms of foregut, midgut, hindgut, and unknown primary. Neuroendocrinology. 2012;95:157–76.

Poitras P, Gingras MH, Rehfeld JF. The Zollinger-Ellison syndrome: dangers and consequences of interrupting antisecretory treatment. Clin Gastroenterol Hepatol. 2012;10:199–202.

Putzer D, Kroiss A, Waitz D, Gabriel M, Traub-Weidinger T, Uprimny C, et al. Somatostatin receptor PET in neuroendocrine tumours: 68Ga-DOTA0,Tyr3-octreotide versus 68Ga-DOTA0-lanreotide. Eur J Nucl Med Mol Imaging. 2013;40:364–72.

Radulova-Mauersberger O, Stelzner S, Witzigmannn H. Rectal neuroendocrine tumors: surgical therapy. Chirurg. 2016;87:292–7.

Ramage JK, De Herder WW, Delle Fave G, Ferolla P, Ferone D, Ito T, et al. ENETS consensus guidelines update for colorectal neuroendocrine neoplasms. Neuroendocrinology. 2016;103:139–43.

Rinke A, Muller HH, Schade-Brittinger C, Klose KJ, Barth P, Wied M, et al. Placebo-controlled, double-blind, prospective, randomized study on the effect of octreotide LAR in the control of tumor growth in patients with metastatic neuroendocrine midgut tumors: a report from the PROMID study group. J Clin Oncol. 2009;27:4656–63.

Sato Y, Hashimoto S, Mizuno K, Takeuchi M, Terai S. Management of gastric and duodenal neuroendocrine tumors. World J Gastroenterol. 2016;22:6817–28.

Sommer WH, Sourbron S, Huppertz A, Ingrisch M, Reiser MF, Zech CJ. Contrast agents as a biological marker in magnetic resonance imaging of the liver: conventional and new approaches. Abdom Imaging. 2012;37:164–79.

Steinmuller T, Kianmanesh R, Falconi M, Scarpa A, Taal B, Kwekkeboom DJ, et al. Consensus guidelines for the management of patients with liver metastases from digestive (neuro)endocrine tumors: foregut, midgut, hindgut, and unknown primary. Neuroendocrinology. 2008;87:47–62.

Strosberg J, El-Haddad G, Wolin E, Hendifar A, Yao J, Chasen B, et al. Phase 3 trial of (177) Lu-Dotatate for midgut neuroendocrine tumors. N Engl J Med. 2017;376:125–35.

Strosberg JR, Halfdanarson TR, Bellizzi AM, Chan JA, Dillon JS, Heaney AP, et al. The north American neuroendocrine tumor society consensus guidelines for surveillance and medical Management of Midgut Neuroendocrine Tumors. Pancreas. 2017;46:707–14.

Anorectal Disorders

4

Timothy K. McCullough and Matthias W. Wichmann

4.1 Fistula-in-Ano and Perianal Abscess

A perianal abscess is effectively an incomplete fistula-in-ano, which is made complete when it drains spontaneously or is incised. This is underpinned by the 'cryptoglandular' aetiology of almost all true perianal abscesses, with a small number being infections or folliculitis of the perianal skin. Microbiology of the drained pus may be instructive. The natural history of abscesses does not always include progression to chronic fistulae, a common estimate is 50% conversion, with men affected twice as often as women. Some fistulae may become apparent without an obvious initial abscess episode, particularly in the setting of perianal Crohn's disease. Abscesses should be drained by incision and rarely treated with antibiotics, except, for example, where there is significant cellulitis or in diabetic patients or other immunosuppressed people, where there is sometimes florid and extensive sepsis. This might exploit the expansile ischiorectal spaces and produce very large abscesses, requiring equally extensive, repeated and prolonged surgical drainage, dressing and debridement procedures. Intersphincteric abscesses may be more difficult to appreciate on inspection but are typically disproportionately painful, with anatomical distortion and asymmetry seen nearer to the anal verge.

If asymptomatic, Crohn's fistulae need no treatment. If the fistulae are suppurative, painful or extensive, management can be challenging. There is an appreciable fistula closure rate with infliximab in Crohn's, and this should be exploited before committing to extensive fistula surgery, with the goal to eliminate sepsis.

The surgical treatment of fistula-in-ano requires accurate assessment of the anatomy, in most cases to decide whether laying open is appropriate. The mainstays of this assessment are examination under anaesthesia and MRI, with extensions of the fistula being an often-neglected aspect of the anatomy. Laying open provides the

T. K. McCullough (✉) · M. W. Wichmann
Department of Surgery, Mount Gambier General Hospital, Mount Gambier, SA, Australia
e-mail: timothy.mccullough@sa.gov.au; matthias.wichmann@sa.gov.au

M. W. Wichmann et al. (eds.), *Gastroenterology For General Surgeons*,
https://doi.org/10.1007/978-3-319-92768-8_4

greatest chance of healing, and in simple intersphincteric and low trans-sphincteric fistulae, it should remain the first choice of therapy. The many proposed treatments for higher fistulae reflect the lack of a successful single strategy in this setting. Seton use remains common. Surgeons' reluctance to lay open arises from the potential to leave insufficient sphincter muscle to preserve continence, with the contribution of the internal sphincter to continence being underestimated. In order to preserve the sphincter, the seton and the profusion of procedures for high fistulae are used. The loose seton is a safe long-term solution for many, which prevents recurrent acute sepsis well but does not eliminate the fistula. The cutting seton avoids section of the sphincter and an acute wound but probably results in similar distortion of the sphincter and impact on continence. Many of the sphincter-preserving operations seek to excise the fistula and close the track by ligation, mucosal advancement or interposition grafting, with or without diversion. Their detailed review is beyond the scope of this chapter, but in the cases of recurrent high fistula where multiple conservative surgical treatments have failed, it may be that laying open provides the only viable alternative and at a time when the fibrosis and contracture of repeated sepsis may mitigate the risk of incontinence somewhat. Incontinence remains the primary concern in procedures to lay open fistula-in-ano, and in extreme cases or a perineum largely destroyed by fistula disease, stoma formation as a final resort may be preferred.

4.2 Fissure-in-Ano

Fissure may be acute or chronic and is often transient, resolving without specific treatment. It is a breach in the anoderm thought to arise from a tear and results in sharp pain on and after defecation, typically in the midline, more often posteriorly. The condition, especially acutely, causes searing pain often likened to razor blade cuts, and there is often bleeding and pruritus. The chronic fissure is easily palpable and may be accompanied by a sentinel pile, the acute less so. With off-midline fissures, an alternate pathological process may be the cause, such as Crohn's disease or anal cancer. The pathophysiology of midline fissures is thought to have to do with the relative paucity of the blood supply to the anoderm midline combined with a spastic/hypertonic sphincter, and the treatments seek to address this.

The acute fissure has historically been treated with fecal softeners and analgesia and may heal without intervention or coming to medical attention. If healing does not occur within 6–8 weeks, a chronic fissure will result which is unlikely to resolve without treatment. In addition to fecal softeners and attention to a problematic bowel habit, the interventions seek to improve blood flow to the fissure by reducing the tone of the internal sphincter, chemically or, if unsuccessful, surgically.

Topical treatment includes GTN ointment and calcium-channel blocker creams such as diltiazem. These are applied to the fissure, and treatment is continuous for

6 weeks typically. The side-effect of headache very commonly reported with GTN often fades early in the treatment or requires change to diltiazem ointment treatment, where it is infrequent. Most reviews find topical treatment to be effective: both GTN and diltiazem treatments result in about two thirds of fissures healing, with some non-discordance, so both treatments undertaken successively in the event of one failing may bring about healing. Botox injection of the internal sphincter also results in the healing of the majority of fissures and is increasingly used before resorting to surgical sphincterotomy.

The surgical operation of choice for chronic fissure is lateral internal anal sphincterotomy. This is a controlled division of the lower portion of the internal sphincter for the length of the fissure, made in a lateral part of the sphincter. Anal stretch procedures achieve the same goal and often more, with incontinence being a significant concern with this less controlled method of sphincter disruption. Sphincterotomy results in resolution of more than 90% of chronic fissures with incontinence to flatus or seepage in perhaps 10%. No medical treatment has any significant permanent incontinence as a complication. In those in whom sphincterotomy fails, curettage and suture (fissurectomy) or mucosal advancement may be tried, though outcome data are relatively lacking. With an apparent accelerating move towards sphincter preservation, more procedures are being put forward for trial.

4.3 Hemorrhoids

The anal canal includes the so-called anal cushions, which are swellings of the lowest rectal and highest anal submucosa, vascular in nature, which may be variously congested or engorged or flat at different times. When they bleed, prolapse, become inflamed or otherwise cause symptoms, they are called hemorrhoids. The threshold for this name change is subjective. It is extremely common, and most people will have symptomatic hemorrhoids at some stage.

Hemorrhoids cause symptoms such as bright red bleeding per anum, the nature of which may be spotting, heavy, intermittent, associated with stool passage or between bowel movements. The blood is described as being separate from the stool, as opposed to being mixed or passed concurrently. Defecation may be painful, usually with an aching quality. They are an important cause of pruritus and may cause mucus seepage particularly when prolapsed. It is prudent to exclude other pathologies with similar presentations in certain age groups, particularly colorectal cancer, with flexible sigmoidoscopy or colonoscopy as appropriate. Anal cancer may resemble a prolapsed haemorrhoid.

The useful descriptors for hemorrhoids include their site and whether are able to prolapse or indeed be reduced. The higher hemorrhoids commonly seen on proctoscopy or retroflexion at flexible scope examination are often called internal. These are the hemorrhoids usually described by grading, according to their propensity to prolapse. Grade 1 represents swellings only, without prolapse. The rest of the stages refer to prolapse, which occurs through the anal canal but which reduces spontaneously with Grade 2, with manual reduction in Grade 3 and not at all in Grade 4. The vascular swellings seen at the anal margin, often purple swellings seen under the skin, are termed external hemorrhoids. These sometimes thrombose, causing intense pain and tense swelling, and may be called perianal hematoma. Thrombosis resolves and may leave a skin tag. Thrombosed hemorrhoids may be incised with good symptomatic relief if thrombus can be expressed. Acute hemorrhoidectomy is difficult because of the anatomical distortion caused by the acute inflammatory process and swelling, and is as painful as the thrombosis, probably ultimately taking longer to heal.

Topical therapies are used widely and may contain local anaesthetic, corticosteroid or antiseptic preparations or combinations thereof. These undoubtedly can provide symptomatic relief, but there is no scientific support for their long-term use nor evidence that they eliminate hemorrhoids. Protracted use of steroid preparations risks thinning and potential breakdown of the perianal skin.

Beyond conservative measures to do with dietary changes and management of bowel habit, avoidance of straining and topical treatments, the mainstays of treatment of hemorrhoids are outpatient procedures. Lead amongst these is suction banding, but others are injection sclerotherapy and infrared coagulation. All aim to reduce tissue and cause fibrosis and to reduce and fix the haemorrhoid. Banding has been popular for more than 50 years and, seems, upon repeated review, to be frequently effective in treating all but the largest prolapsing hemorrhoids. It is safe and well-tolerated by comparison to excision and may be repeated but on a limited basis to avoid excessive scarring of the anorectum. Hazards include bleeding, often after some days when the hemorrhoid separates and is passed, and, more rarely, sepsis. Sclerotherapy with oily phenol may improve symptoms from Grade 1 to 2 hemorrhoids but has no benefit in larger or external hemorrhoids. There is a high recurrence following sclerotherapy, and hazards include sepsis, prostatitis and urinary retention, all of which are rare. Infrared coagulation is easily and safely performed and well-tolerated, but recurrence may be as high as sclerotherapy.

For larger, external or refractory hemorrhoids, excision is effective and remains the most frequent operative procedure for haemorrhoid treatment. Preservation of bridges of the anoderm is protective against stricture of the canal. Postoperative pain is the main detractor. Circumferential, permanently prolapsed hemorrhoids, distinct from rectal mucosal prolapse, have been treated with stapled hemorrhoidopexy which removes a circular cuff of rectal mucosa from well above the dentate line, designed to hitch up the prolapsing mucosa but also to disrupt inflow to the hemorrhoid. The method has had its problems, including chronic pain and induction of a low anterior resection syndrome situation with urgency, and more serious complications such as fistula, pelvic sepsis, stricture and incontinence. Hemorrhoidal artery ligation using a Doppler-equipped proctoscope combined with suture hemorrhoidopexy, provides a less painful alternative to excision; recurrence may be more frequent.

4.4 Fecal Incontinence

Fecal incontinence is a common cause for surgical referral and a very common problem amongst the elderly and nursing home residents. The description covers a large variety of problems which range from small-volume seepage occurring after evacuation to involuntary passage of an entire bowel movement, and incontinence has as many potential causes as the many factors contributing to continence. The complicated mechanism of maintaining continence relies upon the physical integrity of the sphincter, the strength of the muscular squeeze, the angle maintained between anal canal and rectum by the levators and the neurological function of the same sensory function including the sampling mechanism; recto-anal inhibitory reflex; rectal compliance; the consistency of stool; the mode of delivery of stool to the anorectum, i.e. bowel transit; and learned and behavioural elements. The contribution of any single element to the entire process is not always measurable, and the relative importance of one may be compensated for by other factors to maintain continence.

The assessment of fecal incontinence, therefore, best includes a wide view on the influences on it, notably those to do with obstetric or surgical injury or weakening of the sphincter complex or its nerve supply. Bowel habit and any indication of recent change, towards a diarrheal or constipated habit with overflow, are also an important and an easy target for investigation and treatment, as is a medication review. It is an important feature that incontinence may appear once a few contributors take effect, for example, possibly unmasking a much earlier obstetric injury which may have been compensated for, until age-related muscle weakening reveals it in later years. Physical examination should include the broader general assessment but also specifically the inspection of the perineum and perianal areas, with attention to the response to straining. Pelvic floor descent should be sought. Digital anorectal examination might reveal deficient resting tone or voluntary squeeze or an indication of the reflexive sphincter response. Rectocele, rectal compliance and sphincter length and symmetry can be examined, and prolapse, either mucosal or full-thickness, may be elicited or seen. Physical examination may inform the choice of whether and which further investigation may be of use. In the absence of any immediate mechanical cause, it may be advisable to investigate any abnormality of the bowel habit if present, most usually including but not limited to flexible sigmoidoscopy or colonoscopy. In the setting of a likely mechanical cause, anorectal physiology can identify sensory-, muscular- and reflex-related issues, whilst visualization of the sphincters with endo-anal ultrasound might reveal a defect, particularly of the internal sphincter. A more functional assessment may include a defaecating proctogram MRI, which displays much more than a standard contrast x-ray study and better informs the choice of target for treatment.

Surgery for fecal incontinence is seldom the most appropriate first step, but careful and expert sphincter assessment for injury and repair at the time of any obstetric or other episode is protective against incontinence, either in the short- or the longer term. Initially, treatments for incontinence ought to be focused on dietary, behavioural, medical and pharmacological approaches. Addressing a diarrheal bowel habit, after appropriate investigation of cause, is often effective in ameliorating incontinence. The use of fibre as a bulking agent in diarrhea, and as a laxative in constipated bowel habits, may improve voiding sufficiently to also influence continence, especially seepage. Alternatively, loperamide or other pharmacological diarrhea treatments may slow transit enough to reduce urgency and incontinence and also dry the stool and decrease seepage. Scheduling of toilet visits for the very elderly and frail may improve continence. Relearning or training for the bowel and pelvic floor with strengthening of the musculature is the goal of biofeedback, which improves upon simple dietary and lifestyle modifications, and is effective.

Beyond these conservative managements, the surgical treatments have moved gradually away from anatomical correction-type procedures (although these are most appropriate for the comparatively rare isolated sphincter defects) towards interventions to augment anal tone and squeeze. Bulking injections at proctoscopy into the submucosa of the lower rectum are used to improve on the results of biofeedback or conservative measures alone, with some success and with little morbidity. Sacral nerve stimulation is also thought to increase anal tone and squeeze pressures, is relatively low risk and is frequently beneficial.

4.5 Pruritus Ani

Pruritus ani is common and frequently a chronic condition tolerated over decades. It is an itching or prickling sensation with very many potential causes, some of which are outlined in this chapter. Other causes may be chemical, such as detergent or medication, or dietary, such as spicy food, caffeine or citrus. Seepage incontinence or chronic wetness of the perianal skin from diarrheal illness or IBD may be the trigger, or an intrinsic skin problem or malignancy, infection or allergy. Diagnosis might require perianal skin biopsy. The final common symptomatic pathway results from irritation or breakage of the intensely itchy skin by scratching, which is often irresistible or unconscious, but which perpetuates and aggravates the itch and commences a cycle which it is difficult, but necessary, to break. Treatment of the cause is imperative, but the many possible causes confound diagnosis often, and pruritus is not infrequently a matter of chronic symptom treatment and may result in a thickened, ichthyotic perianal skin. Topical steroid is effective in symptom relief, but chronic use is contraindicated. Local desensitization is reportedly effective, using topical capsaicin.

4.6 Anal Cancer

Anal cancer occurs infrequently in the general population but is not infrequently seen in higher-risk groups such as people with HPV-associated genital cancers, the immunosuppressed and men who have sex with men. Overall, it occurs more often in women and is associated with smoking. Most anal cancers are squamous cell carcinoma (SCC), with variants being basaloid cancers and cloacogenic cancers, embryologically and pathologically distinct, but presenting similarly. Anal cancer is prone to misdiagnosis and can be dismissed as a minor condition such as hemorrhoids. Melanoma, lymphoma and adenocarcinoma may occur at the anus. There is benefit in screening high-risk groups with anoscopy and vaccinating for HPV and likely benefit in detecting and managing anal intraepithelial neoplasia, the putative precursor to the majority of anal cancer. SCC of the anus is most commonly treated with combined chemo- and radiotherapy, often as a definitive treatment, or with salvage resection following downstaging. Frequently there is defunctioning with a loop stoma prior to chemoradiotherapy. SCC of the anus is more often survived than not. Other histological types of anal cancer are varied as mentioned before, as is their prognosis and treatment.

Recommended Reading

Acheson AG, Scholefield JH. Management of haemorrhoids. BMJ. 2008;336(7640):380–3.

Foxx-Orenstein AE, Umar SB, Crowell MD. Common anorectal disorders. Gastroenterol Hepatol. 2014;10(5):294–301.

Symer MM, Yeo HL. Recent advances in the management of anal cancer. F1000Res. 2018;7:F1000 Faculty Rev-1572. https://doi.org/10.12688/f1000research.14518.1.

Wald A, Bharucha AE, Cosman BC, Whitehead WE. Clinical guideline: management of benign anorectal disorders. Am J Gastroenterol. 2014;109(8):1141–57.

Colorectal Cancer

5

Matthias W. Wichmann and Timothy K. McCullough

5.1 Epidemiology/Risk Factors/Pathogenesis

The global burden of colorectal cancer (CRC) is expected to increase by 60% by 2030. Currently CRC is the fourth leading cause of cancer death in the world. Incidence and mortality are increasing rapidly in low- and middle-income countries, while stabilizing trends can be seen in highly developed countries.

Colorectal cancer develops under the influence of environmental and genetic factors. The incidence of CRC varies around the world with the highest rates observed in Australia, New Zealand, Europe, and North America. Age and socioeconomic status contribute to the incidence of CRC. The incidence increases significantly after age 40 with more men than women affected by CRC. Lower socioeconomic status results in poorer diet, less physical activity, higher nicotine addiction rates, higher obesity rates, and reduced uptake of screening programs, thus contributing to a up to 30% increased risk of CRC in these patients.

Up to 10% of unselected patients with CRC appear to have one or more genetic mutations contributing to the development of CRC. In patients with early-onset (before the age of 50) CRC genetic counseling and testing should be considered.

5.2 Hereditary CRC

Familial adenomatous polyposis (FAP), Gardner syndrome, Turcot syndrome, and attenuated FAP (AFAP) account for less than 1% of all CRC. FAP and AFAP are caused by germline mutations on Chromosome 5.

Hereditary nonpolyposis colorectal cancer (HNPCC, Lynch syndrome) is an autosomal dominant syndrome and accounts for 3% of CRC. The Lynch syndrome

M. W. Wichmann (✉) · T. K. McCullough
Department of Surgery, Mount Gambier General Hospital, Mount Gambier, SA, Australia
e-mail: matthias.wichmann@sa.gov.au; timothy.mccullough@sa.gov.au

M. W. Wichmann et al. (eds.), *Gastroenterology For General Surgeons*,
https://doi.org/10.1007/978-3-319-92768-8_5

is caused by a defect in one of the DNA mismatch repair genes (hMLH1, hMSH2, hMSH6, hPMS2) resulting in hypermutable and microsatellite unstable CRC. CRC in patients with Lynch syndrome is usually diagnosed before the age of 50 and is predominantly right-sided (70%).

Pancolitis due to ulcerative colitis or Crohn's disease carries an up to 15 times increased risk to develop CRC. Quiescent disease carries a smaller risk than chronically active disease.

Survivors of childhood cancer who received more than 30 Gy abdominal radiation should have surveillance colonoscopy performed every 5 years.

CRC mortality is 25% higher in men than in women, but screening recommendations are not influenced by patient gender.

Metachronous CRC after previous bowel cancer resection can be detected in up to 3% of patients during the first 5 years after initial surgery.

Family history of large bowel cancer influences the individual risk of CRC with a single first-degree relative with CRC doubling the individual's risk to develop CRC. This risk is further increased with more affected relatives or diagnosis in a patient younger than 50 years.

Other risk factors for the development of CRC are obesity, diabetes mellitus, and increased consumption of red or processed meats (mainly left side tumors, inconsistent data). Processed meat (bacon, ham, sausages, etc.) has been classified as a Group 1 carcinogen (such as asbestos, cigarettes, alcohol). The absolute risk of developing cancer due to processed meats however is small and is only seen with daily consumption. Cigarette smoking and moderate (2–3 drinks/d) to heavy (>3 drinks/d) alcohol consumption are also associated with an increased risk of CRC.

Protective factors against the development of CRC have been described in observational studies. These include aspirin, NSAIDS, dietary factors, physical activity, and hormone replacement therapy in postmenopausal women.

- Aspirin/NSAIDS: up to 40% risk reduction in normal risk population.
- Dietary factors with potentially beneficial effects are fruit and vegetables, fiber, dairy products, calcium, vitamin D, magnesium, and omega-3 fatty acids.
- Hormone therapy in women: best protection with the use of combined (estrogen + progesterone) therapy.

The pathogenesis for the development of CRC involves the accumulation of genetic and epigenetic modifications within pathways that regulate cell proliferation, apoptosis, and angiogenesis. There are at least three molecular pathways contributing to the development of colorectal cancer. These are the chromosomal instability (CIN) pathway (familial adenomatous polyposis), the mutator-phenotype/DNA mismatch repair pathway (Lynch syndrome, some sporadic CRCs), and the hypermethylation phenotype hyperplastic/serrated polyp pathway (hereditary and sporadic CRCs).

5.3 Macroscopy/Histology

Tumors of the proximal colon are mainly fungating exophytic masses, whereas distal colon cancers tend to be more annular in appearance. Synchronous disease must be expected in up to 5% of patients, and a complete colonoscopy should always be performed prior to elective surgery or within 3–6 months after emergency surgery for bowel cancer to exclude missed synchronous disease.

Most tumors of the large bowel and rectum are carcinomas, and more than 90% are adenocarcinomas. Low-grade (well- and moderately differentiated) tumors show gland formation on histology, whereas high-grade (poorly differentiated) tumors do not form glandular structures. Mucinous carcinomas (up to 17%) produce large amounts of extracellular mucin and are more common in the ascending colon. It appears that these tumors do not respond well to neoadjuvant and/or adjuvant chemotherapy.

Immune-histochemistry helps to identify cancer of colorectal origin through positivity for the surface antigens CK20 (cytokeratin 20) and CDX2 (caudal-type homebox 2).

5.4 Diagnosis

CRC is usually diagnosed via colonoscopy (Fig. 5.1). Alternatively, CT colonoscopy (Fig. 5.2a) or CT scan with fecal tagging (Fig. 5.2b) may identify CRC prior to histological confirmation (see also Chapter 15). A complete evaluation of the large bowel should be attempted prior to surgery since up to 5% of patients present with synchronous CRC.

Malignant lesions of the appendix are usually identified postoperatively in appendectomy specimen (<0.5% of all appendectomies). Most of these are

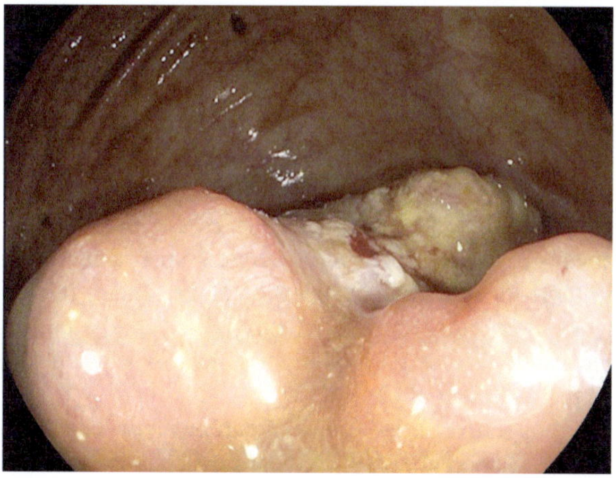

Fig. 5.1 Colonoscopy finding of colon cancer

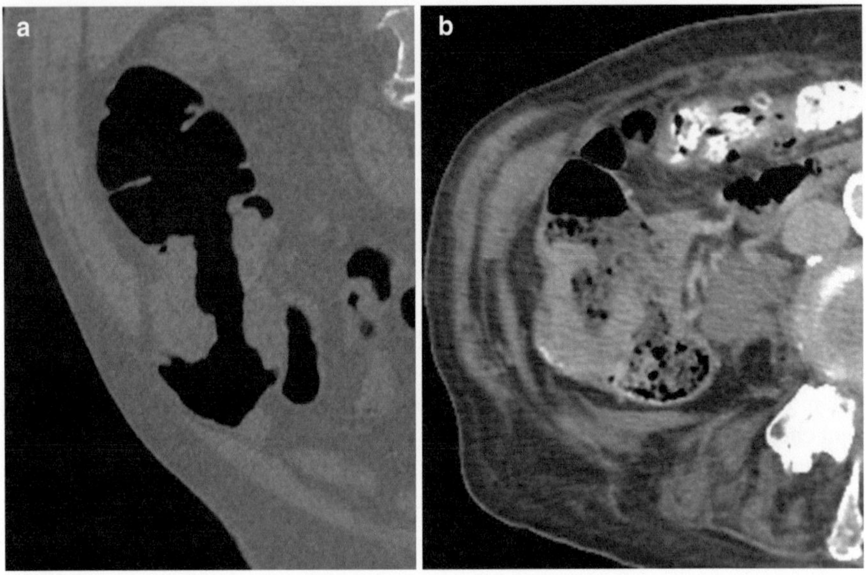

Fig. 5.2 (**a**) CT colonoscopy finding of colon cancer. (**b**) Fecal tagging CT finding of colon cancer

neuroendocrine tumors, but approximately 30% are adenocarcinomas. *Pseudomyxoma peritonei* develops from peritoneal dissemination after rupture of a mucinous cystadenocarcinoma of the appendix.

5.5 Staging

Colorectal cancer has the potential to spread via the lymphatic and venous system as well as through direct invasion of the surrounding tissue and the peritoneum. Most common metastatic stations are the liver, lung, and lymph nodes.

Pre-therapeutic staging of CRC involves computed tomography (*CT*) of the abdomen, pelvis, and chest. For rectal cancer magnetic resonance imaging (*MRI*) is also necessary to establish the potential indication for preoperative neoadjuvant radio-chemotherapy (Fig. 5.3).

The preoperative identification of isolated liver or lung metastases does not always result in a change of surgical approach. Isolated liver metastases may be suitable for synchronous resection at the time of bowel surgery.

Positron emission tomography (*PET*) can be used to determine whether or not metastatic disease is suitable for resection or whether systemic chemotherapy may be the treatment of choice.

Preoperative serum levels of carcinoembryonic antigen (*CEA*) should be determined as a potential aid for identification of recurrent disease during postoperative follow-up.

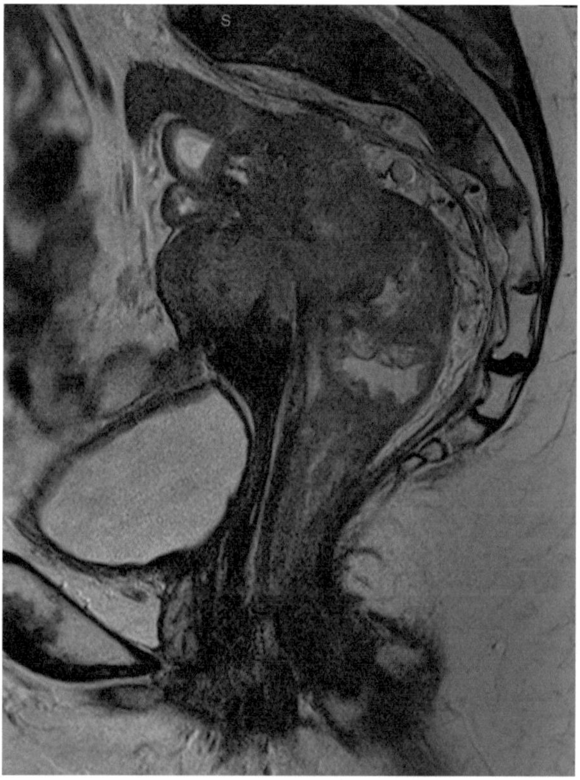

Fig. 5.3 Magnetic resonance imaging (MRI) of rectal cancer

5.6 Treatment

5.6.1 Preoperative (Neoadjuvant) Radiotherapy and Chemotherapy

Randomized trials confirm the benefits of preoperative administration of neoadjuvant chemoradiotherapy in patients with locally advanced rectal cancer. Locally advanced disease is defined via pelvic MRI and/or endorectal ultrasound. If these imaging modalities confirm T3/T4 disease, endangered or involved circumferential resection margin (CRM), enlarged lymph nodes in the mesorectum (N+) neoadjuvant short- or long-course treatment should be offered. Most of our patients receive long-course radio-chemotherapy over 5 weeks with definitive surgery delayed until 10–12 weeks after completion of the neoadjuvant treatment regimen. Alternatively short-course radiation over 5 days can be considered. These patients usually undergo surgery within 1 week after the radiotherapy. This treatment aims at sterilization of perirectal lymph nodes and does not reduce the size of the primary rectal cancer.

Tumor eradication after neoadjuvant radio-chemotherapy is associated with significantly improved survival when compared with patients who are found to have residual disease or positive regional lymph nodes after preoperative chemoradiation.

5.6.2 Adjuvant Chemotherapy

The benefits of adjuvant chemotherapy have been demonstrated in patients with Stage 3 (node positive) disease who can expect a 30% risk reduction for recurrent disease and up to 32% better survival rates. Most of these patients will be offered a 6-month course of oxaliplatin-based chemotherapy (FOLFOX = oxaliplatin+FU + leucovorin; XELOX = oxaliplatin+capecitabine). Treatment must be initiated within a 6–8-week time window after surgical resection, highlighting the importance of a fast and uncomplicated recovery after surgery.

5.7 Nonsurgical Management

Most patients with metastatic colon or rectal cancer cannot be cured. Nonsurgical management is reserved for these advanced stages of colorectal cancer with diffuse, non-resectable metastatic disease. In these patients a palliative approach involving chemotherapy, radiation therapy, and/or best supportive care should be discussed with the patient.

Patients with resectable metastases in the lungs or liver should be assessed for radical surgical resection of both primary cancer and metastatic sites.

In the palliative situation, surgery can be useful for the treatment of complications of progressive disease. These complications include bowel obstruction, gastrointestinal hemorrhage, and bowel perforation due to obstruction or as a consequence of palliative chemotherapy. Surgical options include stent insertion, bypass surgery, stoma formation, or palliative resection (±anastomosis). In order to minimize postoperative complications, laparoscopic surgery should be used for surgical palliation wherever possible.

Asymptomatic patients with unresectable metastatic disease have low risks of bleeding (3%) and obstruction/perforation (14%) and should therefore be managed with a nonsurgical approach.

5.8 Medical Treatment of Metastatic Colorectal Cancer (mCRC)

Contemporary medical treatment of metastatic CRC is based on a wide spectrum of drugs, whereas until 2000, only fluorouracil was available.

The mechanism of cytotoxicity of fluorouracil (FU) is believed to be impaired DNA synthesis (inhibition of thymidylate synthase). Leucovorin (LV) enhances FU cytotoxicity (response rate increases from 11% to 21%), and nowadays a combination of FU/LV with irinotecan or oxaliplatin is considered first-line treatment for metastatic CRC.

Capecitabine is an oral alternative to IV regimens of FU. The final enzymatic step of conversion into FU requires thymidine phosphorylase which is present in higher concentration in tumor tissue. This results in enhanced selectivity of the drug for tumor cells.

Irinotecan is a topoisomerase I inhibitor and is usually used in combination with FU/LV for first-line treatment of mCRC (FOLFIRI). Irinotecan can also be used in combination with targeted agents (Bevacizumab, Cetuximab).

Oxaliplatin is a platinum derivative, and in combination with FU/LV, it is an option for first-line treatment of mCRC (FOLFOX). FOLFOX and FOLFIRI have similar treatment effects in patients with mCRC.

Vascular endothelial growth factor (VEGF) is the dominant factor regulating the development of blood supply for tumor growth. Targeted antitumor therapy aims to inhibit VEGF. Bevacizumab (Avastin) is a humanized monoclonal antibody targeting VEGF. Addition of Bevacizumab to first-line chemotherapy regimens for mCRC improves outcomes (modestly). For surgeons it is important to note that the long half-life of Bevacizumab and the problems of wound healing due to VEGF inhibition must be considered for the planning of elective surgery (minimum 28 days after last administration, better 6–8 weeks).

Epidermal growth factor (EGF) and its receptor (EGFR) are involved in the control of colorectal cancer growth, angiogenesis, and metastatic spread. Monoclonal antibodies blocking EGFR can be used for treatment of mCRC and have been observed to be only effective in patients who suffer from wild-type (WT) RAS cancer. BRAF mutations also make response to these EGFR-targeting drugs very unlikely. Cetuximab (Erbitux) is a mouse/human chimeric antibody binding to the EGFR, and it is useful in combination with irinotecan but has also been shown to be effective as monotherapy (versus best supportive care). Panitumumab (Vectibix) is a fully human antibody targeting the extracellular domain of EGFR. Both monoclonal antibodies are effective as monotherapy and recent evidence supports their addition to first-/second-/third-line treatment regimens for mCRC provided biomarker analysis does not exclude the effectiveness of these drugs (wild-type RAS cancer, absence of BRAF mutations).

Currently initial combination chemotherapy should be considered for most patients especially if an initial response to chemotherapy may result in a potentially resectable stage of disease.

5.9 Surgical Management

Approximately 80% of colon cancers are limited to the bowel walls and have not metastasized beyond the regional lymph nodes. Surgical resection of the bowel together with the lymphatic and vascular pedicle is the only curative approach. Resectable structures adherent to or invaded by the cancer should be removed en bloc with the affected bowel. The plane of adherence should not be opened during surgery (>40% malignant adhesions). If R1 resection appears to be likely, the surgeon should place metal clips and an omental flap into the area of resection to allow for postoperative radiation of the area.

Most CRCs arise from adenomas (adenoma-carcinoma sequence: adenoma → dysplasia → in situ cancer → invasive cancer), and invasive malignancy can be prevented by polypectomy. The transformation to invasive cancer is believed to take many years (up to 15).

Malignant polyps (without evidence of invasive cancer) can be treated with polypectomy only. No further bowel resection is necessary unless histology shows poor differentiation, lymphovascular invasion, involved resection margin, and T2 disease or a flat/sessile polyp was identified. If there is a risk for perforation during endoscopic resection of a possibly malignant polyp, it is important to only take biopsies. The lesion is then tattooed and the patient can be prepared for elective radical surgery.

Most common surgical procedures for the treatment of CRC are right and left hemicolectomy, sigmoid colectomy, (low) anterior resection, Hartmann procedure, and abdominoperineal resection (APR). We do not advocate transverse colectomy as a treatment option for cancers within the transverse colon. Most cancers are localized either right or left of the midline, and an extended (right or left) hemicolectomy should be performed instead.

There is Level 1 evidence (meta-analyses of prospective randomized trials) confirming faster recovery of patients after laparoscopic surgery for colorectal cancer without compromising oncological results (lymph node yield, recurrence, survival). Provided expertise in advanced laparoscopic colorectal surgery is available, this approach should therefore be offered rather than open surgery for uncomplicated CRC. The faster recovery after laparoscopic surgery results in a 5% higher uptake of adjuvant chemotherapy following surgical resection in these patients.

Whether open or laparoscopic surgery is performed, proximal and distal margins should be at least 5 cm (different margins apply to the rectum), and a minimum of 12 lymph nodes should be available for histological evaluation. There is a close relationship between the number of lymph nodes evaluated and long-term survival. If fewer than 12 lymph nodes are available for pathological evaluation, adjuvant chemotherapy should be offered. Other reasons to consider adjuvant chemotherapy in Stage 2 (node negative) disease are T3/T4 lesion, bowel perforation, bowel obstruction, poorly differentiated cancer, lymphovascular or perineural invasion, and young patient age.

In patients with synchronous cancers of the large bowel (app 5% of all patients), a subtotal/total colectomy should be performed. In female patients with HNPCC, a total colectomy should be combined with hysterectomy and bilateral salpingo-oophorectomy.

Complete tumor resection is the goal of curative surgery, and residual tumor is a poor prognostic factor. The clearance of malignant disease is classified as:

- R0: complete resection
- R1: microscopic residual disease
- R2: macroscopic incomplete tumor resection

The circumferential resection margin (CRM) is of significant importance for the prognosis after rectal cancer resection. If the distance between the primary cancer and the CRM is less than 1 mm (positive CRM), this has been shown to negatively influence local and distant recurrence as well as survival.

Involvement of regional lymph nodes is one of the strongest factors influencing survival after surgical resection of colorectal cancers. Presence of distant metastatic disease is the only more relevant prognostic factor. Due to the prognostic relevance of the lymph node status, it is recommended that at least 12 lymph nodes should be examined to accurately determine the postoperative N status. After neoadjuvant radio-chemotherapy for rectal cancer, it has been observed that 12 lymph nodes can often not be found in the specimen—in this setting a lower lymph node count has not been associated with poorer survival.

Currently there are only few molecular markers influencing treatment decisions in colorectal cancer. The most relevant is MMR (mismatch repair) deficiency. Patients with MMR-deficient tumors have better chances of long-term survival; the biological basis for this observation is not known. RAS mutations are used to identify tumors that are not suitable for the treatment with biological agents targeting the epidermal growth factor receptor (EGFR). BRAF mutations have also been shown to have prognostic and predictive relevance. BRAF mutation favors a sporadic tumor. Mutations of the RAS and BRAF oncogenes lead to activation of the EGFR pathway even if the receptor itself is blocked.

5.10 Follow-up

The most important factor affecting long-term survival is the pathological stage at presentation. For patients receiving neoadjuvant therapy (chemo- and/or radiotherapy), it is important to perform a complete restaging after completion of neoadjuvant treatment since the post-neoadjuvant treatment disease stage is a better prognostic factor than the original tumor stage at the time of diagnosis.

Local and/or regional recurrent disease develops in up to 12% of patients after curative resection. Early detection of recurrent disease is possible with regular follow-up examination, and if R0 resection of recurrent disease can be performed, a 5-year survival of more than 50% can be observed.

We recommend a close follow-up after CRC surgery for at least 5 years after surgery. Currently we perform regular blood tests, physical examination, scans, and colonoscopies at varying time points until 10 years after surgery (similar to the surveillance protocol suggested by the American Society of Clinical Oncology). Follow-up results are collected in a departmental follow-up database (Fig. 5.4). In smaller surgical centers, postoperative follow-up should remain within the surgical department, and we strongly recommend establishing a departmental follow-up database.

The most important prognostic factor for postoperative long-term survival is the pathological stage (TNM classification, Table 5.1) at the time of diagnosis (Fig. 5.4). The risk of recurrent disease and cancer-related death decreases significantly at

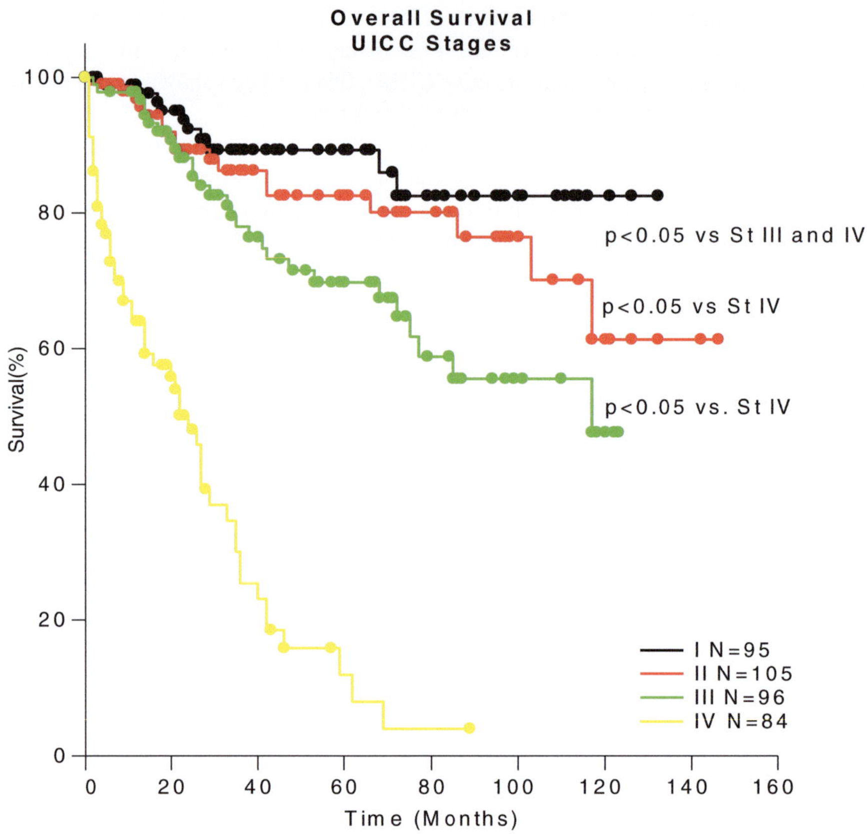

Fig. 5.4 Follow-up results—Mount Gambier Hospital

5 years after surgery, but there still is a risk of 8% in men and of 5% in women after curative resection to develop recurrent disease between 5 and 10 years after surgery. This should be considered when establishing postoperative follow-up protocols, and we recommend yearly follow-up in years 5 to 10 after surgery.

5.11 When to Transfer

Management of colorectal cancer requires a multidisciplinary care approach, and this should be available to all patients diagnosed with CRC in developed countries. Fast and uncomplicated recovery after surgery is essential for the optimal timing of adjuvant (chemo-) therapy. If multidisciplinary treatment or adequate surgical and nursing/allied health care cannot be provided in a smaller surgical center, patients requiring elective resection should be transferred. The authors however favor implementation and provision of the necessary infrastructure and resources as close to home as possible for CRC patients. Emergency surgery may require postoperative

Table 5.1 TNM classification (seventh edition) and colorectal cancer stages

T	Depth of invasion	N	Number of nodes involved	M	Distant metastasis
In situ	Lamina propria	0	0	0	No
1	Submucosa	1	1–3	1	Yes
2	Muscularis propria	1a	1	1a	1 organ
3	Pericolorectal tissue	1b	2–3	1b	More than one organ
4a	Penetrates visceral peritoneum	1c	Deposits in subserosa, mesentery, pericolic/perirectal tissue		
4b	Other organs/structures	2	≥4		
		2a	4–6		
		2b	≥7		
Stage	Dukes				
0	–	Tis	N0	M0	
I	A	T1–2	N0	M0	
IIa	B	T3	N0	M0	
IIb	B	T4a	N0	M0	
IIc	B	T4b	N0	Mo	
IIIa	C	T1–2	N1/N1c	M0	
	C	T1	N2a	M0	
IIIb	C	T3–4a	N1/N1c	M0	
	C	T2–3	N2a	M0	
	C	T1–2	N2b	M0	
IIIc	C	T4a	N2a	M0	
	C	T3–4a	N2b	M0	
	C	T4b	N1–2	M0	
IVa	–	Any T	Any N	M1a	
IVb	–	Any T	Any N	M1b	

care in high-dependency or intensive care units. If this cannot be provided and the patient can still be transferred, this should be considered prior to surgical intervention.

Recommended Reading

Brenner H, et al. The colorectal cancer epidemic: challenges and opportunities for primary, secondary and tertiary prevention. Br J Cancer. 2018;119(7):785–92. [Epub ahead of print]

Kim BJ, et al. The role of targeted agents in the adjuvant treatment of colon cancer: a meta-analysis of randomized phase III studies and review. Oncotarget. 2017;8(19):31112–8.

Matsuda T. Recent updates in the surgical treatment of colorectal cancer. Ann Gastroenterol Surg. 2018;2(2):129–36.

Meyers BM, et al. Adjuvant chemotherapy for stage II and III colon cancer following complete resection: a cancer care ontario systematic review. Clin Oncol (R Coll Radiol). 2017;29(7):459–65.

Oki E, et al. Recent advances in multidisciplinary approach for rectal cancer. Int J Clin Oncol. 2015;20(4):641–9.

UpToDate®: Acute colonic diverticulitis: Surgical Management.
UpToDate®: Overview of the management of primary colon cancer.
UpToDate®: Pathology and prognostic determinants of colorectal cancer.
UpToDate®: Surgical resection of primary colon cancer.
UpToDate®: Systemic chemotherapy for metastatic colorectal cancer: Completed clinical trials.
Vennix S. Laparoscopic versus open total mesorectal excision for rectal cancer. Cochrane Database Syst Rev. 2014;15(4):CD005200.
Wu C. Systemic therapy for colon cancer. Surg Oncol Clin N Am. 2018;27(2):235–42.

Inflammatory Bowel Disease: Diagnosis and Management

6

Madeleine Gill and Robert V. Bryant

6.1 Pathogenesis and Epidemiology

The pathogenesis of Inflammatory Bowel Disease (IBD) is complex, multifactorial and incompletely understood. Factors thought to play a role in IBD pathogenesis are host genetics, immune dysregulation, abnormal composition and function of the gut microbiome and environmental factors. An aberrant immune response to the gut's commensal bacteria with associated disturbance of intestinal barrier function underpins the inflammatory process in IBD. Genome-wide association studies (GWAS) have identified >250 risk loci for IBD, many of which overlap with other autoimmune disorders. A 'dysbiosis' of the gut microbiome in IBD has been characterised by a reduction in the diversity of microbial communities in patients with IBD as compared to healthy individuals.

Twin concordance studies show 35% of monozygotic twins are concordant for Crohn's Disease (CD), compared with 3% of dizygotic twins. Twenty to thirty percent of CD patients have a family history of IBD; children of an affected parent have a 5% chance of having CD. The genetic component of UC is less strong than CD with only 10–15% having family history.

Multiple putative environmental factors influence the susceptibility and disease course of IBD, including dietary factors (in particular a typical Western diet consisting

M. Gill
Department of Gastroenterology and Hepatology, The Queen Elizabeth Hospital, Adelaide, SA, Australia
e-mail: Madeleine.Gill@sa.gov.au

R. V. Bryant (✉)
Department of Gastroenterology and Hepatology, The Queen Elizabeth Hospital, Adelaide, SA, Australia

School of Medicine, Faculty of Health Sciences, University of Adelaide, Adelaide, SA, Australia
e-mail: Robert.Bryant@sa.gov.au

M. W. Wichmann et al. (eds.), *Gastroenterology For General Surgeons*,
https://doi.org/10.1007/978-3-319-92768-8_6

of processed foods, animal fats and refined sugars), enteric infections, medications and lifestyle factors. Smoking confers increased risk of a more severe CD phenotype (stricturing and fistulising), whereas conversely for Ulcerative Colitis (UC), active smoking reduces disease susceptibility and severity. Early-life antibiotic therapy and hygiene have also been implicated in risk of IBD, whereas breast-milk appears to be protective. The prevalence of IBD varies according to latitude with lowest rates reported in hotter equatorial climates, implicating sunlight exposure and vitamin D levels as possible factors in susceptibility. Interestingly, appendicectomy confers a protective effect for UC when performed for acute appendicitis in young patients.

IBD typically presents in late adolescence to early adulthood, although there is a small rise in incidence in later life. IBD tends to affect men and women equally. The global prevalence of IBD has trebled over the last 30 years. Australia has one of the highest rates of IBD in the world with an estimated 1:250 Australians affected. Although the prevalence of IBD is highest in developed countries, there has been a rapid increase in the incidence of IBD in developing countries, where environmental factors and a Western lifestyle are implicated in observed trends.

6.2 Definitions

The term IBD encompasses both UC and CD. UC is characterised by chronic non-granulomatous inflammation that is limited to the colonic mucosa, typically involving the rectum and a variable proximal extent of the colon in continuity. CD is characterised by transmural, often granulomatous inflammation, and can involve any part of the gastrointestinal tract from the mouth to anus. CD most frequently involves the terminal ileum and perianal regions, and stricturing and fistulising disease behaviour is common. A small proportion of patients are affected by predominant oral or upper gut inflammation. IBD-unclassified (IBD-U or IBD-hi yet to be classified) is a label applied when a clear distinction between UC and CD cannot be readily made and is more common in pediatric patients.

6.3 Clinical Presentation

The clinical presentation of UC is typified by bloody diarrhea with associated urgency, tenesmus and lower abdominal pain. Around 25% of patients with UC initially present with acute severe colitis requiring hospitalisation. In terms of disease extent, around 50% of patients with UC have disease involving the left side of the colon, and around 30% have extensive disease (extending beyond the splenic flexure). Distal colitis may present with symptoms of urgency and tenesmus, whereas in pancolitis, bloody diarrhea and abdominal pain may be more prominent. Up to 10% of patients with proctitis or left-sided colitis can suffer from paradoxical constipation.

The clinical presentation of CD varies widely according to disease behaviour and phenotype but is typically one of abdominal pain, diarrhea and weight loss. Perianal disease affects around one-third of patients with CD and can present with fistulising disease, fibrostenosing disease or perianal sepsis with abscess formation. Obstructive symptoms may result from small bowel stricturing disease and include cramping abdominal pain (especially in the hours after eating), nausea and vomiting, diarrhea and bloating. Constitutional symptoms of weight loss, anorexia and fatigue are common in CD, as are extra-intestinal manifestations (EIMs) (Table 6.1).

EIMs are common and affect up to half of patients with IBD, more often in CD than in UC. EIMs may precede the diagnosis of intestinal inflammation in some instances. The range of EIMs is broad and includes arthropathy, skin disease (pyoderma gangrenosum and erythema nodosum), eye inflammation (iritis uveitis and episcleritis), venous thromboembolic disease (VTE) and metabolic bone disease.

Table 6.1 Extra-intestinal manifestations of IBD

System	Manifestation	Clinical presentation
Joints	Type 1 arthropathy	Pauciarticular (< five joints), large joints (hips, knees, shoulders)
	Type 2 arthropathy	Polyarticular (> five joints), symmetric, small joints of hands
	Spondyloarthropathy	Inflammatory back pain, prolonged stiffness in back and/or buttocks
Eyes	Episcleritis	Acute redness of one or both eyes; pain, irritation, itching or burning with injection and tenderness Does not impair vision
	Uveitis	Anterior uveitis may produce pain and redness; posterior uveitis is more likely to be painless and visual loss
	Scleritis	Severe, constant, boring pain that worsens at night or in the early morning hours and radiates to the face and periorbital region. Redness, watering and photophobia may be present Can impair vision
Skin	Erythema nodosum	Raised, tender, red subcutaneous nodules 1–5 cm in diameter. Commonly located on the extensor surfaces or the extremities, particularly the anterior tibial area
	Pyoderma gangrenosum[a]	Single or multiple erythematous papules or pustules that are often preceded by trauma to the skin. Most common on the legs
	Psoriasis	Sharply defines erythematous plaques with overlying silvery scale on the scalp, extensor elbows, knees and back
	Sweet syndrome	Acute inflammatory dermatitis characterised by tender papules, plaques and nodules on the face, arms and trunk
Other	Osteoporosis Primary sclerosing cholangitis[a] Venous thromboembolic disease Vitamin D deficiency Anxiety and depression Fatigue	

[a]More common in UC than CD

IBD-associated arthropathy is one of the most common extra-intestinal manifestations of IBD. Type 1 arthropathy is pauciarticular, involves large joints, parallels disease activity and responds to optimising disease control. Type 2 arthropathy is polyarticular, symmetrical, involving small joints and is unrelated to disease activity.

Primary sclerosing cholangitis (PSC) is a hepatobiliary manifestation of IBD, affecting up to 5% of patients with IBD, typically those with milder forms of UC. PSC can damage hepatic tissue to the extent that a liver transplant is indicated, and also carries a high risk of progression to cholangiocarcinoma. The co-existence of PSC and IBD also conveys a higher risk of colonic malignancy requiring more frequent colonic surveillance.

A healthy index of suspicion is required to investigate for and identify IBD, with many patients suffering from symptoms for many months to years prior to formal diagnosis and commencement of therapy.

6.4 Diagnosis and Work-Up

There is no single gold standard for the diagnosis of IBD. Rather, it is based on a composite assessment, incorporating clinical, endoscopic, histological and radiological factors (summarised in Table 6.2).

Table 6.2 Diagnosis of IBD

Diagnostic features	Crohn's Disease	Ulcerative Colitis
Clinical	Abdominal pain, weight loss, diarrhea or obstructive symptoms Extra-intestinal manifestations	Colitis symptoms: bloody diarrhea, urgency, tenesmus Extra-intestinal manifestations
Endoscopy	Discontinuous inflammation with mucosal cobblestoning, anal involvement, terminal ileal inflammation Endoscopic score: CDEIS or SES-CD	Continuous inflammation from rectum extending proximally with mucosal friability, spontaneous bleeding and ulceration Endoscopic score: Mayo Score or Ulcerative Colitis Endoscopic Index of Severity (UCEIS)
Histology	Patchy inflammation, crypt architectural disturbance, granulomatous inflammation (30%)	Confluent inflammation, basal plasmacytosis, cryptitis, architectural disturbance, crypt abscess formation, goblet cell depletion
Imaging	Plain abdominal film in acute presentations to exclude bowel obstruction MRE to assess extent of small bowel disease and nature of strictures (inflammatory vs. fibrostenotic). CTE can also be used, but cumulative radiation exposure must be considered Gastrointestinal ultrasound to identify extent of small and large bowel involvement, confirm transmural inflammation, exclude collections or phlegmon	Plain abdominal film in acute presentation to exclude toxic megacolon Gastrointestinal ultrasound to identify proximal extent of disease

6.4.1 Clinical History and Examination

A detailed clinical history (as outlined above) coupled with a thorough physical examination is the first step to diagnosis. The clinical history should include bowel habit (including incontinence and nocturnal bowel actions), per-rectal bleeding (mixed with stool or separate from stool), abdominal pain and obstructive symptoms, perianal symptoms, weight loss and constitutional symptoms. Features of EIMs (as outlined above) should also be included in the clinical history. Physical examination should include abdominal, perianal and oral examination, alongside examination of the skin, eyes and joints for EIMs.

6.4.2 Laboratory Tests

Laboratory markers of inflammation, nutrition and anemia are useful in the work-up of possible IBD.

Blood tests. C-reactive protein (CRP) is a biomarker of systemic inflammation that can indicate the presence of active inflammation. It is worth noting that CRP is often normal in mild-to-moderate UC, and a normal CRP therefore does not exclude a diagnosis of IBD. CRP correlates only modestly with endoscopic disease activity in IBD and may not be reliable in interpreting response to therapy in some patients.

A full blood count is useful and may reveal the presence of anemia (in the setting of inflammation and/or iron deficiency). An elevated white cell count may indicate active inflammation and infection (in particular perianal sepsis) or may be elevated in the context of corticosteroid use. Biochemical analysis may reveal hypoalbuminemia due to acute inflammation (with contribution of malnutrition). Cholestatic liver enzyme derangement warrants further investigation to exclude the presence of underlying PSC. Hypokalemia may be the result of profuse diarrhea.

A nutritional screen is an important part of the diagnostic work-up of IBD. Iron deficiency is common in IBD even in the absence of overt bleeding, both due to chronic occult mucosal blood loss and malabsorption. Interpretation of iron studies in the setting of inflammation can be difficult due to hyperferritinemia. Anemia of chronic disease is also common in IBD, and many patients present with both anemia of chronic disease and functional iron deficiency anemia. A comprehensive approach to interpreting iron studies is therefore advised, incorporating hematinics, full blood picture and markers of inflammation. Involvement of a gastroenterologist or hematologist can also be of assistance. Further nutritional screening should include vitamin B12, folate and vitamin D at a minimum.

Stool tests. A stool pathogen screen is important to exclude the possibility of an infectious aetiology and should include microscopy, culture and sensitivities, parasitology, viral studies and testing for *Clostridium difficile* toxin.

Fecal calprotectin, a test measuring neutrophil breakdown products in the bowel, has become a commonly used surrogate marker for bowel inflammation. Fecal calprotectin is a very sensitive test for inflammation; a normal fecal calprotectin (<50 μg/g) has a strong negative predictive value for IBD and is a useful test to differentiate between possible IBD and functional gastrointestinal symptoms. Fecal calprotectin also has a role in monitoring IBD disease activity and response to therapy.

6.4.3 Endoscopy

For UC, a diagnosis is established using colonoscopy, with consistent features including continuous and confluent rectal and colonic mucosal friability, spontaneous bleeding and ulceration.

Colonoscopy will also establish a diagnosis of CD, with consistent features including discontinuous inflammation, cobblestoning, anal lesions and ileal involvement of disease.

Several endoscopic scoring systems exist for both UC and CD. The Mayo Index endoscopic subscore is most commonly used for UC:

- Mayo 0: normal or inactive disease
- Mayo 1: mild disease (erythema, decreased vascular patent, mild friability)
- Mayo 2: moderate disease (marked erythema, absent vascular pattern, friability, erosions)
- Mayo 3: severe disease (spontaneous bleeding, ulceration)

The endoscopic findings in CD are most often reported descriptively in practice, but Crohn's Disease Endoscopic Index of Severity (CDEIS) and the Simplified Endoscopic Score for Crohn's Disease (SES-CD) are useful in clinical trials and may help in providing a more objective tool for disease monitoring in practice.

6.4.4 Histology

Histology is essential to demonstrate chronicity of colonic inflammation and to distinguish IBD from other acute causes of colitis. It does not always, however, distinguish between CD and UC. Mucosal biopsy features of UC include changes of chronicity, basal plasmacytosis, cryptitis, crypt architectural distortion and crypt abscess formation.

Mucosal biopsies in CD typically show features of chronicity with crypt architectural distortion, patchy inflammation, and the presence of granulomas. It is worth noting that granulomatous inflammation is evident in only around 30% of patients with CD.

6.4.5 Imaging

Cross-sectional imaging is important to evaluate for small bowel CD involvement, beyond the reaches of the endoscope. Enterography describes imaging performed after ingestion of oral contrast to distend and enhance views of the small bowel and is generally preferred to enteroclysis (where the contrast agent is administered through an enteric tube). Enterography may be performed using both magnetic resonance imaging (MRI) and computed tomography (CT). Given the IBD cohort is typically young and may require frequent imaging over time, MRI is preferred over CT to avoid cumulative radiation exposure. Although CT can be helpful when an intrabdominal abscess or phlegmon is clinically suspected, the use should be strongly justified in IBD patients and CT generally avoided where possible. Magnetic resonance enterography (MRE) is useful in the assessment of small bowel CD and helps to differentiate inflammatory strictures from fibrostenotic disease. Pelvic MRI is essential for the diagnosis and characterisation of perianal CD.

In UC, plain abdominal X-ray is imperative in the work-up of acute severe colitis (ASUC) to exclude toxic megacolon. Colonic 'thumb-printing' may be seen in acute colitis, and a lead pipe appearance due to loss of haustration is suggestive of long-standing and severe disease. Plain abdominal X-rays can also be helpful in the setting of potential obstructive symptoms in CD to evaluate for dilatation of small bowel loops.

Gastrointestinal ultrasound is emerging as a useful modality in IBD imaging, in visualising the colon (above the rectum) and the small bowel. Its use in point-of-care assessment and the absence of radiation make it a very appealing modality for both initial diagnosis and assessment of disease activity; however, it is operator dependent and not widely available outside of tertiary centres as yet.

6.4.6 Distinguishing CD and UC

Differentiating between CD and UC can be difficult, and 5–10% of patients initially classified as UC might eventually have their diagnosis changed to CD. Crohn's colitis and UC may be difficult to distinguish clinically; however, relative rectal sparing, endoscopic features of cobblestoning and skip lesions and granulomatous inflammation on biopsies would make CD more likely. Backwash ileitis in the setting of UC can confound endoscopic diagnosis as it may be interpreted as terminal ileitis. Similarly, a cecal patch of inflammation in UC is common and may be confused as a CD lesion because it is discrete from distal confluent disease.

6.5 Classification of IBD

IBD can be classified according to the age of onset, natural history of disease, distribution of disease, activity of disease and response to therapy. The Montreal classification and its later Paris modification for pediatric patients are the most widely used classification systems for IBD, incorporating age of onset, disease distribution and phenotype (behaviour) (Table 6.3). It is worth noting that most current classification systems only take into account disease activity at a moment in time and fail to account for the long-term burden of disease, complications and the impact on the patient.

Table 6.3 Montreal classification system for Crohn's disease and ulcerative colitis

Age at diagnosis	A1: <16 years A2: 17–40 years A3: >40 years
UC distribution	E1: Ulcerative proctitis E2: Left-sided UC (distal to splenic flexure) E3: Extensive (proximal to splenic flexure)
CD distribution	L1: Ileal L2: Colonic L3: Ileocolonic L4: Isolated upper digestive
CD behaviour	B1: Non-stricturing, non-penetrating B2: Stricturing B3: Penetrating P: Perianal disease

6.5.1 Disease Activity Assessment in IBD

Disease activity in IBD can be measured using clinical, endoscopic, histological or radiological assessment tools, as well as using biomarkers of inflammation and quality of life. Each of these domains of disease activity assessment in IBD has its merits, although none are perfect. Clinical symptoms are known to correlate poorly with objective measures of inflammation in IBD. Up to 40% of patients with IBD suffer from concurrent irritable bowel syndrome, which leads to symptoms in the absence of inflammation. Conversely, insidious progression of IBD can occur in the absence of symptoms. Therapeutic decisions in IBD are best made adjusting for objective measures of inflammatory activity.

Within each domain of disease activity assessment in IBD, there is a multitude of scoring systems. Most of these have not been validated and are cumbersome for use in routine practice. Nonetheless, indices of disease activity are important metrics in IBD care, in that they are repeatable and responsive to change and thereby allow objective longitudinal assessment of therapeutic efficacy.

Several clinical scoring systems exist for CD, the most commonly used of which is the Crohn's Disease Activity Index (CDAI), which is required to apply for biologic agents through the Pharmaceutical Benefits Scheme (PBS). The Mayo Score is most commonly used activity index for UC; it includes stool frequency, rectal bleeding, mucosal appearance at endoscopy and physician rating of disease.

6.5.2 Natural History and Burden of IBD

The natural history of IBD is one of the relapsing and remitting diseases, although some patients experience an unremitting disease course from the outset. Half of patients with CD will experience a stricturing or penetrating complication within 20 years of diagnosis, and more than half will undergo surgery in a similar time period. Proximal extension occurs in 30% of patients with UC, and around 10% will undergo a colectomy within 10 years of diagnosis.

The socioeconomic burden of IBD on affected individuals, their family units/communities and the healthcare system is substantial. Although patients with IBD have a normal life expectancy, they are burdened with physical and psychological morbidity, with accordingly high rates of disability and loss of work-related productivity. The overall cost of IBD to healthcare systems is driven by healthcare, surgery and hospitalisation as well as the high cost of biologic therapies.

6.5.3 Medical Management of IBD

6.5.3.1 Therapeutic Considerations in IBD

Most patients with IBD require lifelong medical therapy, and treatment decisions must be strategic, balancing drug efficacy, side effects and the likely duration of therapy. IBD management has two phases: remission induction and maintenance. Corticosteroids have a role in induction of remission only but should not be used in the long term. The early use of 'aggressive' combined immunosuppression (with subsequent de-escalation if possible) is referred to as the 'top-down' approach, aiming to prevent permanent damage by achieving early mucosal healing. The more conventional 'step up' approach is also still used in practice, now with more accelerated progression through therapeutic options with the aim of achieving mucosal healing.

Using patient- and disease-related factors to guide approach to therapy is essential, in particular, predicting those who may have a more severe disease phenotype. In CD, perianal and ileal disease are associated with higher risk of complicated disease. Patients with penetrating or stricturing CD who are active tobacco smokers also have more severe disease. Patients with prior surgery are also a group in whom avoidance of further surgery is paramount and for whom a more aggressive medical approach is more appropriate. In UC, the extent of disease (pancolitis) is associated with a higher rate of colectomy.

Prognostic factors at IBD diagnosis should also be considered, including age (younger age at diagnosis associated with a more complicated disease course), requirement for steroids, weight loss and baseline malnutrition. Treatment decisions in IBD should be personalised and tailored to individual goals and treatment acceptability.

6.5.4 Goals of IBD Therapy

Treatment targets have evolved with major therapeutic advances. A 'treat to target' approach to IBD management has been proposed, which advocates striving not only for resolution of symptoms but also objective resolution of inflammation. This involves achieving clinical, endoscopic and histologic biomarker and imaging targets of remission. The pursuit of remission in all these domains needs to be balanced with the risk of therapy and pragmatic concerns, but this paradigm should underpin the medical, surgical and supportive management of IBD patients.

The short-term goal of therapy is to induce remission of IBD and, in so doing, relieve symptoms and improve life quality. The long-term goal is to maintain steroid-free remission with objective control of inflammation, so as to prevent cumulative bowel damage and disability and normalise quality of life.

6.5.5 Conventional Management of IBD

Corticosteroids remain an important option for the induction of remission in IBD. 5-aminosalicylates (5-ASAs), including sulfasalazine and mesalazine, are anti-inflammatory therapies that are the foundation of therapy for UC. Many patients with IBD require immunomodulator therapy; the most commonly used are thiopurines (azathioprine (AZA) or mercaptopurine (6-MP)) and methotrexate (MTX). The advent of effective biologic therapies, in particular the antitumour necrosis factor-alpha (anti-TNF) agents, has revolutionised the management of IBD. Since the arrival of anti-TNFs, other biologicals have emerged such as anti-integrin agents (i.e. vedolizumab) and cytokine inhibitors (such as the IL 12-1 L-23 inhibitor ustekinumab). Figure 6.1 outlines the stepwise therapeutic choices in both UC and CD, and Table 6.4 summaries the safety profile and monitoring of these agents.

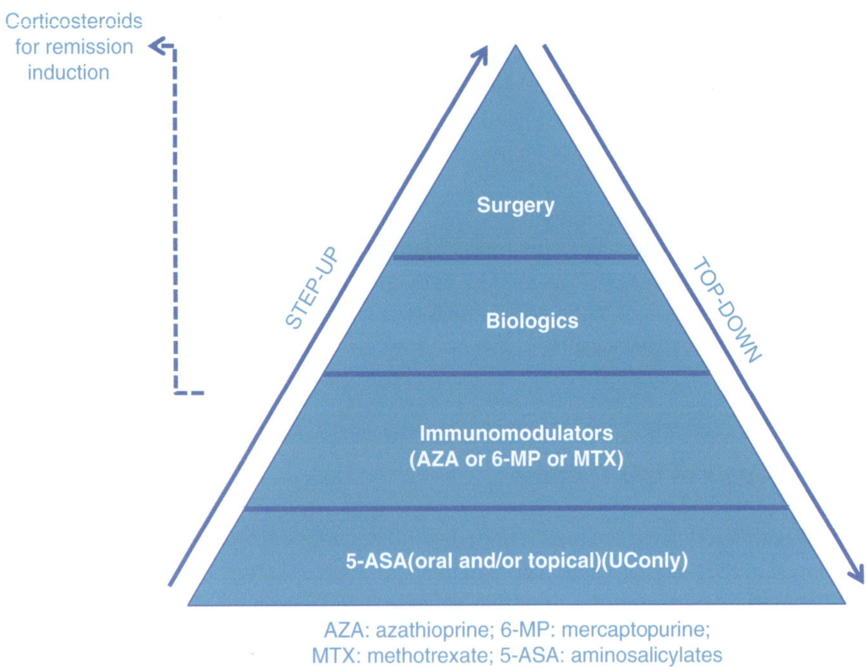

Fig. 6.1 Treatment pyramid for UC and CD. *AZA* azathioprine, *6-MP* 6-mercaptopurine, *MTX* methotrexate, *5-ASA* 5 aminosalicylic acid

Table 6.4 Summary of adverse events and monitoring for common IBD medications

Drug	Use	Adverse events	Monitoring
5-aminosalicylic acid therapy (sulfasalazine and mesalazine)	Induction and remission maintenance in UC	Common: diarrhea, headache, nausea, rash, flatulence, abdominal pain Rare: interstitial nephritis, marrow suppression, hepatotoxicity, alveolitis	Sulfasalazine: full blood count and liver enzymes ever 6–12 months 5-ASA: renal function every 6–12 months
Thiopurines (azathioprine and mercaptopurine)	Remission maintenance in UC and CD	Common: nausea, hepatotoxicity, myelotoxicity, non-melanoma skin cancers Rare: pancreatitis, lymphoma	Weekly full blood count and liver enzymes for 4 weeks, then three monthly thereafter Metabolite testing (6TG and 6MMP) after 6–8 weeks of stable therapy Sun protection and annual skin checks Annual pap smear Annual influenza vaccination and five yearly pneumococcal vaccination
Methotrexate	Remission induction and maintenance in CD	Common: nausea, headache, fatigue, hepatotoxicity Rare: liver fibrosis, pneumonitis	Weekly full blood count and liver enzymes for 4 weeks, then three monthly thereafter
Anti-TNF-α agents	Remission and induction maintenance in CD and UC Rescue therapy for acute severe colitis (IFX)	Infusion reactions Serious infections	Prescreening: viral hepatitis serology, HIV, varicella serology, TB screening
Corticosteroids	Remission induction in UC and CD	Early: acne, moon face, oedema, striae, sleep and mood disturbance, dyspepsia, glucose intolerance Late (>12 weeks): cataracts, osteoporosis, osteonecrosis, myopathy	Bone mineral density two yearly Calcium and vitamin D supplementation

6.5.6 Aminosalicylates

Efficacy and dosing. Sulfasalazine, which is metabolised to 5-ASA, along with mesalazine, is the first-line therapy for both induction and maintenance of UC. Sulfasalazine has similar efficacy to other 5-ASAs such as mesalazine but is generally less well tolerated due to the sulphur moiety. 5-ASAs may be administered orally (tablets or granules) and/or rectally (suppositories or enemas), with the route of administration dependent on extent of disease.

For distal UC, topical therapy is preferred, given that the 5-ASA agent is directly applied to the inflamed mucosa. Suppositories can be used for proctitis; however, enemas are preferred for disease beyond the rectosigmoid junction if tolerated. For pancolitis and left-sided disease, oral 5-ASA therapy is appropriate, with 5-ASA doses of ≥4 g typically used to induce remission and ≥ 2 g to maintain remission. Combined oral and topical therapy is more effective than either alone and should be used for moderate to severe UC. Corticosteroid therapy should be introduced if rectal bleeding persists for >10–14 days after initiation of 5-ASA therapy for patients with active UC.

5-ASAs have limited efficacy in CD, and their use is generally not recommended as they have not been shown to influence disease course.

Safety. 5-ASA therapy is generally well-tolerated, although side effects are more common with sulfasalazine necessitating a switch to mesalazine. Common adverse events include, diarrhea, headache, nausea, rash, flatulence and abdominal pain. Serious adverse effects are rare and include renal failure (interstitial nephritis), marrow suppression, pancreatitis, liver failure and alveolitis. Patients managed with 5-ASA therapy should undergo testing for renal function every 6–12 months. Patients managed with sulfasalazine should additionally undertake full blood count and liver function testing every 3–6 months.

6.5.7 Corticosteroids

Efficacy and dosing. Corticosteroids, such as oral prednisolone, intravenous or rectal hydrocortisone, have long been used in the management of IBD. Steroids, oral and rectal, are used to induce remission for both CD and UC. Prednisolone is a commonly used oral corticosteroid for IBD. The optimal starting dose of prednisolone is 50 mg/day with a 6–8-week taper as shorter courses may result in a rebound of inflammation. Steroid therapy is used as a bridge to maintenance therapy, and long-term use should be avoided due to adverse effects.

Budesonide is a synthetic steroid with low systemic bioavailability due to inactivation by first-pass hepatic metabolism. In standard form, budesonide is released in the small bowel and may be used for remission induction of mild-to-moderate CD. A novel multi-matrix system of budesonide (MMX) has been developed to extend release to the colon, which is useful for mild-to-moderate UC. Rectal steroids are not as effective as rectal mesalazine in remission induction but can be used as an adjunct if required.

Safety. Systemic corticosteroids cause early side effects including acne, moon face, oedema, skin striae, sleep and mood disturbance, dyspepsia and glucose intolerance. Prolonged use (>12 weeks) can lead to cataracts, osteoporosis, osteonecrosis and myopathy. Osteoprotective therapy with calcium and vitamin D supplementation is advised for all patients where steroid therapy for >8 weeks is planned. Budesonide is associated with few adverse effects due to limited systemic bioavailability.

6.5.8 Thiopurines

Efficacy and dosing. AZA and 6-MP are thiopurine antimetabolite therapies. Each are metabolised to the active metabolite, 6-thioguanine (6-TG), which inhibits cell growth and interferes with nucleic acid synthesis. They are efficacious in both UC and CD for remission maintenance; however, they are not effective for remission induction as their full effect is not seen until 8–12 weeks. A therapeutic 'bridge', such as corticosteroids, is therefore required whilst awaiting thiopurine effect. The dose range for AZA is 2–2.5 mg/kg/day; patients who do not tolerate AZA will often tolerate 6-MP at a dose of 1–1.5 mg/kg/day. Dosing should begin at 50–75 mg depending on weight and can be up-titrated on a weekly basis if tolerated (both clinically and biochemically). TPMT genotyping should be routinely performed prior to initiation of AZA or 6-MP so as to better predict the likelihood of toxicity. 'Shunting' of AZA refers to the preferential metabolism of the prodrug to the inactive metabolite 6-methylmercaptopurine (6MMP) (which is hepatotoxic) rather than 6-TG. Shunting can be overcome through addition of allopurinol; however, this should only be undertaken with the oversight of an experienced gastroenterologist with appropriate thiopurine dose reduction (typically to a quarter of the dose or 25 mg daily).

Safety. Common side effects include nausea, flulike symptoms and a rash (around 20%). Hepatotoxicity (due to inactive metabolite 6-MMP) and myelotoxicity (due to active metabolite 6-TG) are also relatively common. Pancreatitis is a reported idiosyncratic reaction, and non-Hodgkin lymphoma and hepatosplenic T-cell lymphoma are relatively rare. The risk of non-melanomatous skin cancers is increased with thiopurines, and sun protection should be encouraged as well as annual skin checks.

Monitoring. Liver enzymes and full blood count should be monitored closely (at least weekly) after thiopurine initiation until 4 weeks after a stable dose is reached. Ongoing blood monitoring during the treatment duration of thiopurine therapy is imperative at a minimum of three monthly (including liver enzymes and full blood count). Thiopurine metabolite testing (6-TG and 6-MMP) is routine to ensure optimised dosing of thiopurine therapy and should be performed 6–8 weeks after a stable dose of therapy is reached. Additional preventative measures include annual skin checks and cervical cancer screening (for women) as well as annual flu vaccination and five-yearly pneumococcal vaccination.

6.5.9 Methotrexate

Efficacy and dosing. MTX is a dihydrofolate reductase inhibitor, which may be administered via oral, subcutaneous or intramuscular routes. MTX is an option for both induction and maintenance of CD, typically at a dose of 15–25 mg/week subcutaneously. There is insufficient evidence to support the use of MTX in UC. As described below, MTX is not an option in either sex when planning conception or pregnancy.

Safety. Common side effects include nausea, headache, fatigue and hepatotoxicity. Pneumonitis and liver fibrosis are rare complications.

Monitoring. Liver enzymes and full blood count should be monitored closely (at least weekly) after MTX initiation until 4 weeks after a stable dose is reached. Ongoing blood monitoring during the treatment duration of MTX therapy is imperative at a minimum of three monthly (including liver enzymes and full blood count). If concerns regarding liver fibrosis arise, particularly if there is a cofactor such as alcohol or non-alcoholic fatty liver disease, transient elastography can be used to monitor for liver fibrosis.

6.5.10 Biologics

6.5.10.1 Anti-TNF Agents

Efficacy and dosing. There are two anti-TNF agents available in Australia: infliximab (IFX) and adalimumab (ADA). Both have been shown to be highly efficacious for both remission induction and maintenance for both UC and CD and are amongst the most effective medications currently available for IBD.

IFX (5 mg/kg IV) is indicated for remission induction (at 0, 2 and 6 weeks) and maintenance (8 weeks) in both CD and UC. ADA is also indicated for remission induction (160/80 mg SC) and maintenance (40 mg SC fortnightly). Both agents are only available on the Australian Pharmaceutical Benefits Scheme (PBS) if there has been failure of or intolerance to conventional therapy, i.e. thiopurines. The route of administration may influence the choice of therapy; ADA may be self-administered subcutaneously and may be preferred by patients living remotely. In obese patients, IFX is preferred as it calculated as a weight-based dose.

Safety. Anti-TNF therapy is better tolerated than immunomodulators. Anaphylaxis has been reported following administration of anti-TNF therapy. To reduce the likelihood of infusion reaction, a slow IFX infusion is performed during induction with hydrocortisone and antihistamine coadministration. Active malignancy and prior melanoma are absolute contraindications to anti-TNF therapy. Anti-TNF must be used with caution in patients with a prior history of solid organ malignancy, and any such decision should be made in conjunction with a gastroenterologist and oncologist. There are other less common risks with anti-TNF therapy including lymphoma, demyelinating disease and congestive cardiac failure.

There is an increased risk of serious infections on anti-TNF therapy, and active infection is a contraindication to treatment. A 'biologic' prescreen involves tuberculosis (TB) assessment (usually interferon gamma release assay (IGRA test)) with or without chest X-ray depending on pretest probability). A clinical history is the most important screening tool for the risk of TB. If latent TB is suspected, prophylactic treatment regimens can be administered concurrently to reduce the risk of reactivation.

Other tests to be performed prior to therapy include hepatitis B core antibody (surface antibody and surface antigen), hepatitis C antibody, HIV serology, Epstein-Barr virus serology, cytomegalovirus (CMV) serology and varicella serology.

Live vaccines (measles, mumps, rubella, polio, yellow fever, varicella) are contraindicated during anti-TNF therapy.

6.5.11 Vedolizumab

Efficacy and dosing. Vedolizumab (300 mg IV at 0, 2 and 6 weeks for induction then every 8 weeks for maintenance) is a $\alpha 4\beta 7$ integrin inhibitor and reduces inflammation by inhibiting the adhesion of T lymphocytes to gastrointestinal tissues. There is strong evidence for efficacy for both UC and CD.

Safety. As vedolizumab is gut-specific, it does not share the adverse safety profile of the systemically acting anti-TNF agents. There is a theoretical risk of posterior multifocal leukoencephalopathy (PML) from reactivation of the John Cunningham virus; this risk has been extrapolated from natalizumab, an agent in the same class used in multiple sclerosis; however, this has not been established with vedolizumab in IBD.

6.5.12 Ustekinumab

Efficacy and dosing. Ustekinumab (weight-based IV initial dose following by SC dosing eight weekly) is a monoclonal antibody directed against IL-12 and IL-23. It is currently only approved for use in Australia for severe CD.

Safety. Ustekinumab's safety profile is similar to the anti-TNF agents, with infusion reactions possible and serious infection or reactivation of TB or viruses being the major reported adverse effects.

6.6 Exclusive Enteral Nutrition

Exclusive enteral nutrition (EEN) is first-line therapy for remission induction in CD in the pediatric population. EEN entails intake of a medical liquid nutrition formula (typically polymeric for palatability), excluding table foods, for 6–8 weeks. EEN is more effective than corticosteroids for remission induction in pediatric CD. In adults, the same premise of efficacy exists; however, EEN is less well tolerated, and data are of poorer quality. In the perioperative setting, EEN can be used to reduce inflammatory burden prior to surgery, which has been shown to improve nutrition status and surgical outcomes in adult CD patients. It has also been shown to downstage disease such that surgery may be avoided all together. EEN is also useful in patients in whom immunosuppression with steroids or biologicals is contraindicated, often because of concurrent sepsis. For example, in patients with penetrating small bowel CD with abscess or phlegmon, it can be used for remission induction as either a bridge to surgical resection or immunosuppression.

6.6.1 Surgical Management

Surgery is not curative in CD and should be judiciously approached. Specific indications for surgery include abscesses, complex perianal or internal fistulae or fibrostenotic strictures. In localised ileocecal disease, surgery can be considered an alternative to medical management in selected cases. The decision to start or continue medical therapy to prevent postoperative recurrence is guided by phenotype, disease severity, smoking status and previous small bowel surgery. Metronidazole is routinely used for 3 months following ileocecal resection to prevent recurrence.

Indications for surgical management in UC include refractory ASUC or medically refractory disease. The most commonly performed elective surgery for UC is proctocolectomy with ileal pouch-anal anastomosis; this is typically a staged procedure with the initial formation of a temporary ileostomy to decrease the risk of immediate postoperative complications such as anastomotic leak. Pouchitis is a common complication, occurring in almost half of patients at least once, and should be treated with antibiotics (ciprofloxacin and metronidazole for 2–4 weeks). 10–15% of patients develop chronic pouchitis. Residual rectal tissue, the 'rectal cuff', can also become inflamed, leading to cuffitis. This can be treated with topical 5-ASA. Another common concern with pouch surgery is decreased fertility and erectile dysfunction. In patients in whom pouch surgery is not appropriate or completion proctectomy is required, a permanent colostomy or ileostomy may be performed.

6.6.2 Other Factors in IBD Care

Beyond medical and surgical management of inflammatory disease, there are multiple other factors that need to be addressed in routine IBD care (as summarised in Table 6.5).

6.7 Special Concerns

6.7.1 Acute Presentations

Acute presentations of IBD can occur at diagnosis or throughout the disease course; they include ASUC, acute bowel obstruction and intrabdominal collection and sepsis.

ASUC is a life-threatening emergency, and approximately 30% of patients admitted with ASUC will proceed to colectomy within 12 months of presentation. ASUC is defined by Truelove and Witt's criteria (see Table 6.6). Immediate management should include correction of dehydration and/or electrolyte imbalance, intravenous hydrocortisone 100 mg 6 hourly, deep venous thrombosis prophylaxis, stool specimens to exclude infection and plain abdominal film to exclude toxic megacolon. Biologic prescreening (see below) should be performed early in

Table 6.5 Supportive care in IBD

Domain	Description	Management
Mental health	Anxiety and depression is common in IBD and may affect clinical outcome. Symptom-related anxiety and abnormal illness behaviour may be observed	Clinical psychology Specialised hypnotherapy
Venous thromboembolic disease (VTE)	Active IBD is a risk factor for incident and recurrent VTE	Prophylaxis with low-molecular-weight heparin during hospitalisation with acute flares
Opioid use	Opioid use and dependence can be high in IBD patients particularly those with complicated or long-standing disease. Contributes to mortality	Limit commencement of short- or long-term opioids during hospital admissions Engage GP in opioid avoidance or weaning strategies
Sarcopaenia and malnutrition	Patients suffer from sarcopaenia because of disease activity prior to diagnosis or because of ongoing symptoms	Clinical dietician Dietary supplements Enteral feeding as required Exercise physiologist, physiotherapy, rehabilitation programmes
Metabolic bone disease	IBD patients are at risk because of increased bone turnover driven by chronic inflammation and steroid use	Bone mineral density scans as required, with anti-resorptive therapy as needed Calcium and vitamin D supplementation with steroid use >12 weeks
Vitamin D	Vitamin D deficiency is associated with IBD disease activity and contributes to fatigue	Regular monitoring and supplementation as required
Vaccinations	All patients on immunomodulators or biologics	Annual influenza vaccination Five yearly pneumococcal vaccination
Cancer surveillance	All patients AZA can increase incidence of cervical cancer and non-melanomatous skin cancers	Age-appropriate cancer screening as per national guidelines for breast and prostate cancer Colorectal cancer surveillance is dependent on chronicity, severity and type of IBD (see below) On AZA: annual pap smears and skin checks

Table 6.6 Scoring systems for acute severe colitis

Truelove and Witt criteria	Oxford criteria
>6 bloody stools/day plus one or more of the following: • Temperature > 37.8 °C • Pulse >90 bpm • Haemoglobin <10.5 g/dL • Erythrocyte sedimentation rate (ESR) >30 mm/h	If assessed on day 3: • >8 stools/day, OR • >3 stools/day if CRP >45 mg/L If assessed on day 7: • >3 stools/day with visible blood

all patients. Flexible sigmoidoscopy is often performed within 24 hours to assess the severity of disease and for biopsies to exclude primary or secondary infection from CMV or *Clostridium difficile*. Failure to achieve an adequate response to steroid treatments is defined by the Oxford criteria, which should be applied on day 3 of admission (with day of admission being labelled as day 1) (see Table 6.5). The Oxford criteria is useful to guide the need for medical or surgical rescue therapy, given that 85% of patients who meet the criteria will come to colectomy during admission without rescue. The most commonly used medical rescue therapy is IFX, although cyclosporine therapy is also used and has similar efficacy. Decisions in ASUC are best made in collaboration between gastroenterologist and surgeon.

CD patients may present with small or even large bowel obstruction from stricturing disease. Strictures may be inflammatory or fibrostenotic or both; this will determine response to steroid treatment in the immediate phase. Patients with a significant inflammatory component are more likely to respond to medical management, whereas those with predominantly fibrostenotic disease will often require surgical management. Inflammatory markers and MRE are helpful in delineating this. Endoscopic balloon dilatation is possible for short predominantly fibrotic CD-related strictures.

Abscess or phlegmon formation occurs with penetrating CD, and patients can present with local peritonitis or sepsis. The mainstay of management is antibiotics and surgical drainage where possible and appropriate. Where there is high inflammatory disease burden, EEN is an option to induce remission with immunosuppression or to reduce inflammatory burden prior to surgery.

6.7.2 Perianal Disease

Perianal disease is common in CD, especially in those with proctitis. Perianal fistulae can be classified into:

- Simple: low fistulae that involve superficial tissue and include subcutaneous and intersphincteric and intrasphincteric fistulae that remain below the dentate line, have a single opening and are not associated with perianal complications
- Complex: high intersphincteric, high transphincteric, suprasphincteric and extrasphincteric. May have multiple openings, be associated with abscess, proctitis, stricture or connection with the bladder or vagina

Symptomatic simple fistula can be managed with seton placement and antibiotics, with recurrent simple fistula requiring thiopurine and/or anti-TNF therapy. In complex fistulising disease, perianal sepsis should be identified early, and urgent drainage performed with seton placement as appropriate. Anti-TNF therapy is first line after surgical drainage in complex perianal disease. There is not a strong evidence to guide antibiotic choice and duration of therapy, but a combination of oral ciprofloxacin and metronidazole for 2–6 weeks is often used.

6.7.3 Bowel Cancer in IBD

The risk of colorectal cancer (CRC) is increased in both CD and UC; it develops at a younger age and prognosis is worse than non-IBD CRC. Factors that increase the risk include extent and duration or disease, severity of inflammation and the presence of PSC or a family history or CRC. National screening guidelines should be closely adhered to.

6.7.4 Pregnancy and Family Planning

IBD commonly affects women in their child-bearing years, and counselling patients about family planning is essential. Active disease as the time of conception predicts poor outcomes; it is ideal to have disease in remission prior to conception. Many IBD therapies are safe during pregnancy, including 5-ASAs and thiopurines, and the biggest risk to pregnancy is in fact active IBD rather than medical therapy. MTX is contraindicated during pregnancy. Of the biologicals, IFX has the best evidence regarding safety during pregnancy, and the decision to stop IFX in the third trimester can be made on a case-by-case basis depending on disease control and risk of flare. Other biological agents such as vedolizumab are likely safe, but long-term data are not yet available.

Fertility in males can be affected by medication such as sulfasalazine, which reduces sperm motility, as well as MTX, which may affect pregnancy outcomes.

6.8 Summary

IBD is a complex and heterogeneous disease, requiring a collaborative multidisciplinary management approach. Modern medical management targets mucosal healing so as to avoid cumulative disability and normalise quality. Judicious, appropriate and timely surgical intervention is complementary to medical management to achieve the best outcomes for patients with IBD.

Recommended Reading

- European Crohn's and Colitis Guidelines
- Gastroenterological Society of Australia Inflammatory Bowel Disease Surveillance Guidelines

Disorders of Motility

7

Paul Kuo and Ian C. Roberts-Thomson

Normal motor function in the gastrointestinal tract is essential for the transit of food and fluids from the mouth to the rectum. Central to this process is a branch of the peripheral nervous system called the enteric nervous system. This is composed of two concentric rings of nerve ganglia: an outer ring located between the longitudinal and circular smooth muscle layers called the myenteric plexus and an inner ring called the submucosal plexus. These nerve plexuses contain neurons with both excitatory and inhibitory motor functions as well as neurons with various sensory functions, reflex activity and effects on glands and blood vessels. Superimposed on this complex arrangement are the interstitial cells of Cajal that are coupled to smooth muscle cells and generate pacemaker activity.

The enteric nervous system can also be influenced by the central nervous system, largely through the activities of the sympathetic and parasympathetic nervous systems. Sympathetic activation usually downregulates gastrointestinal motility but can enhance the contraction of sphincters. In contrast, parasympathetic activity is largely mediated by the vagus nerve and pelvic splanchnic nerves and usually enhances gastrointestinal motility. Both pathways have additional effects on intestinal blood flow and on secretions from epithelial cells and various glands. Various neurotransmitters such as serotonin, noradrenaline [norepinephrine], adrenaline [epinephrine] and dopamine can also have effects, not only on blood flow and motility but on nutrient absorption, the intestinal microbiome and mucosal immunity.

Changes in gastrointestinal motility are a normal part of human life. For example, changes in bowel habit can often be linked to changes in diet [fibre, alcohol and coffee] or to psychological factors such as stress. Chronic diarrhea has many causes

P. Kuo (✉)
Department of Gastroenterology and Hepatology, Royal Adelaide Hospital, Adelaide, SA, Australia
e-mail: paul.kuo@sa.gov.au

I. C. Roberts-Thomson
School of Medicine, University of Adelaide, Adelaide, SA, Australia
e-mail: ian.robertsthomson@adelaide.edu.au

M. W. Wichmann et al. (eds.), *Gastroenterology For General Surgeons*,
https://doi.org/10.1007/978-3-319-92768-8_7

including infections, non-infectious gastrointestinal disease, hyperthyroidism and disorders of uncertain cause such as the irritable bowel syndrome. The latter is discussed in more detail in Chapter 1. Other disorders such as colonic diverticulosis, diverticula in other parts of the gastrointestinal tract, reflux oesophagitis and non-ulcer dyspepsia seem likely to involve motility but have not been traditionally categorized as motility disorders. In this chapter, we will focus on motility disorders likely to be encountered by the general surgeon and have included achalasia, gastroparesis and slow-transit constipation. Motility disorders of the sphincter of Oddi and motility disorders induced by opioids have been discussed in Chapters 17 and 23, respectively.

7.1 Achalasia

Achalasia has been chosen for more detailed discussion in this review as the disorder is a well-recognized example of hypermotility and at least some information is available regarding pathogenesis. However, other motor disorders of the esophagus have been described including the hypercontractile [jackhammer] esophagus, distal esophageal spasm, absent contractility and motility changes associated with scleroderma and Chagas disease.

7.1.1 Pathogenesis

The pathogenesis of achalasia involves the loss of myenteric ganglion cells in the distal esophagus including the lower esophageal sphincter. This appears to be caused by inflammation around ganglion cells [plexitis] that is mediated by T-cells and eventually results in neuronal loss. A possible etiology is an autoimmune process as a minority of patients have neural antibodies and there is a higher than expected frequency of other autoimmune disorders. However, triggers for the autoimmune process remain unclear, and there are no apparent reasons for the focus on ganglion cells in the lower esophagus. In addition, no major susceptibility genes have been identified. Inflammation in the myenteric plexus appears to have a particular effect on inhibitory postganglionic neurons leading to unopposed cholinergic stimulation with hypercontractility. Interestingly, achalasia can also be one manifestation of Chagas disease, an infection caused by *Trypanosoma cruzi* that causes widespread damage to the myenteric plexus.

7.1.2 Clinical Features

Achalasia has an annual incidence of approximately 1/100,000 and a prevalence of approximately 10/100,000. The disease has a similar incidence in males and females. The onset of symptoms is usually in midlife but ranges from adolescence to old age. For most patients, the initial symptom is dysphagia for solid foods, but this can also be accompanied by dysphagia for liquids. Additional symptoms include heartburn [70–80% of patients], regurgitation or vomiting

[40–50% of patients] and a minority of patients with chest pain, epigastric pain and odynophagia. Symptoms may also include a chronic cough, chronic aspiration, sore throat, hoarseness and asthma.

7.1.3 Investigations

The diagnosis of achalasia is usually straightforward but may be delayed in those with atypical symptoms or early disease. For most patients, the first investigation is upper gastrointestinal endoscopy. Positive features include a dilated esophagus, food and fluid in the lower esophagus and resistance to passage of the endoscope into the stomach. Of equal importance is the exclusion of causes of pseudo-achalasia such as peptic strictures in the lower esophagus, cancer in the gastric fundus, eosinophilic esophagitis and oesophageal webs [Schatzki rings]. A barium esophagram can also be helpful, particularly if the esophagus is dilated with a "bird's beak" appearance in the region of the diaphragm (Fig. 7.1). However, investigation in most

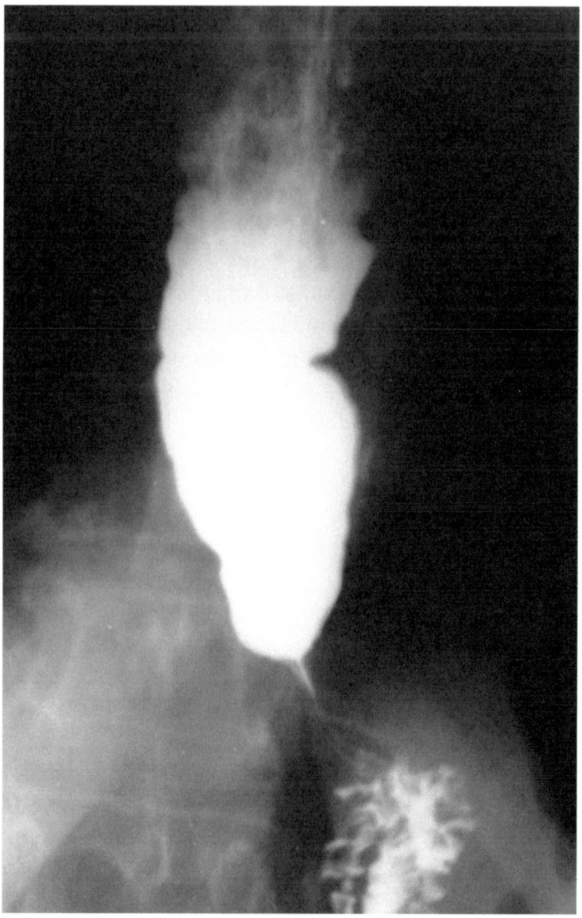

Fig. 7.1 Typical barium esophagram in achalasia showing a dilated esophagus with narrowing at the cardio-esophageal junction with a "bird's beak" appearance

if not all patients should now include esophageal manometry. For the general surgeon, this will usually involve referral of the patient to a tertiary centre for either a water-perfused or strain-gauge study or, hopefully, a contemporary high-resolution study. The latter is more accurate and reproducible and permits categorization of achalasia into different clinical phenotypes. A detailed discussion of manometric features is beyond the scope of this review, but typical abnormalities in achalasia include impaired relaxation of the lower esophageal sphincter and absent peristalsis in the lower esophagus. Some patients also have an elevated resting pressure in the lower esophageal sphincter.

7.1.4 Medical and Surgical Management

The definitive treatment for achalasia involves disruption of the lower esophageal sphincter. However, drugs such as calcium channel blockers, nitrates and sildenafil are of temporary benefit in some patients, largely by reducing the lower esophageal sphincter pressure. Another option is injections of botulinum toxin into the lower esophageal sphincter at endoscopy. This results in improvement in dysphagia in two-thirds of patients, but the benefit only lasts for 6–12 months. Repeat injections can also be helpful but may make a subsequent Heller's myotomy more difficult.

Methods for disruption of the lower esophageal sphincter include pneumatic dilatation, operative Heller's myotomy [usually laparoscopic] and peroral endoscopic myotomy [POEM]. None of these procedures have an ideal outcome with resolution of symptoms and absence of significant esophageal reflux. However, comparisons of pneumatic dilatation with laparoscopic Heller's myotomy appear to show similar frequencies of substantial symptom improvement [approximately 80%] after 5 or more years of follow-up. Some authors prefer Heller's myotomy for younger patients and include a modified antireflux fundoplication to reduce the risk of symptomatic reflux. Thus far, no randomized trials have compared POEM to other treatment modalities. Patients with achalasia require regular follow-up as up to 20% need additional therapy within 5 years and there is a minor increase in risk for the development of squamous carcinoma.

7.2 Gastroparesis

Gastric motor function can be broadly divided into two parts: the proximal stomach which serves as the initial reservoir for food and fluids and later acts as a pump to drive gastric content out of the stomach into the duodenum and the distal stomach which acts as a grinder that breaks food into small particles and mixes them with gastric secretions. Anatomically, the proximal stomach has relatively thin walls, whilst the distal stomach has thick, muscular walls. The pyloric sphincter acts as a "brake" to gastric emptying that is regulated by neural and hormonal feedback mechanisms generated by nutrient-gut interactions in the small intestine including in the ileum. The sphincter relaxes intermittently to control the rate of gastric emptying to

Table 7.1 Causes and risk factors for gastroparesis

Diabetes mellitus
Abdominal or esophageal surgery (vagal nerve injury)
Infection (usually viral)
Critical illness
Medications, e.g. opiates, anticholinergic drugs
Scleroderma (or other connective tissue diseases)
Amyloidosis
Malignancy (as a part of paraneoplastic syndrome)
Nervous system diseases, e.g. Parkinson's disease, multiple sclerosis
Vascular disorders, e.g. history of mesenteric ischaemia
Cardiac ablation for arrhythmia (vagal nerve injury)

2–3 kcal per minute, thus avoiding a rush of nutrients into the small bowel that might overwhelm the normal digestive process.

Delay in gastric emptying is relatively common and is briefly discussed in Chapter 1 in relation to non-ulcer dyspepsia. In most patients, a minor delay in gastric emptying is unlikely to result in symptoms. Gastroparesis describes a more severe variant where gastric emptying is objectively delayed by greater than two standard deviations from mean values in healthy individuals. This delay can be caused by neuropathy, myopathy or a mixture of both disorders. One important aspect of neuropathy is loss of the interstitial cells of Cajal. Approximately one-third of patients with gastroparesis have diabetes, and a further third are of unknown cause [idiopathic]. Another significant group have post-operative issues, sometimes related to division or damage to the vagus nerve. These and other causes of gastroparesis are listed in Table 7.1.

7.2.1 Clinical Features

The symptoms of gastroparesis include nausea, vomiting, retching, anorexia, epigastric fullness, abdominal bloating, inability to finish a normal meal and excessive fullness after meals. For research studies, these symptoms can be quantified using the Gastroparesis Cardinal Symptom Index that is listed in Suggested Reading. Physical signs include abdominal distension, a succession splash, weight loss and muscle wasting.

Gastroparesis needs to be considered in the differential diagnosis of upper gastrointestinal symptoms as there are overlapping symptoms with several other disorders such as non-ulcer dyspepsia and peptic ulceration. In addition, recurrent vomiting, a major symptom of gastroparesis, can also occur in severe reflux disease, cyclical vomiting syndrome, rumination syndrome and the cannabinoid hyperemesis syndrome [see Chapter 23]. A further difficulty is that the nature and severity of symptoms correlate poorly with the actual rate of gastric emptying. For example, some patients with severe symptoms show only a minor delay in gastric emptying, whilst others can have severe gastroparesis but little in the way of symptoms.

7.2.2 Investigations

For most patients, the first investigation is upper gastrointestinal endoscopy to exclude a mechanical gastric outlet obstruction and other causes for gastrointestinal symptoms. This can then be followed by scintigraphy or a breath test, but both investigations will normally require referral to a major centre. Scintigraphy is the gold standard for the quantitation of gastric emptying. For measurement of both solid and liquid emptying, a dual isotope study is performed with the patient sitting in front of a gamma camera. Images are collected for 2–4 h to track the movement of isotopes through the stomach into the small bowel. The rate of gastric emptying is then calculated according to the scintigraphic count remaining inside the stomach relative to the original count at the beginning of the study and expressed as a percentage. The commonest measure of gastric emptying is the half-emptying time (T 1/2), meaning the time it takes for half of the stomach contents to leave the stomach.

The ^{13}C-breath test measures the quantity of $^{13}CO_2$ in breath samples as a surrogate marker of gastric emptying. The test requires the patient to ingest a ^{13}C-labelled solid or liquid meal after which multiple breath samples are collected at different time points over the subsequent 4–6 h to measure the amount of $^{13}CO_2$ contained within the breath. As with all breath test techniques, the accuracy of the test relies on gastric emptying being the rate-limiting step and involves a number of assumptions including normal intestinal absorption, normal portal venous circulation and relatively normal liver and lung function to metabolize and release the ^{13}C into the exhaled breath. The test does not require a nuclear medicine facility, and results appear to be similar to those from scintigraphy. Newer techniques for the assessment of gastric emptying such as the wireless motility capsule [SmartPill] and three-dimensional ultrasonography are currently in the research phase.

7.2.3 Medical Management

The management of gastroparesis should aim to improve symptoms and, hopefully, to improve gastric emptying. There is little joy in achieving a normalized gastric emptying rate, whilst the patient is no better symptomatically. Dietitians need to be part of the team for nutritional assessments and advice on feeding strategies and nutritional supplements. Common strategies include smaller and more frequent meals, administration of more calories in liquid form, sitting or standing for 1–2 h after meals and use of prokinetic drugs 15–30 min prior to meals. Short-term inpatient management will be necessary for those who need post-pyloric feeding tubes [usually placed endoscopically], a feeding jejunostomy or total parenteral nutrition.

Drug therapy has traditionally been based on the use of prokinetic agents and anti-emetics. The traditional prokinetic agents include erythromycin, cisapride, metoclopramide and domperidone. These agents have all been shown to have a prokinetic effect on the stomach but little or no activity on other parts of the gastrointestinal tract. Erythromycin is sometimes used for short-term therapy, often in the setting of critical illness. Cisapride, a 5-hydroxytryptamine 4 agonist, is an effective prokinetic agent but is currently restricted to the Special Access Scheme in Australia because of prolongation of the Q-T interval and reports of cardiac arrhythmias. Metoclopramide and domperidone have both prokinetic and anti-emetic activity but have been associated with adverse effects on the central nervous system when used for prolonged periods. Domperidone has not been approved for use in the USA.

Several newer prokinetic agents are under evaluation but have not, as yet, shown efficacy in gastroparesis. Anti-emetic drugs such as phenothiazines (prochlorperazine), antihistamines (promethazine), 5-hydroxytryptamine 3 receptor antagonists (ondansetron, granisetron), antidepressants (mirtazapine) and a neurokinin receptor antagonist (aprepitant) can also be prescribed in combination with prokinetics for better control of symptoms.

7.2.4 Surgical Management

Treatment of gastroparesis by endoscopic and surgical interventions should be restricted to tertiary centres. One approach is ablation of the pylorus muscle which is seen as the main rate-limiting step to gastric emptying. A relatively simple option is the injection of botulinum toxin into the pylorus. This is helpful in approximately 50% of patients, but benefit is usually short-term in the order of months. Another option is a fully covered metallic stent across the pylorus. This is also helpful in the short-term, but there is a significant risk of stent migration. Other options include gastric surgery [pyloroplasty, partial gastrectomy or gastric bypass] and endoscopic myotomy of the pylorus [performed in a similar way to POEM]. Gastric electrical stimulation using an implantable Enterra device is also available in some countries. These various procedures have not been compared, but, thus far, none have been associated with high success rates after longer-term follow-up.

7.3 Slow-Transit Constipation

The normal range for stool frequency is generally considered to be between three times per day and three times per week. However, reduced stool frequency per se, in the absence of other symptoms, is inadequate to make a diagnosis of constipation. In the Rome III report, chronic constipation is defined as having a symptom onset more than 6 months prior to the diagnosis with at least two of the following criteria fulfilled in the past 3 months:

- Fewer than three bowel movements per week
- Hard or lumpy stools more than 25% of the time
- Straining with defaecation more than 25% of the time
- Sensation of incomplete evacuation more than 25% of the time
- Manual manoeuvres necessary to facilitate defaecation more than 25% of the time
- Sensation of anorectal obstruction more than 25% of the time

Risk factors for constipation include lower socioeconomic status, lower parental education rates, low physical activity, depression, medications, history of abuse and stressful life events. A low intake of dietary fibre was a risk factor in some but not all studies. Some medical disorders as well as medication associated with constipation are listed in Tables 7.2 and 7.3. The assessment of colonic transit and anorectal function permits the classification of constipation into three groups: normal-transit constipation, pelvic floor dysfunction and slow-transit constipation. This section will be restricted to the latter disorder.

7.3.1 Pathogenesis

Slow-transit constipation is characterized by reduced motility of the colon including a reduction in propagating contractions and pressure generation in the colonic lumen. It is often accompanied by passage of hard and lumpy stools. Some patients have an elongated colon, whilst in others, slow-transit constipation is combined with obstructive defaecation. The pathogenesis is still poorly understood but some patients have a reduction in colonic intrinsic nerves and interstitial cells of Cajal. There is also evidence that elongation of the colon inhibits colonic propulsive activity via increased release of nitric oxide.

Table 7.2 Common medical disorders associated with constipation

Mechanical obstruction
Colon cancer
Other malignant strictures
Benign colonic strictures
Megacolon
Rectocoele
Chronic anal fissure
Metabolic disorders
Diabetes mellitus
Hypothyroidism
Hypercalcemia
Hypomagnesemia
Hypokalemia
Uremia
Neurogenic disorders
Parkinson's disease
Multiple sclerosis
Spinal cord injury
Cerebrovascular disease
Autonomic neuropathy
Myopathies
Muscular dystrophies
Scleroderma
Other disorders
Pregnancy
Depression
Dementia
Immobility [various causes]

Table 7.3 Commonly used medications that may cause constipation

Analgesics
Various opioids including morphine and codeine
Various nonsteroidal, anti-inflammatory agents
Medications with anticholinergic activity
Tricyclic antidepressants
Parkinson's disease medication
Some antipsychotic medication
Some antihistamines
Antispasmodic drugs including mebeverine
Medication for hypertension
Calcium channel blockers
Some diuretics
Anti-arrhythmic agents such as amiodarone
Some beta-blocking drugs
Anticonvulsant agents
Carbamazepine
Cation-containing medication
Calcium
Aluminium
Lithium
Chemotherapeutic agents
Vinca alkaloids such as vincristine
Alkylating agents such as cyclophosphamide
Other agents
Oral contraceptives

7.3.2 Clinical Features

The symptoms of constipation include bloating, fullness, reduced appetite, nausea, abdominal pain and difficulty in evacuating stool. The Bristol stool scale can be a useful tool in helping the patient to accurately describe their stool form. The symptoms of slow-transit constipation tend to be stable over prolonged periods [usually years], although intermittent acute exacerbations may induce more severe symptoms, sometimes to the point of being mistaken for a surgical abdomen. Physical signs include abdominal distension, palpable loops of the colon that can be firm and sausage-shaped and abdominal tenderness on palpation.

7.3.3 Investigations

The diagnosis of slow-transit constipation is often made on the basis of clinical features, after the exclusion of secondary causes. However, it is often helpful to objectively measure transit time using radio-opaque markers or scintigraphy. The motility capsule [SmartPill] can also be used for this purpose. Among the functional causes of constipation, it is important to exclude pelvic floor dysfunction [dyssynergia] which can be diagnosed with either anorectal manometry or a defecating proctogram.

The simplest test for intestinal transit is the use of radio-opaque markers as it is low-cost and requires only plain abdominal radiographs. The technique has been used since the 1960s and allows measurement of both total and segmental colonic transit times. However, its interpretation is based on the assumption that the locations of the markers are representative of a physiological meal. The markers are either plastic rings or beads that are ingested in capsule(s) containing 20–50 markers (e.g. sitz markers). There is the single- and multiple-capsule technique. The single-capsule technique requires ingestion of all markers in a single capsule, followed by either serial abdominal radiographs until all markers have passed or a single radiograph at day 5 (120 h) after ingestion. The multiple-capsule technique involves the ingestion of one capsule per day for 3 days, followed by radiographs on day 4 and day 7 [or only on day 7].

Interpretation is based on the distribution and number of markers seen on the radiographs (Fig. 7.2). In the single-capsule technique, delayed transit is defined as >20% of the markers remaining in the abdomen at day 5. In the multiple-capsule technique, colonic transit time in each segment and for the whole colon is calculated by multiplying the number of markers by 1.2 (or 1.0 if capsule contains 24 markers).

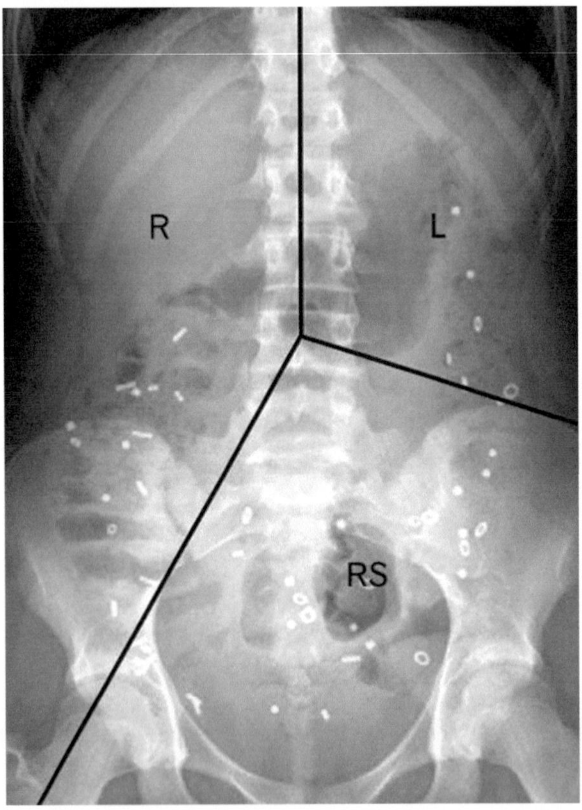

Fig. 7.2 Radio-opaque markers for measuring colonic transit. The abdomen is divided into three areas which roughly correlate with the right colon, left colon and rectosigmoid colon. The number of plastic rings is manually calculated to reflect regional and whole colon transit

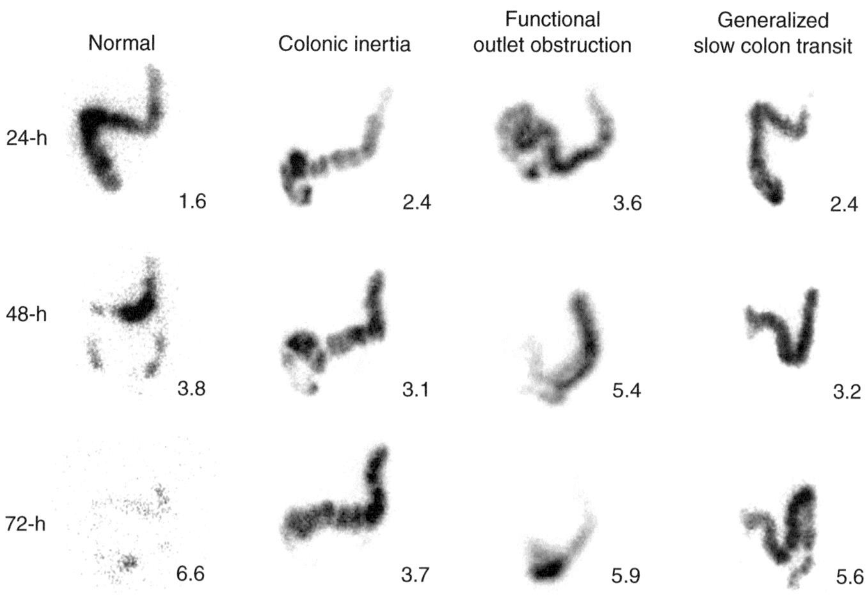

Fig. 7.3 Scintigraphic measurement of colonic transit. The distribution of intensity of scintigraphic count across the colon offers a measure of regional and whole colon transit

The mean colonic transit time is 30–40 h in Western populations and 20–30 h in Asian populations and is influenced by the menstrual cycle in women.

Scintigraphy is able to measure the transit time for various segments of the gastrointestinal tract including the colon. It is more laborious and costly compared to other techniques and requires the presence of a nuclear medicine facility. The technique involves the ingestion of a radionuclide-labelled meal or a radionuclide contained inside a pH-sensitive capsule, followed by acquisition of scintigraphic images of the abdomen at 24 and 48 h after ingestion (Fig. 7.3). The geometric centre is the weighted average of the radioisotope distribution within the colon and stool and is calculated according to a mathematical equation that provides an indication of overall colonic transit. The measurement of proximal colonic transit and the geometric centre can help differentiate slow colonic transit and pelvic outlet obstruction, with the former showing delayed transit in both the proximal colon and geometric centre, whilst the latter has delayed transit in the geometric centre but normal proximal colonic transit.

7.3.4 Medical Management

Treatment of slow-transit constipation starts with strategies that are similar to treating any other cause of chronic constipation. These include an adequate intake of dietary fibre (18–30 g per day for adults), regular exercise (e.g. walking) and good toileting habits such as attempting to evacuate stool at the same time each day (ideally after breakfast due to a more active colon in the morning and the gastrocolic reflex). Advice may also include a relaxed environment during evacuation, avoidance of straining and the adoption of a slightly forward leaning posture with knees slightly elevated (sometimes with the help of placing a block under the feet) during evacuation to help straighten the anorectal angle.

Laxatives can also be used at the lowest dose necessary if the above-mentioned measures are inadequate. The choice of laxatives is wide and includes bulking agents [psyllium, ispaghula husk and sterculia], osmotic laxatives [sorbitol, lactulose, glycerol, macrogol and saline laxatives], stool softeners [docusate, liquid paraffin and poloxamer] and stimulant laxatives [senna and bisacodyl]. In general, combining laxatives with different mechanisms of action appears more effective than increasing the dose of laxatives within the same class although there is wide interindividual variability in terms of which laxatives work best. Osmotic laxatives, especially the saline laxatives and stimulant laxatives, are more potent choices and should be used more sparingly. Suppositories and enemas are appropriate in those with distal colonic faecal loading, often in combination with oral laxatives to maximize efficacy. Adverse effects from chronic laxative use that were thought to include megacolon and a "lazy bowel" have not been supported by recent studies. In recent years, a number of newer pharmacological agents have become available such as prucalopride, lubiprostone and linaclotide. Of these, only prucalopride is currently available in Australia. Prucalopride is a selective 5-hydroxytryptamine receptor agonist that has been shown in randomized trials to increase the number of spontaneous bowel motions per week. Thus far, the drug has only been approved for use in women, and longer-term efficacy beyond 12 weeks remains unclear. However, the drug is a promising agent for use in patients with chronic constipation who are refractory to more conventional treatment. Lubiprostone and linaclotide have also been helpful for difficult constipation in preliminary studies. Finally, there are also reports that patients with slow-transit constipation may benefit from faecal microbial transplantation.

7.3.5 Surgical Management

Although most patients with slow-transit constipation can be managed adequately with a combination of dietary, lifestyle modifications and pharmacological therapies, a small proportion continue to have severe and debilitating symptoms. In this group, surgical therapy appears to be of some help although the preferred operation remains unclear. Options include a total colectomy with ileostomy, colectomy with ileosigmoid anastomosis and colectomy with cecorectal anastomosis. One retrospective study preferred the ileosigmoid anastomosis to the cecorectal anastomosis. However, a recent systematic review did not identify any factor to guide the selection of patients or procedures. One study also found colectomy for slow-transit constipation failed to reduce healthcare utilization. Another surgical procedure is that of sacral nerve stimulation using implanted electrodes, but, thus far, results have been disappointing.

Recommended Reading

Bassotti G, Blandizzi C. Understanding and treating refractory constipation. World J Gastrointest Pharmacol Ther. 2014;5:77–85.

Bharucha AE, Pemberton JH, Locke GR 3rd. American Gastroenterological Association technical review on constipation. Gastroenterology. 2013;144:218–38.

Camilleri M. Novel diet, drugs and gastric interventions for gastroparesis. Clin Gastroenterol Hepatol. 2016;14:1072–80.

Dinning PG, Di Lorenzo C. Colonic dysmotility in constipation. Best Pract Res Clin Gastroenterol. 2011;25:89–101.

Jones MP, Maganti K. A systematic review of surgical therapy for gastroparesis. Am J Gastroenterol. 2003;98:2122–9.

Knowles CH, Grossi U, Chapman M, et al. Surgery for constipation: systematic review and practice recommendations: Results I: colonic resection. Colorectal Dis. 2017;19(Suppl 3):17–36.

Kuo P, Rayner CK, Jones KL, Horowitz M. Pathophysiology and management of diabetic gastropathy: a guide for endocrinologists. Drugs. 2007a;67:1671–87.

Kuo P, Rayner CK, Horowitz M. Gastric emptying, diabetes, and aging. Clin Geriatr Med. 2007b;23:785–808.

Liu N, Abell T. Gastroparesis updates on pathogenesis and management. Gut Liver. 2017;11:579–89.

Mittai R, Debs LH, Patel AP, et al. Neurotransmitters: the critical modulators regulating gut-brain axis. J. Cell Physiol. 2017;232:2359–72.

Pandolfino JE, Gawron AJ. Achalasia: a systematic review. JAMA. 2015;313:1841–52.

Rao SS, Camilleri M, Hasler WL, et al. Evaluation of gastrointestinal transit in clinical practice: position paper of the American and European Neurogastroenterology and Motility Societies. Neurogastroenterol Motil. 2011;23:8–23.

Revicki DA, Rentz AM, Dubois D, et al. Gastroparesis Cardinal Symptom Index [GCSI]: development and validation of a patient reported assessment of severity of gastroparesis symptoms. Qual Life Res. 2004;13:833–44.

Gallstones

8

Gian A. Prevost, Harsh A. Kanhere, and Guy J. Maddern

8.1 Epidemiology, Risk Factors and Pathogenesis

Gallstone disease is a major health problem in developed countries and one of the most common causes of surgical hospital admissions. Cholesterol stones account for about 90% of all gallstones in Western populations and form when bile is supersaturated with cholesterol. The remaining 10% are black or brown pigment stones consisting of calcium salts of bilirubin. Black pigment stones are more common in patients with cirrhosis or chronic haemolysis, whereas brown pigment stones are usually associated with infection and originate mostly in bile ducts.

The prevalence of gallstones increases with age and differs between ethnic populations. In people aged 60 and above, prevalence ranges from 8% (Asian population) to 75% (Native American populations) with an incidence of around 20% in Western populations. The prevalence of gallstone disease has increased in recent years, probably due to an increasingly older population and high prevalence of obesity. It is estimated that 1–4% of patients with gallstones develop biliary symptoms per year with 0.1–0.3% suffering from complications. Interestingly, once a person develops biliary symptoms, the risk for recurrent symptoms is greater than 50%. Multiple stones increase the risk for complications such as acute cholecystitis or symptomatic gallstone disease. Acute cholecystitis is the most common complication of gallstone disease, occurring in about 10% of patients with symptomatic gallstones.

Females are more prone to develop gallstones than males, especially in their younger years. Pregnancy and hormonal changes are postulated to be the reason for increased prevalence in younger women. With increasing age, the gender difference in prevalence decreases. Obesity and rapid weight loss are both known causative factors.

G. A. Prevost (✉) · H. A. Kanhere · G. J. Maddern
Discipline of Surgery, University of Adelaide, Adelaide, SA, Australia
e-mail: Gian.Prevost@sa.gov.au; Harsh.Kanhere@sa.gov.au; guy.maddern@adelaide.edu.au

M. W. Wichmann et al. (eds.), *Gastroenterology For General Surgeons*,
https://doi.org/10.1007/978-3-319-92768-8_8

The risk of developing gallstones is 2–4 times higher in first-degree relatives compared to non-related controls. Familial clustering suggests that genetics, diet and environmental factors may have a significant role in the development of gallstones. Conditions resulting in bile stasis such as spinal cord injuries, prolonged fasting, use of total parenteral nutrition, somatostatin administration and postvagotomy status are associated with a higher prevalence of gallstones. Finally, cirrhotic patients suffer from a significantly higher risk, due to factors such as reduced hepatic synthesis, reduced transport of bile salts, nonconjugated bilirubin, high oestrogen levels and impaired gallbladder contraction in response to food intake.

8.2 Primary Prevention

There is no validated means for primary prevention of cholesterol stones. Hypothetically, a healthy diet and lifestyle should reduce the risk as elevated body mass index and diabetes mellitus are associated with gallstones, and recent evidence suggests that physical activity may be protective. It needs to be noted that rapid weight loss is associated with increased risk of developing gallstones. A regular eating pattern which allows regular gallbladder emptying (allowing for decreased gallbladder stasis) may reduce stone formation. Regular vitamin C supplementation or a vitamin C-enriched diet might also have a protective effect on gallstone formation because of its role in the conversion of cholesterol to bile acids. Statins may also have a protective effect on gallstone formation especially in higher doses. Ursodeoxycholic acid can be tried in high-risk groups; however there is no clear evidence to support its use in primary prevention.

8.3 Diagnosis of Gallbladder Stones and Cholecystitis

Symptomatic gallbladder stones typically cause episodic attacks of severe pain in the right upper abdominal quadrant or epigastrium, radiating to the right back or shoulder and lasting for variable amounts of time. Concomitant nausea or vomiting can also occur, and signs of a food or fat intolerance are common.

Acute cholecystitis should be considered if there are signs of local infection with local tenderness (positive Murphy's sign) and systemic signs (fever, tachycardia) with elevated C-reactive protein (CRP) and leucocytosis. Further liver function evaluations, including bilirubin, gamma-glutamyl transferase (GGT), alkaline phosphatase (AP), alanine aminotransferase (ALT) and lipase, should always be undertaken.

Abdominal ultrasonography is the gold standard for diagnosing gallbladder stones with a sensitivity >95% and a specificity of almost 100%. It is also the investigation of choice to diagnose cholecystitis. In cholecystitis, typical sonographic appearances are thickening of the gallbladder wall (>4 mm), pericholecystic fluid, gallbladder distension and sonographic Murphy's sign (intensified pain upon probe pressure directly over the gallbladder). Computed tomography (CT) and magnetic resonance imaging (MRI) have similar sensitivity and specificity to confirm or exclude cholecystitis but are not preferred as first-line investigations because of radiation exposure, limited availability and high costs. These modalities should be reserved for cases where there is a diagnostic dilemma, or equivocal findings on clinical and ultrasound examinations, or where there is a suspicion of bile duct calculi. Gallbladder wall thickening can be caused by cholecystitis but also as a consequence of viral hepatitis, other viral diseases with liver involvement or abdominal infections. Fluid retention as part of liver cirrhosis, cardiac failure, renal failure, protein deficiency and shock can also lead to significant thickening of the gallbladder wall. In these cases a cholecystectomy is not indicated, and it is crucial to differentiate these cases from acute cholecystitis.

A CT and MRI (especially magnetic resonance cholangiopancreatography, MRCP) are the investigations of choice if there is a suspicion of bile duct stones as alluded to in the following text.

8.4 Treatment

Asymptomatic gallstones: Asymptomatic gallbladder stones are not an indication for cholecystectomy. The risks associated with surgery (although very small) are still greater than adopting a wait-and-see policy in asymptomatic patients.

Surgery should be considered in asymptomatic patients if stones are bigger than 3 cm or concomitant gallbladder polyps are greater than 1 cm, or in the presence of porcelain gallbladder and non-circumferential calcifications of the wall as these conditions are associated with gallbladder cancer. Similarly, immune compromised patients and those undergoing bariatric surgery may be considered for a prophylactic cholecystectomy in the presence of asymptomatic gallstones.

Biliary colic and acute cholecystitis: Laparoscopic cholecystectomy is the gold standard for the treatment of biliary colic and cholecystitis. Laparoscopic cholecystectomy has the advantages of shorter hospital stay and recovery period than open cholecystectomy. Elective laparoscopic cholecystectomy can be performed in most patients as day surgery. The standard laparoscopic cholecystectomy procedure is a four-trocar technique. There is no evidence available showing benefit of single incision technique (SILS) or natural orifice transluminal endoscopic surgery (NOTES). As such, these approaches are not the standard of care in most Western countries.

Injury to the bile ducts is the most important complication of a laparoscopic cholecystectomy. The risk can be minimized by performing a standard dissection of the cystic artery and the cystic duct. The incidence of such injuries is about 0.1–0.5%. Should a bile duct injury be suspected, the patients must be managed in a tertiary centre by experienced hepatobiliary surgeons. Interventional radiology input may be valuable. When an intraoperative injury is suspected, the area should be assessed with intraoperative cholangiogram if available and feasible, followed by sub-hepatic drain insertion, and the patient transferred to a specialized centre.

It is important to note that up to a third of patients have persistent unspecific abdominal complaints after cholecystectomy.

Timing of cholecystectomy in acute cholecystitis: Several studies, including the well-known ACDC study, have shown the benefit of early cholecystectomy within the first 24 h after admission, in most acute cholecystitis presentations. It is accepted that cholecystectomy performed during the initial acute cholecystitis admission reduces the readmission rates due to recurrent symptoms. Concerns regarding increased risk of open conversion or higher rates of bile duct injury and higher morbidity are not supported by available evidence. It is likely that a cholecystectomy done within 72 h of diagnosis of acute cholecystitis has the best outcomes. Mandatory demonstration of the so-called Critical View of Safety has resulted in reduced risk of common bile duct injury and surgical morbidity (Fig. 8.1).

In acute cholecystitis patients who carry high operative risks and severe comorbidities, conservative treatment is an option but must be considered with the knowledge that over a third of these patients will develop further complications. Percutaneous gallbladder drainage can be performed as an alternative treatment option in such instances. This should be performed by an experienced interventional radiologist using a trans-hepatic approach to minimize the risk of intraperitoneal biliary leak. In difficult cases with inflammatory-obscured biliary anatomy, subtotal cholecystectomy may be favoured to reduce the risk of injury to the common bile duct, portal vein and hepatic arteries. Randomized controlled trials show no need for continued postoperative antibiotic treatment for patients with acute cholecystitis. Only patients with severe infection (septic shock, impaired consciousness or organ failure) are known to benefit from such treatment.

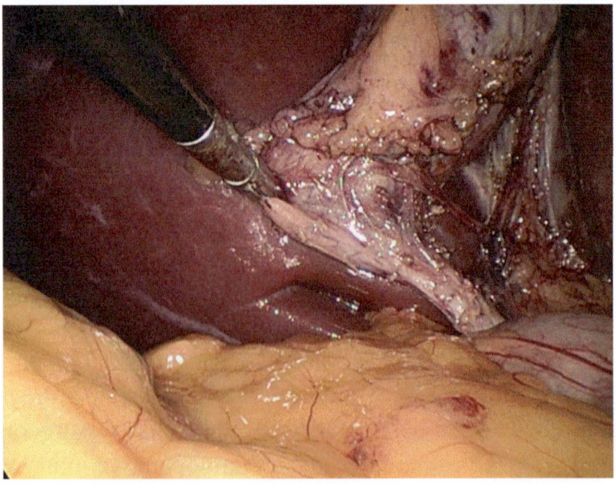

Fig. 8.1 Critical View of Safety

8.5 Management of Bile Duct Stones

Concomitant choledocholithiasis with cholelithiasis has a high probability (>50%) in patients with:

- Dilated bile ducts (>7 mm) and hyperbilirubinemia and elevation of GGT, AP, ALT or aspartate aminotransferase (AST)
- Clinical signs and biochemical blood tests suggesting ascending cholangitis
- Sonographic proof of choledocholithiasis

There is medium (5–50%) probability if one or two of high-probability criteria are fulfilled.

Concomitant choledocholithiasis is unlikely and has a low probability (<5%) in patients with:

- Non-dilated bile ducts (<7 mm)
- Normal liver biochemical tests (bilirubin, GGT, AP, ALT)
- Lack of episodes of biliary pancreatitis, acholic feces and dark urine

In patients with a low probability for bile duct stones, the above-mentioned predictors can exclude choledocholithiasis with similar certainty to endoscopic retrograde cholangiopancreatography (ERCP) or intraoperative cholangiogram. These patients can therefore safely proceed to a laparoscopic cholecystectomy without additional investigations.

In patients with a medium probability for bile duct stones, further investigations are recommended. Trend for bilirubin levels, serum transaminases, AP and GGT should be monitored. A rising trend and/or persistently high levels are an indication of persistent outflow obstruction. A decline in transaminases and cholestasis parameters may be a sign of passage of a stone.

In cases where the diagnosis is not clear, MRCP has high sensitivity and specificity rates though small stones (<5 mm) may sometimes be missed. Endoscopic ultrasound (EUS) where available is an excellent option due to sensitivity of up to 100% and a specificity of >93%. EUS is more sensitive, especially in detecting small gallstones (<4 mm) and pre-papillary stones, and has a lower intervention risk compared to ERCP. ERCP has a risk of 5–10%, of which post-interventional pancreatitis is the leading complication. Intraoperative cholangiography and laparoscopic sonography have a sensitivity of 87% and a specificity of almost 100%. In summary, patients with a medium probability for bile duct stones should undergo MRCP or EUS to determine if therapeutic ERCP is required. If bile duct stones are diagnosed on these investigations, a preoperative ERCP should be undertaken to clear the bile duct.

Some surgical units favour performing an intraoperative bile duct exploration. This can be safely and effectively undertaken via a laparoscopic approach in experienced hands. A transcystic route can be used to retrieve small stones in a narrow duct. A formal common bile duct (CBD) exploration with a choledochotomy can be carried out laparoscopically as well especially for larger stones and a widened duct. Most surgeons prefer leaving a T-tube to drain the CBD in these instances. The T-tube allows access for postoperative cholangiogram to ascertain ductal clearance and ensure that there are no residual stones or distal ductal obstruction. A transductal biliary stent can be used with a primary closure of the duct. The stent can be removed endoscopically after a few weeks.

In patients with a high probability for bile duct stones, therapeutic ERCP is a reasonable first-line treatment. However, EUS is recommended prior to ERCP to exclude patients who present with high-probability symptoms but do not have gallstones (roughly 50%). An added advantage of EUS is the high sensitivity and specificity for the diagnosis of non-gallstone causes of biliary obstruction.

Sensitivity of abdominal ultrasonography is reported in different studies with variable values; however the specificity of abdominal ultrasonography is one of the highest of the available radiological investigation methods. Pre-papillary stones and small stones (<5 mm) are often missed in abdominal ultrasonography. The detection of a dilated CBD (>7 mm) in abdominal ultrasonography has a sensitivity of around 40% and a specificity of over 95% for existence of bile duct stones. Multiple small gallstones increase the risk of bile duct stones fourfold compared to single or fewer and larger stones.

Bile duct stones should be treated irrespective of symptom severity due to the high risk of pancreatitis and cholangitis. ERCP is the gold standard for the treatment of bile duct stones, but a surgeon with high expertise can conduct a laparoscopic bile duct exploration with the same complication rates as ERCP. If logistically possible, an intraoperative ERCP is a viable option. It has the advantage allowing antegrade cannulation of a guidewire through the cystic duct into the duodenum, thus reducing the risk of post-ERCP pancreatitis. In patients with altered anatomy, e.g. after Roux-en-Y gastric bypass, a percutaneous trans-hepatic cholangiography or surgical exploration may be required.

In patients with simultaneous gallbladder and bile duct stones, early laparoscopic cholecystectomy should be performed within 72 h of preoperative ERCP if there is no evidence of post-procedural pancreatitis. Cholecystectomy should be performed as soon as the patient recovers from pancreatitis. This progressive approach leads to significantly less recurrent biliary events compared to delayed laparoscopic cholecystectomy (after 6–8 weeks). Again, there are no differences in conversion rate, operation time or surgical complications with the straightforward approach. In elderly patients with severe comorbidities, ERCP and papillotomy alone may be a favoured strategy in patients with known persistent cholecystolithiasis.

Prevalence of intrahepatic stones or recurrent bile duct stones in young patients should raise suspicion of haemolytic anaemias, bile acid malabsorption syndrome, parasitic or bacterial infection or low phospholipid-associated cholelithiasis (ABCB4 gene mutation) and should warrant further investigations.

8.6 Cholangitis and Biliary Pancreatitis

Acute cholangitis derived from bile duct obstruction and consecutive infection is a feared complication of bile duct stones, with a mortality rate of 3–10%. Choledocholithiasis is the main cause for biliary outflow obstruction followed by malignant stenoses, benign strictures, (Mirizzi's syndrome, postinflammatory stenosis, iatrogenic injuries) and rare causes like intraductal parasitosis, e.g. liver flukes. Cholangitis is traditionally diagnosed in the presence of right upper quadrant pain, fever and obstructive jaundice (Charcot's triad).

However the Tokyo guidelines, released in 2018, are much more sensitive and are the superior diagnostic criteria. The guidelines encompass systemic inflammation (fever, chills or increased inflammatory markers), cholestasis (jaundice or abnormal liver function tests) and imaging (biliary dilation or evidence of stricture, stone or stent). Diagnosis can be suspected in cases of systemic inflammation and one of the two other parameters. Diagnosis is confirmed if all three parameters are present. If abdominal ultrasonography does not confirm bile duct dilatation, choledocholithiasis or other causes for outflow obstruction, further investigation with CT, EUS or MRCP is warranted.

Aggressive resuscitation with intravenous broad-spectrum antibiotic treatment should be commenced as soon as possible after diagnosis of acute cholangitis. Endoscopic treatment with either stone extraction or stent insertion to drain an obstructed duct should be performed in a timely manner depending on the severity of cholangitis. If endoscopic decompression is not successful, other interventional procedures, e.g. percutaneous trans-hepatic cholangio drainage (PTCD), or surgical intervention should be considered.

Hyperlipasaemia and appropriate clinical signs in the context of known cholelithiasis should lead to suspicion of biliary pancreatitis. Gallbladder stones or sludge in combination with elevated liver function tests have a high predictive value for a biliary genesis of pancreatitis.

EUS has a high sensitivity to detect biliary genesis of pancreatitis and can refute undiagnosed biliary genesis of pancreatitis in up to 50% of patients with negative abdominal ultrasonography, CT and even MRCP findings.

In cases of uncomplicated biliary pancreatitis, with no evidence of choledocholithiasis on EUS or MRCP, cholecystectomy should be performed as soon as possible, rather than ERCP (PONCHO study).

In cases of severe pancreatitis and known bile duct stones without cholangitis, ERCP with papillotomy should be performed within 72 h of symptoms appearing. In these cases, cholecystectomy is performed after recovery from pancreatitis. In patients with concomitant cholangitis, ERCP should be performed as soon as possible.

8.7 Special Circumstances: Pregnancy

Laparoscopic cholecystectomy can be performed during pregnancy if the indication is urgent, regardless of trimester. Symptomatic patients in the first trimester should be operated early because of high recurrence rate.

Similar to symptomatic gallbladder stones, complicated choledocholithiasis should be addressed by ERCP and papillotomy during pregnancy.

Recommended Reading

Afdhal NH et al. Epidemiology of and risk factors for gallstones. UpToDate® 2018; https://www.uptodate.com/contents/epidemiology-of-and-risk-factors-for-gallstones. Accessed 28 Apr 2018.

Da Costa DW, et al. Same-admission versus interval cholecystectomy for mild gallstone pancreatitis (PONCHO): a multicentre randomised controlled trial. Lancet. 2015;386(10,000):1261–8. https://doi.org/10.1016/s0140-6736(15)00274-3.

EASL Clinical Practice Guidelines on the prevention, diagnosis and treatment of gallstones. J Hepatol 2016;65(1):146–81. https://doi.org/10.1016/j.jhep.2016.03.005.

Gutt CN, et al. Acute cholecystitis: early versus delayed cholecystectomy, a multicenter randomized trial (ACDC study, NCT00447304). Ann Surg. 2013;258(3):385–93. https://doi.org/10.1097/SLA.0b013e3182a1599b.

Lammert F, et al. S3-guidelines for diagnosis and treatment of gallstones. German Society for Digestive and Metabolic Diseases and German Society for Surgery of the Alimentary Tract. Z Gastroenterol. 2007;45(9):971–1001. https://doi.org/10.1055/s-2007-963437.

Strasberg SM, Brunt LM. Rationale and use of the critical view of safety in laparoscopic cholecystectomy. J Am Coll Surg. 2010;211(1):132–8. https://doi.org/10.1016/j.jamcollsurg.2010.02.053.

Takada T. Tokyo Guidelines 2018: updated Tokyo Guidelines for the management of acute cholangitis/acute cholecystitis. J Hepatobiliary Pancreat Sci. 2018;25(1):1–2. https://doi.org/10.1002/jhbp.526.

Venneman NG, van Erpecum KJ. Pathogenesis of gallstones. Gastroenterol Clin N Am. 2010;39(2):171–83. https://doi.org/10.1016/j.gtc.2010.02.010.

Spleen

9

Matthias W. Wichmann and Timothy K. McCullough

9.1 Introduction

The spleen is of interest to the general surgeon when dealing with:

- Patients after blunt or penetrating abdominal trauma
- Splenic laceration during/after abdominal surgery or colonoscopy
- Indications for elective splenectomy

Normal splenic function is of significant importance for host immunity, and the consequences of splenectomy are complex. A "cowboy approach" to the spleen and its removal should be considered obsolete—every effort should be made to preserve splenic function whenever possible.

9.2 Normal Splenic Function

The spleen is part of the erythroid, myeloid, megakaryocytic, lymphoid, and monocyte-macrophage systems. The spleen is a lymphopoietic organ and contains 1/4 of the lymphoid mass (white pulp of the spleen) of the body. In addition to this, about 1/3 of the platelets are "stored" in the normal spleen.

The white pulp of the spleen contains B-lymphocytes, plasma cells, and T-lymphocytes—these cells mount an immune response to foreign antigens in the circulation. Antibody production in patients without a functional spleen can be significantly decreased. Splenic sinusoids course through the white and red pulp and are lined with macrophages. These cells act as antigen-presenting cells and also remove aged/damaged red cells from the circulation.

M. W. Wichmann (✉) · T. K. McCullough
Department of Surgery, Mount Gambier General Hospital, Mount Gambier, SA, Australia
e-mail: matthias.wichmann@sa.gov.au; timothy.mccullough@sa.gov.au

M. W. Wichmann et al. (eds.), *Gastroenterology For General Surgeons*,
https://doi.org/10.1007/978-3-319-92768-8_9

9.3 Abnormal Splenic Conditions

9.3.1 Splenomegaly

Enlargement of the spleen is usually associated with liver disease (1/3 of all cases), hematologic disorders (1/4 of all cases), infection (1/4 of all cases), or inflammatory conditions. Non-hematologic metastases are rarely localized in the spleen. The spleen has to increase in size by at least 40% before it is palpable.

In children splenomegaly is most commonly associated with infection (Epstein-Barr virus, cytomegalovirus), hematologic malignancy, immune dysfunction (systemic lupus erythematosus, rheumatoid arthritis), and hemolytic anemia.

Splenomegaly can result in about 90% of all platelets being sequested in the spleen, leading to relative thrombocytopenia in the circulating blood.

If no underlying condition for splenomegaly is established, patient work-up should include accurate history, physical examination, blood count with white blood cell differential, peripheral blood smear, liver function studies, urinalysis, and chest X-ray. Imaging studies can include ultrasound, CT scan, MRI, and Tc-99m sulfur colloid scintigraphy. If these investigations are not sufficient to establish a diagnosis and the patient is symptomatic, splenectomy can be considered. Outcomes of this procedure are usually better with the laparoscopic approach. It is important to note that splenectomy can only be considered curative if isolated splenic lesions are present; in all other circumstances, the splenectomy is diagnostic in nature.

Splenosis describes implants of splenic tissue in the abdominal cavity due to blunt/penetrating trauma or surgical intervention. Return of normal splenic function is usually incomplete, and normal splenic function can only be expected with a minimum volume of 20 cm^3 of splenic tissue.

Splenic infarction occurs after occlusion of the splenic artery or one of its sub-branches. It presents with acute left upper quadrant pain and can occur in a variety of settings such as hypercoagulable states (malignancy), embolic disease, hemoglobinopathy, and splenomegaly.

Splenic artery aneurysms are the third most common aneurysms within the abdominal cavity and can be treated with embolization, stenting, or vascular reconstruction.

Atraumatic splenic rupture is uncommon. It can be observed due to neoplasm, infection, and pregnancy.

Splenic abscess is an uncommon infection and typically results from endocarditis.

Accepted indications for elective splenectomy include thrombocytopenia, hemolytic anemia, hemolytic neutropenia, pain due to enlarged spleen, splenic artery aneurysm, cytopenia due to hypersplenism, splenic vascular/parenchymal lesions, and splenomegaly of unknown cause. In patients suffering from immune thrombocytopenia (ITP) or autoimmune hemolytic anemia, the spleen is responsible for clearing antibody-coated platelets or red cells.

The spleen has important functions but can be removed in part, or completely, via open laparotomy or laparoscopy. Only isolated splenic lesions can be cured by splenectomy. Postoperative morbidity can be as high as 40% and the mortality up to 6% in these patients.

Long-term risks of splenectomy include infection (pneumococcal pneumonia, meningitis, sepsis), thromboembolism (DVT, PE), and malignancy (13% of splenectomized patients).

9.3.2 Splenic Trauma

The spleen is a frequently injured intra-abdominal organ, and this can result in life-threatening blood loss (approximately 6–7% of cardiac stroke volume perfuses the spleen). The decision to remove the spleen should not be made without an attempt of complete or partial salvage (leaving approximately 1/3 of the spleen with an intact blood supply), but this has to be abandoned if other life-threatening injuries require treatment or if blood loss from the spleen cannot be controlled.

Blunt abdominal trauma (motor vehicle accidents, falls, sport-related) more commonly affects the spleen rather than penetrating trauma. Iatrogenic traumatic injuries include surgical or endoscopic handling of the colon, stomach, pancreas, kidney, and proximal aorta. Colorectal surgery has been reported to carry a 1% risk of splenic laceration.

Splenic trauma is assessed using ultrasound (hypoechoic rim around the spleen, fluid in Morrison's pouch = hepatorenal space) and computed tomography (hemoperitoneum, hypodense regions in the spleen, contrast blush/extravasation). Splenic lacerations are graded from I (hematoma, <10% of surface area) to V (shattered spleen) depending on the extent and depth of splenic hematoma/laceration. Management of splenic injury includes observation, embolization, or surgery depending on hemodynamic stability, grade of injury, presence of other injuries, as well as comorbidities. Surgery is indicated if the patient cannot be adequately monitored, if comorbidity does not allow a period of hypotension, or if nonsurgical management fails. Nonsurgical management is successful in up to 70% of all patients with splenic injury. Patients with splenic trauma should be observed in an intensive care or high-dependency unit. During the initial 24 h, strict bed rest and serial hemoglobin testing (every 6 h) are recommended. The patient should remain fasted during this period due to the potential need for emergency surgery. If conservative management fails, this can be expected to occur in most patients within 4 days after trauma, and more than half of the conservative treatment failures develop within 24 h. In hospital, observation should last for approximately 1 week, and limited activities (sport, work with risk of repeat trauma, travelling to areas with limited access to surgery) should be recommended for approximately 6 weeks. Re-imaging after 3 months is not generally recommended; if done it should document complete healing of the laceration.

9.4 Hyposplenism, Functional/Surgical Asplenia

Patients without functional splenic tissue have increased risks of infection (pneumococcal pneumonia, pneumonia of other causes, meningitis, septicemia), thromboembolism (DVT, PE), and malignancy (liver, pancreas, lung, NHL, leukemia).

Poor or non-existing splenic function can result in:

- Sepsis with encapsulated organisms
- Thrombocytosis and leukocytosis
- Howell-Jolly bodies in circulating red cells, erythrocyte pits, and Heinz bodies

Patients after splenectomy are at risk of *fulminant sepsis* caused by encapsulated organisms (*Streptococcus pneumonia*, *Haemophilus influenzae*, *Neisseria meningitidis*). The most important pathogen is *S. pneumonia*, and the highest risk for fulminant sepsis has been observed during the initial 5 years after surgery.

Prophylactic immunization after splenectomy is ideally delayed until 14 days after surgery to allow for an optimal antibody response. This is not always feasible (lack of patient compliance) and must then be done at the time of discharge from hospital. Recommended immunizations for patients after splenectomy are against *Streptococcus pneumonia*, *Neisseria meningitidis*, and *Haemophilus influenza* type B. If the postoperative vaccination is performed prior to day 14 after splenectomy, repeating postsplenectomy vaccination at 8 weeks after the initial immunization is recommended. Yearly influenza vaccinations are also necessary in these patients.

In children, daily oral antibiotic prophylaxis until age 5 is indicated (penicillin VK or amoxicillin). In adults, routine antibiotic prophylaxis is not recommended.

Fulminant asplenic sepsis must be assumed when the patient presents with acute onset of extreme malaise, high fever, rigors, hypotension, and signs of bacteremia (petechiae, purpura, meningitis). Broad-spectrum antibiotic treatment and organ support measures must be started immediately in these patients. Vancomycin (adults: 15–20 mg/kg i.v. every 12 h; children: 60 mg/kg i.v. in 4 doses; adjust to vancomycin serum through concentration of 15–20 mcg/mL) and ceftriaxone (adults: 2 g i.v. every 12 h; children: 100 mg/kg i.v. in 2 doses) or cefotaxime (adults: 2 g i.v. every 6 h; children: 300 mg/kg i.v. in 4 doses) are given empirically. For patients with hypersensitivity to beta-lactam antibiotics, vancomycin should be combined with moxifloxacin (adults: 400 mg i.v. every 24 h; children: 5 mg/kg every 24 h).

9.5 Prevention of Sepsis in Asplenic Patients

Adherence to prevention requires education of the patient and his/her carers about the situation. Furthermore, a systemic approach within a hospital/healthcare unit can contribute to better sepsis prevention. This systemic approach should include a registry of patients after splenectomy.

Immunization with pneumococcal, meningococcal, and *Haemophilus influenzae* type B vaccines must be done. Inactivated influenza vaccinations should be repeated annually.

Only asplenic children should receive daily antibiotic prophylaxis (penicillin VK, amoxicillin) until age 5 and for at least 1 year after splenectomy. Routine antibiotic prophylaxis in adults after splenectomy is not recommended (antibiotic resistance, side effects of treatment). In immunocompromised adults or adults who survived pneumococcal sepsis, oral antibiotics can be discussed.

9.6 When to Transfer

Elective surgery of the spleen should be minimally invasive and performed by surgeons with adequate experience in this field. Systemic disease affecting the spleen may require specialist input, and this can be provided via telemedicine or through patient transfer if not available locally. Conservative management of splenic injury requires 24 h access to operating theatres and adequate monitoring (ICU, HDU). If this cannot be provided locally, patient transfer must be considered if it is safe to do so. Alternatively prophylactic splenectomy may be necessary.

Patients presenting with postsplenectomy sepsis must be resuscitated, and empiric broad-spectrum antibiotic treatment must be initiated immediately. Adequate long-term patient care requires an intensive care unit, and patient transfer must be arranged if this is not available in the hospital providing the initial emergency care.

Recommended Reading

Hildebrand DR, et al. Modern management of splenic trauma. BMJ. 2014;348:g1864.
Rodeghiero F, et al. Short- and long-term risks of splenectomy for benign haematological disorders: should we revisit the indications? Br J Haematol. 2012;158:16.
Rubin LG, et al. Clinical practice. Care of the asplenic patient. N Engl J Med. 2014;371:349.
Sun LM, et al. Splenectomy and increased subsequent cancer risk: a nationwide population-based cohort study. Am J Surg. 2015;210:243.
Theilacker C, et al. Overwhelming postsplenectomy infection: a prospective multicenter cohort study. Clin Infect Dis. 2016;62:871.
UpToDate®: approach to the adult with splenomegaly and other splenic disorders
UpToDate®: approach to the child with an enlarged spleen
UpToDate®: clinical features and management of sepsis in the asplenic patient
UpToDate®: liver, spleen, and pancreas injury in children with blunt abdominal trauma
UpToDate®: management of splenic injury in the adult trauma patient
UpToDate®: prevention of sepsis in the asplenic patient

Acute Pancreatitis, Chronic Pancreatitis and Pancreatic Neoplasms

10

Ali Arshad and Ashley Dennison

10.1 Acute Pancreatitis

10.1.1 Definition

A condition in which there is acute inflammation of the pancreas, which leads to cell damage and local release of digestive enzymes, and may lead to local and systemic complications.

10.1.2 Epidemiology

The incidence of acute pancreatitis is rising, with approximately 30 cases per 100,000 per year or 18,000 new diagnoses in the UK each year.

10.1.3 Etiology

Gallstones account for up to 40% of cases, with alcohol responsible in 25%. Other rarer causes of hyperlipidemia (10%), trauma (1.5%), hypercalcemia (0.6%), autoimmune pancreatitis, cystic fibrosis, prior ERCP and malignancy should also be considered. Gallstones lodged just above the ampulla of Vater, cystic fibrosis and malignancy all cause pancreatitis by obstruction of the pancreatic duct. This leads

A. Arshad
Department of Surgery, Southampton General Hospital, Southampton, UK
e-mail: ali.arshad@doctors.org.uk

A. Dennison (✉)
Department of Hepatobiliary and Pancreatic Surgery, University Hospitals of Leicester, Leicester, UK
e-mail: ashley.dennison@ulh-tr.nhs.uk

M. W. Wichmann et al. (eds.), *Gastroenterology For General Surgeons*,
https://doi.org/10.1007/978-3-319-92768-8_10

to impaired drainage of exocrine enzymes into the duodenum and subsequent autodigestion of the pancreas, with the subsequent cascade and cycle of inflammation and further autodigestion and necrosis. Alcohol causes direct damage to pancreatic acinar cells with the release of pro-inflammatory cytokines and upgrading of the local and systemic inflammatory response.

10.1.4 Diagnosis

To diagnose acute pancreatitis, it is necessary to fulfil at least two of the following criteria:

1. A history of acute abdominal pain, usually with vomiting
2. An elevated serum amylase or lipase greater than 3 times the laboratory reference range
3. Typical features on CT imaging

There may be a history of alcohol excess or prior known gallstones. If there is diagnostic doubt, cross-sectional imaging, such as CT, is indicated to confirm the diagnosis. This is particularly important where a modestly elevated amylase is present in an unwell patient. The differential diagnosis then includes perforated gastric or duodenal ulcer, perforated gallbladder or a leaking abdominal aortic aneurysm, all of which require urgent operative management.

10.1.5 Assessment of Severity

Various scoring systems have been devised including Ranson, Glasgow, Apache II, CRP and physiological early warning scores. Of these the most sensitive predictor of future severe pancreatitis is CRP alone. Apache II is the most sensitive predictor of current severe pancreatitis, which is defined as pancreatitis with evidence of end organ dysfunction. A more useful bedside tool for the assessment of severity and subsequent triage of patients is the early warning score. Patients with severe pancreatitis should be managed in a level 1 or 2 facility. The mortality from severe pancreatitis is 30%.

10.1.6 Management

10.1.6.1 Fluid Management

Pancreatitis should be thought of as a systemic disease, requiring active physiological support. The multi-system sequelae of severe acute pancreatitis includes adult respiratory distress syndrome (ARDS), renal failure, cardiorespiratory instability and disseminated intravascular coagulation. All patients should have meticulous fluid balance monitoring with aggressive replacement of intravenous fluid, as fluid losses and intracellular shifts may be dramatic. Urinary catheterisation should be strongly considered to aid fluid management and is mandatory in those with renal failure or cardiovascular instability. Patients with severe pancreatitis should have invasive haemodynamic monitoring including central venous access and continuous arterial pressure measurement.

10.1.6.2 Antibiotics

As pancreatitis is an inflammatory condition, rather than an infective one, there is no indication for antibiotic therapy. The exception is where there is confirmed concurrent infection, such as in the respiratory, biliary, or urinary tracts, or proven infected necrosis of the gland. Infected necrotic collections appear as localized areas of fluid with pockets of gas or an enhancing wall.

10.1.6.3 Drainage of Collections

The majority of patients with acute pancreatitis will have a minor degree of fluid adjacent to the pancreas demonstrated on CT, either in the lesser sac or in the peritoneal cavity. These sterile acute fluid collections resolve spontaneously in the majority of cases but may develop into sterile pseudocysts after a number of weeks. The temptation to drain these collections radiologically or via endoscopic ultrasound (EUS) must be resisted as iatrogenic infection is then inevitable, with a resulting cycle of superimposed infection, sepsis, further drains and deterioration. Percutaneous drainage purely to reduce intra-abdominal pressure "caused" by the acute fluid collections is also rarely rewarding or effective. The only indication for drainage is unequivocally infected fluid collections with CT appearances as described previously. The days of open pancreatic necrosectomy appear to be over, and a step-up approach with minimally invasive techniques reduces major complications over open surgical debridement of the pancreas. If anatomically suitable and mature, then these can be drained into the posterior wall of the stomach via EUS guided cyst-gastrostomy stenting, with repeated washout and pancreatic necrosectomy through the stent as required. If the infected collections track inferiorly or posteriorly, optimal drainage may be achieved by percutaneous approach through the flank. This tract can be dilated and fluoroscopically accessed for minimally invasive pancreatic necrosectomy using an operative nephroscope. There is equipoise as to whether endoscopic or surgical drainage is superior, although there is recent randomized controlled trial data indicating a reduction in the rates of pancreatic fistulae and length of stay in endoscopically treated patients.

10.1.6.4 ERCP

The only role for ERCP in the treatment of pancreatitis is where there is a proven, obstructing stone lodged in the common bile duct. In this situation, ERCP and sphincterotomy can be employed as a treatment to prevent further attacks of pancreatitis in patients who are unfit for cholecystectomy.

10.1.6.5 Nutrition

It is now clear that early enteral nutrition is a key step in the successful treatment of acute pancreatitis, and there is no role for "gut rest". Trials of nasojejunal over nasogastric feeding have failed to demonstrate the superiority of one approach over the other. Where nasogastric aspirates are persistently high, total parenteral nutrition (TPN) is indicated although there is some concern that the pro-inflammatory lipids used in most TPN preparations may worsen the systemic inflammatory response.

10.2 Chronic Pancreatitis

10.2.1 Definition

Chronic pancreatitis is a pathologic, fibro-inflammatory syndrome of the pancreas in individuals with genetic, environmental and/or other risk factors who develop persistent pathologic responses to parenchymal injury or stress. Common features of established and advanced chronic pancreatitis include pancreatic atrophy, fibrosis, pain syndromes, duct distortion and strictures, calcification, pancreatic exocrine dysfunction, pancreatic endocrine dysfunction and dysplasia.

10.2.2 Diagnosis

The majority of patients present with upper abdominal pain, usually epigastric, dull and constant in nature. Some patients may present with the classical "erythema ab igne" sign of skin discoloration from a hot water bottle applied to provide temporary relief by the technique of counterirritation. A subset of patients may present with silent endocrine or exocrine dysfunction. Radiological features on CT are typical with atrophy of the gland, pancreatic duct dilatation and calcification being almost universal, although some patients may present with a discrete mass which can be extremely difficult to distinguish from carcinoma. EUS examination offers close proximity imaging of the pancreas and surrounding structures in great detail and also the opportunity to take fine needle aspiration or a biopsy of any mass. In addition, the Rosemont EUS criteria for diagnosis of chronic pancreatitis can be used:

1. Hyperechoic foci with shadowing and main pancreatic duct (PD) calculi.
2. Lobularity with honeycombing.
3. Minor criteria for chronic pancreatitis are cysts, dilated ducts ≥3.5 mm, irregular PD contour, dilated side branches ≥1 mm, hyperechoic duct wall, strands, non-shadowing hyperechoic foci and lobularity with noncontiguous lobules.

The APA stepwise (STEP-wise; S, survey; T, tomography; E, endoscopy; and P, pancreas function testing) approach to diagnosis with increasing invasiveness has been proposed for determining the presence of chronic pancreatitis.

10.2.3 Medical Treatment

The mainstay of treatment is symptomatic control. This involves a step-up approach to pain relief, beginning with simple non-opioid analgesia in combination with weak opiates and moving up as necessary to stronger opiates. Patients may require advanced anaesthetic pain management with splanchnic nerve blocks, EUS-guided coeliac plexus block or thoracic splanchnicectomy. It is crucial to aggressively manage exocrine dysfunction with pancreatic enzyme supplementation. The minimum starting dose of enzyme supplements should be 200,000 lipase units divided amongst meals and snacks, although some patients will require 10 times this amount. Close control of blood sugars in diabetic patients is also of paramount importance in order to prevent hyperglycaemic complications.

10.2.4 Endoscopic Treatment

EUS-guided coeliac plexus block can provide highly effective short- to medium-term relief in patients with chronic pain. In symptomatic patients with a dilated main pancreatic duct, it is our practice to insert a pancreatic ductal stent (7 French straight stent) at ERCP to aid future decision-making. Those patients with symptomatic benefit from the stent may be candidates for surgical drainage.

10.2.5 Surgical Treatment

Surgical treatment for chronic pancreatitis can be drainage procedures, resectional procedures or a combination of the two.

10.2.5.1 Drainage Procedures

These include lateral pancreaticojejunostomy (Puestow or Partington-Rochelle procedures) or pancreaticogastrostomy. The aim of the procedure is to create a wide anastomosis through which the pancreas can drain. In the lateral pancreaticojejunostomy, the anterior surface of the pancreas immediately anterior to the duct, which is located by intraoperative ultrasound, is incised. A Roux loop of jejunum is brought up and anastomosed onto the pancreatic duct.

10.2.5.2 Resectional and Combination Procedures

Pancreaticoduodenectomy, distal pancreatectomy or even total pancreatectomy can be employed to excise focal areas of chronic pancreatitis or the whole gland.

In the early days of these procedures, morbidity and mortality rates were determined to be inappropriate for benign disease, and alternatives for disease confined to the head of the gland were developed to ensure the duodenum was preserved. Beger's procedure involves dissection of the neck of the pancreas at the level of the portal vein. The pancreatic head is excavated, leaving a thin layer of pancreatic tissue on the duodenum. The reconstruction consists of two pancreatic anastomoses on the same jejunal Roux limb. The first is a duct to mucosa anastomosis to drain the distal pancreas remnant, and the second is onto the excavated pancreatic head. In the Bern modification of Beger's procedure, the pancreas is not divided over the portal vein and so remains in continuity. The pancreatic head is excavated as before and then a single anastomosis performed onto a Roux loop of jejunum. Frey's procedure involves excavation of the pancreatic head combined with a continuous longitudinal dissection of the pancreatic duct towards the tail. Reconstruction involves a single anastomosis onto a Roux loop of jejunum. A recent large randomized controlled trial has demonstrated no difference in quality of life or adverse events between partial pancreaticoduodenectomy and duodenum-preserving pancreatic head resection for chronic pancreatitis.

10.2.5.3 Total Pancreatectomy and Islet Autotransplantation

Patients with a non-dilated main pancreatic duct, with features such as calcification of the gland, and those who suffer from intractable pain refractory to all other treatments may be candidates for total pancreatectomy. This major procedure inevitably renders the patient a brittle insulin-dependent diabetic, and so the modification of pancreatic islet autotransplantation has been devised to address this. Non-diabetic patients who are candidates for the procedure are meticulously worked up. This includes consultations with the surgeon, anaesthetist, diabetologist, psychologist, dietician, nurse specialist and other patients who have had the procedure. The total pancreatectomy procedure is usually much more difficult than one done for cancer as the gland is often very inflamed and adherent to surrounding major vascular structures. Any element of portal hypertension caused by portal or splenic vein thrombosis also greatly increases the difficulty of the procedure and may even result in abandonment. The excised gland is digested and islets isolated in a local laboratory. The resulting digest containing the insulin producing pancreatic islets and a small amount of parenchymal tissue can then be infused into the portal circulation with the intention of islet implantation into the liver and consequent autonomous function.

10.3 Pancreas Cancer

10.3.1 Epidemiology

Malignant tumours of the pancreas are relatively common with 15 new cases per 100,000 in the UK each year (9600 new diagnoses per year). The predominant type of cancer is primary pancreatic adenocarcinoma, although squamous cell cancer and metastatic cancers are also described. Unfortunately, approximately 80% of patients have inoperable disease at presentation, either from distant metastatic spread or locally advanced disease which cannot be resected. Median survival for surgically resected patients with best current adjuvant chemotherapy is 28 months. Median survival for patients with unresectable disease having the currently most effectively available palliative chemotherapy is 11.1 months.

10.3.2 Diagnosis

Most patients who present with surgically resectable disease present with jaundice from a head of pancreas tumour or as an incidental finding from a CT scan of the abdomen performed for another indication. Patients with unresectable disease typically present with weight loss and vague abdominal discomfort or back pain which has often been present for a number of months. All too frequently they have presented to non-specialist physicians who have been reassured by a normal ultrasound examination.

Full staging of the patient with CT thorax is mandatory to exclude extra-pancreatic disease. The role of laparoscopy, liver MRI and PET to detect occult extra-pancreatic disease, which would preclude successful resection, is controversial, but there is some data to support their use in ongoing clinical trials.

10.3.3 Definition of Resectability

We now know that metastatic pancreatic cancer is incurable. There have been a number of published reports from around the world and case series of surgical resection of liver metastases which were almost universally associated with dismal outcomes.

Traditionally, pancreatic tumors which were confined to the gland, without involvement of the nearby vascular structures (portal vein, superior mesenteric vein, superior mesenteric artery and common hepatic artery), were deemed resectable. Evidence has emerged, albeit from non-randomized case series, that survival outcomes for patients with portal vein resection are similar to those without portal vein resection and significantly superior to palliative surgical bypass. Resection of the involved superior mesenteric artery or common hepatic artery with anastomosis, however, carries no proven survival benefit at the expense of considerable perioperative mortality and morbidity, and it is the authors' view that there is no indication for this outside of randomized controlled trials.

Disease patterns with involvement of the portal vein, or contact with a named first- or second-order arterial branch, which could potentially respond to chemotherapy, are termed borderline resectable. This term encompasses all patterns from minor contact with the portal vein to 180 degree contact of the portal vein, superior mesenteric vein and arteries. Certainly those with more extensive involvement, but in whom surgery is still considered as a future option, should be offered neoadjuvant chemotherapy with intention to resect if there is lack of progression after an initial course. Those with vein involvement alone present a more controversial challenge of whether to proceed directly to surgery and vein resection, ideally without preoperative biliary drainage, or to offer neoadjuvant chemotherapy followed by surgery if there is demonstrated stable disease or response. The ideal approach has not been defined, and a well-designed randomized controlled trial is urgently needed.

10.3.4 Surgery for Tumors of the Pancreas

Tumors in the head of the pancreas are resected by a pancreaticoduodenectomy. Pylorus-preserving pancreaticoduodenectomy confers the advantage of shorter operative time and blood loss without compromising surgical outcomes. It also means that if the reduced hepaticojejunostomy and gastrojejunostomy are placed on the same enteric limb (as is the authors' practice), gastric biliary reflux is abrogated. Classic Whipple's operation involving resection of the antrum of the stomach should in the authors' view be reserved for tumours of the second part of the duodenum for which the proximal duodenal resection margin would be compromised by leaving the pylorus. The jaundiced patient with a resectable mass in the head of the pancreas presents a further dilemma. Randomized controlled trial data suggests that surgery without preoperative biliary drainage results in fewer septic complications than surgery after drainage, although survival is unaffected. Logistic difficulties and pressures on operating theatre space however make this impossible to offer in the majority of pancreatic units, and so patients are stented to then wait for their surgery.

Tumors in the body or tail of the pancreas are resected with distal pancreatectomy. For suspected adenocarcinoma, the spleen is always resected "en bloc" with the pancreatic specimen. More radical distal pancreatectomy, taking the line of resection posterior to the pre-renal fascia once the pancreas has been divided, has been described (**R**adical **A**nterior **M**odular **P**ancreatic **S**urgery—RAMPS), which can be further extended to include the left adrenal gland in case of local invasion of the fascia. There are no current convincing data in favour of this approach in terms of outcomes over classical distal pancreatectomy. There is considerable interest in the laparoscopic approach to distal pancreatectomy, and there are several international case series and one randomized controlled trial of laparoscopic versus open pancreaticoduodenectomy. Unequivocal data however remains lacking, and there are several trials currently recruiting which are hoping to answer definitively whether there is any benefit to this over the open approach, particularly in terms of length of in-hospital stay and pain scores. Reported operating time is longer, but blood loss is lower and length of stay is shorter for the laparoscopic group. Whether this can be reproduced in large Western series where length of stay for open pancreaticoduodenectomy is typically 8–9 days remains to be seen.

10.3.4.1 Vascular Resection

For tumors involving the mesenteric-portal venous system, vascular resection may be appropriate. This may involve a small cuff of vein which is oversewn, a wedge resection of the vein with primary anastomosis, a complete resection of part of the vein with end to end anastomosis, or an interposition graft. Autografts may be harvested from the saphenous, jugular or renal veins, or alternatively in a transplant centre, blood-group matched cadaveric iliac vein is usually readily available and may prove useful.

10.3.4.2 Postoperative Care

All patients should be managed in at least a level 1 or level 2 environment for the first 24 h as there is potential for major secondary haemorrhage, particularly if there is a leak from the anastomosis to the pancreatic remnant. Practice amongst surgeons differs in terms of whether to leave drains or not. While there is some evidence that drainage may increase the risk of complications, most surgeons will drain the abdomen to mitigate the effects of an anastomotic leak, particularly as this will involve tissue-catabolic enzymes found in pancreatic exocrine secretions. There is also heterogeneous practice around early versus delayed introduction of oral feeding, timing of drain removal, use of somatostatin analogues to reduce postoperative pancreatic fistula, anastomotic techniques, and type of incision. There is limited data to suggest superiority of one approach over another, and although postoperative pancreatic exocrine enzyme supplementation has been shown to be an independent factor in prolonging survival after resection, even this is yet to be universally adopted.

10.3.5 Adjuvant Chemotherapy

There is now good evidence from the ESPAC (European Study Group for Pancreatic Cancer) trials that postoperative chemotherapy confers a significant survival benefit over chemoradiotherapy. Furthermore, adjuvant couplet chemotherapy in terms of gemcitabine and capecitabine confers a survival advantage over single agent gemcitabine. The role of more aggressive adjuvant chemotherapy, FOLFIRINOX (**FOL**, **fol**inic acid; **F**, **f**luorouracil (5FU); **IRIN**, **irin**otecan; **OX**, **ox**aliplatin) which has shown a survival benefit in the palliative setting, has yet to be evaluated, although several clinical trials are currently recruiting.

10.3.6 Radiotherapy

In a palliative setting, several trials conducted in the USA have shown a survival benefit of chemoradiotherapy over standard chemotherapy, and there is some interest in neoadjuvant chemoradiotherapy, but to date there is no convincing randomized controlled trial data to support its use.

10.3.7 Palliative Chemotherapy for Advanced Pancreatic Cancer

Patients with locally advanced unresectable (rather than borderline resectable) and metastatic pancreatic cancer who are of ECOG performance status 0, 1 or 2 are candidates for palliative chemotherapy. The first chemotherapy agent to show benefit in pancreatic cancer was the nucleoside analogue gemcitabine. It was then 10 years before any further advances were made, with the EGF receptor antagonist erlotinib showing very marginal improvement in survival in a large cohort of randomized trial patients. Further recent advances with the addition of nab-paclitaxel to gemcitabine and complete substitution of the regimen to FOLFIRINOX have almost doubled the median survival to 11 months but at the expense of greater adverse events. There is no doubt that the newer regimens are only suitable for the fittest of patients which are uncommon with this particular disease process. Patients who progress on gemcitabine chemotherapy are usually unfit for FOLFIRINOX. The nanoliposomal irinotecan preparation, in combination with fluorouracil and folinic acid, has shown survival benefit in these patients.

10.3.8 The Future

It is clear that there is more than one type of ductal adenocarcinoma of the pancreas, yet current practice is to offer the same chemotherapy treatment to all.

The authors are confident that the evolution of personalized medicine will allow administration of individually tailored treatments which target specific receptors, adjustable for the varying disease patterns in different patients.

Whether surgery will stand the test of time as the mainstay of treatment for localized disease confined to the gland remains to be seen.

10.4 Neuroendocrine Tumors of the Pancreas

The variety of cell types in the pancreas can sometimes develop into neuroendocrine tumors (NETs) which may present as an incidental finding on CT scan or with the sequelae of the active molecules which are secreted into the blood by the tumor. These are termed functional tumors.

Insulinomas arising from the beta cells hypersecrete insulin, and the patient usually presents with neuroglycopenic symptoms. Most insulinomas are benign. Glucagonomas form from the alpha cells which produce glucagon and are more difficult to diagnose as the resulting hyperglycaemia is usually clinically silent. Most glucagonomas are malignant. Gastrinomas form in pancreatic G cells, secreting excess gastrin and stimulating hypersecretion of gastric acid. Where severe gastric ulceration is present, this is known as Zollinger Ellison Syndrome. Most pancreatic gastrinomas form in the head of the gland and like glucagonomas are malignant.

Rarer types of pancreatic neuroendocrine tumor include VIPomas (**v**asoactive **i**ntestinal **p**eptide; also known as Verner-Morrison syndrome, after the physicians who first described it) which may cause profuse diarrhoa and somatostatinomas, a malignant tumor of the pancreatic delta cells. Carcinoid tumors which secrete serotonin may also arise in the pancreas and are generally asymptomatic unless they become very large and create local pressure symptoms or metastasise to the liver, where they may result in "carcinoid syndrome". This is a constellation of symptoms caused by excessive plasma serotonin, including flushing, diarrhoa, wheezing, tachycardia and dizziness caused by hypotension.

Non-functional NETs are usually diagnosed incidentally or where they cause local pressure or obstructive symptoms resulting in further investigations.

10.4.1 Diagnosis

The mainstay in the diagnosis of pancreatic NETs is cross-sectional imaging (such as CT or MRI) and EUS. Occasionally, angiography and arterial stimulation selective vein sampling may be required to localize a tumor. Octreotide scanning and FDG PET both have a role in diagnosis and localization of primary disease and identification of sites outside the primary location.

10.4.2 Treatment

Surgical resection is the only chance of cure and is indicated where symptoms are present or in the case of non-functional NET where there is concern over malignant potential. The type of surgery is identical to that for adenocarcinoma with the exception that the spleen can be preserved for benign NETs. Functional NETs, particularly carcinoids, may require perioperative treatment with octreotide infusion in order to abrogate the effects of massive hormonal release caused by tumor handling. For concurrent liver resection in the case of metastatic disease, this is mandatory, and failure to do so may have fatal intraoperative consequences for the patient, including circulatory collapse and bronchospasm.

10.5 Cystic Lesions of the Pancreas

These may arise from the main ductal system (main duct intraductal papillary mucinous neoplasm – IPMN), the side branches of the ductal system (side-branch IPMN), as a serous cystic neoplasm (SCN) or mucinous cystic neoplasm (MCN). Pancreatic pseudocysts are considered separately.

10.5.1 Main Duct IPMN

Main Duct IPMNs may present as incidental findings or as obstructive jaundice due to pressure effects on the common bile duct. There is always direct connection to the main pancreatic duct generally demonstrated on MRCP or EUS. The only indication on cross-sectional imaging may be a dilated pancreatic duct without mass. Cannulation of the pancreatic duct at ERCP or fine needle aspiration at EUS with demonstration of mucus in either case is pathognomonic. They have malignant potential (up to 50% may harbour invasive adenocarcinoma), and therefore resection is the treatment of choice if the patient is fit enough. Following surgical resection of main duct IPMN, patients must undergo regular radiological surveillance as the risk of invasive IPMN recurrence is up to 38% at 10 years.

10.5.2 Side-Branch IPMN

Side-branch IPMNs have a significantly lower malignant potential than main duct IPMNs, and a surveillance approach is valid for the majority. There are now well-defined "worrisome features" on cross-sectional imaging: cyst size >30 mm, enhancing mural nodule <5 mm, thickened enhanced cyst walls, main pancreatic duct (MPD) size 5–9 mm, abrupt change in MPD calibre with distal gland atrophy, lymphadenopathy, elevated serum CA19–9 and rapid rate of cyst growth >5 mm in 2 years. Any cyst without worrisome features should undergo radiological surveillance. If there are no changes to the lesion over a 5-year period, surveillance can be ceased. Those with worrisome features must have further evaluation with EUS. Cysts with "high-risk stigmata", which are again well-defined: a cystic lesion in the head of the pancreas causing biliary obstruction, enhancing mural nodule >5 mm or MPD >10 mm, are candidates for resection in fit patients without any further evaluation.

10.5.3 Serous Cystic Neoplasm

Serous cystic neoplasms (SCN) are almost invariably benign, with only a small number of isolated reports of serous cystadenocarcinoma. The only indication for resection is local pressure symptoms if the tumour grows large enough; otherwise a surveillance approach is appropriate. EUS can be a valuable adjunct to diagnosis.

10.5.4 Mucinous Cystic Neoplasm

Mucinous cystic neoplasms (MCN) occur almost exclusively in women, in the pancreatic body or tail, and are almost invariably an incidental finding on CT examination for another indication. They produce mucin but do not communicate with the pancreatic ductal system, which is how they are distinguished from side-branch IPMN at EUS examination. They may be benign, borderline or malignant, and up to 34% of resected MCNs are found to have undergone malignant change. CEA levels in the cyst, which can be evaluated by EUS-FNA, are typically raised, which may also aid in diagnosis. There is conflicting evidence regarding the sensitivity of cyst fluid CEA and CA19–9 for the detection of malignancy within a cyst. Due to their increased malignant potential, surgical resection is the optimal treatment for MCNs over 4 cm in fit patients. Below this size, rates of malignant transformation are exceptionally low, and radiological follow-up following resected benign MCN is not required. Five-year survival following resection of malignant MCN is approximately 60%.

10.5.5 Pancreatic Pseudocysts

Pancreatic pseudocysts develop following an attack of acute pancreatitis and should be distinguished from acute fluid collections which lack a cyst wall. They may be completely asymptomatic or may cause local pressure effects, particularly compression of the stomach, which usually results in nausea, vomiting or early satiety. Infection within a pseudocyst may cause septic episodes or abdominal pain. Bleeding into a pseudocyst may cause life-threatening haemorrhage and is usually the result of a ruptured pseudoaneurysm caused by compromise of the gastroduodenal, splenic or pancreaticoduodenal arteries. Asymptomatic pseudocysts do not need to be treated but should be followed up radiologically to ensure resolution or shrinkage. Diagnostic doubt can be solved with EUS which demonstrates a cyst which may or may not communicate with the pancreatic duct. FNA of the cyst will reveal a high amylase content and low CEA and CA19–9. Symptomatic or infected pseudocysts can be drained into the stomach with stenting at EUS. Percutaneous drainage of symptomatic or infected pseudocysts is reserved in the modern era for those unsuitable for EUS drainage. Hemorrhage into a pseudocyst usually presents with hypovolaemic shock and abdominal pain. This should be rapidly diagnosed in conjunction with aggressive resuscitation, with CT angiography followed by immediate transfer to the angiography suite where the bleeding vessel can be targeted for angioembolisation. Medical treatment with intravenous proton pump inhibitor infusion may also be useful. Failure of embolization with continued hemodynamic instability is an indication for surgery although outcomes following surgical intervention are poor.

Recommended Reading

Besselink M, van Santvoort H, Freeman M, Gardner T, Mayerle J, Vege SS, et al. IAP/APA evidence-based guidelines for the management of acute pancreatitis. Pancreatology. 2013;13(4 Suppl 2):e1–15.

Bramis K, Gordon-Weeks AN, Friend PJ, Bastin E, Burls A, Silva MA, Dennison AR. Systematic review of total pancreatectomy and islet autotransplantation for chronic pancreatitis. Br J Surg. 2012;99(6):761–6.

Brugge WR. Diagnosis and management of cystic lesions of the pancreas. J Gastrointest Oncol. 2015;6(4):375–88.

Burris HA 3rd, Moore MJ, Andersen J, Green MR, Rothenberg ML, Modiano MR, et al. Improvements in survival and clinical benefit with gemcitabine as first-line therapy for patients with advanced pancreas cancer: a randomized trial. J Clin Oncol. 1997;15(6):2403–13.

Conroy T, Desseigne F, Ychou M, Bouché O, Guimbaud R, Bécouarn Y, et al. FOLFIRINOX versus gemcitabine for metastatic pancreatic cancer. N Engl J Med. 2011; 364(19):1817–25.

Conwell DL, Lee LS, Yadav D, Longnecker DS, Miller FH, Mortele KJ. American Pancreatic Association Practice Guidelines in Chronic Pancreatitis: evidence-based report on diagnostic guidelines. Pancreas. 2014;43(8):1143–62.

Diener MK, Hüttner FJ, Kieser M, Knebel P, Dörr-Harim C, Distler M, et al. Partial pancreatoduodenectomy versus duodenum-preserving pancreatic head resection in chronic pancreatitis: the multicentre, randomised, controlled, double-blind ChroPac trial. Lancet. 2017;390(10,099):1027–37.

Drewes AM, Bouwense SAW, Campbell CM, Ceyhan GO, Delhaye M, Demir IE, et al. Guidelines for the understanding and management of pain in chronic pancreatitis. Pancreatology. 2017;17(5):720–31.

Evans RP, Mourad MM, Pall G, Fisher SG, Bramhall SR. Pancreatitis: preventing catastrophic haemorrhage. World J Gastroenterol. 2017;23(30):5460–8.

He J, Cameron JL, Ahuja N, Makary MA, Hirose K, Choti MA, et al. Is it necessary to follow patients after resection of a benign pancreatic intraductal papillary mucinous neoplasm? J Am Coll Surg. 2013;216:657e65.

Jones MJ, Neal CP, Ngu WS, Dennison AR, Garcea G. Early warning score independently predicts adverse outcome and mortality in patients with acute pancreatitis. Langenbeck's Arch Surg. 2017;402(5):811–9.

Moore MJ, Goldstein D, Hamm J, Figer A, Hecht JR, Gallinger S, et al. Erlotinib plus gemcitabine compared with gemcitabine alone in patients with advanced pancreatic cancer: a phase III trial of the National Cancer Institute of Canada Clinical Trials Group. J Clin Oncol. 2007;25(15):1960–6.

Morgan KA, Lancaster WP, Owczarski SM, Wang H, Borckardt J, Adams DB. Patient selection for total pancreatectomy with islet autotransplantation in the surgical management of chronic pancreatitis. J Am Coll Surg. 2018;226(4):446–51. pii: S1072–7515(17)32181–6

Neoptolemos JP, Dunn JA, Stocken DD, Almond J, Link K, Beger H, et al. Adjuvant chemoradiotherapy and chemotherapy in resectable pancreatic cancer: a randomised controlled trial. Lancet. 2001;358(9293):1576–85.

Neoptolemos JP, Palmer DH, Ghaneh P, Psarelli EE, Valle JW, Halloran CM, et al. Comparison of adjuvant gemcitabine and capecitabine with gemcitabine monotherapy in patients with resected pancreatic cancer (ESPAC-4): a multicentre, open-label, randomised, phase 3 trial. Lancet. 2017;389(10,073):1011–24.

Nilsson LN, Keane MG, Shamali A, Millastre Bocos J, Marijinissen van Zanten M, Antila A, et al. Nature and management of pancreatic mucinous cystic neoplasm (MCN): a systematic review of the literature. Pancreatology. 2016;16(6):1028–36.

Plagemann S, Welte M, Izbicki JR, Bachmann K. Surgical treatment for chronic pancreatitis: past, present, and future. Gastroenterol Res Pract. 2017;2017:8418372. https://doi.org/10.1155/2017/8418372. Epub 2017 Jul 27

Roberts KJ, Schrem H, Hodson J, Angelico R, Dasari BVM, Coldham CA, et al. Pancreas exocrine replacement therapy is associated with increased survival following pancreatoduodenectomy for periampullary malignancy. HPB (Oxford). 2017;19(10):859–67.

Roberts SE, Morrison-Rees S, John A, Williams JG, Brown TH, Samuel DG. The incidence and aetiology of acute pancreatitis across Europe. Pancreatology. 2017;17(2):155–65.

Rockacy M, Khalid A. Update on pancreatic cyst fluid analysis. Ann Gastroenterol. 2013;26(2):122–7.

Suker M, Beumer BR, Sadot E, Marthey L, Faris JE, Mellon EA, et al. FOLFIRINOX for locally advanced pancreatic cancer: a systematic review and patient-level meta-analysis. Lancet Oncol. 2016;17(6):801–10.

Tanaka M, Fernández-Del Castillo C, Kamisawa T, Jang JY, Levy P, Ohtsuka T, et al. Revisions of international consensus Fukuoka guidelines for the management of IPMN of the pancreas. Pancreatology. 2017;17(5):738–53.

van Brunschot S, van Grinsven J, van Santvoort HC, Bakker OJ, Besselink MG, Boermeester MA, et al. Endoscopic or surgical step-up approach for infected necrotising pancreatitis: a multicentre randomised trial. Lancet. 2018;391(10,115):51–8.

van der Gaag NA, Rauws EA, van Eijck CH, Bruno MJ, van der Harst E, Kubben FJ, et al. Preoperative biliary drainage for cancer of the head of the pancreas. N Engl J Med. 2010;362(2):129–37.

van Santvoort HC, Besselink MG, Bakker OJ, Hofker HS, Boermeester MA, Dejong CH, et al. A step-up approach or open necrosectomy for necrotizing pancreatitis. N Engl J Med. 2010;362(16):1491–502.

Von Hoff DD, Ervin T, Arena FP, Chiorean EG, Infante J, Moore M, et al. Increased survival in pancreatic cancer with nab-paclitaxel plus gemcitabine. N Engl J Med. 2013;369(18):1691–703.

Wang-Gillam A, Li CP, Bodoky G, Dean A, Shan YS, Jameson G, et al. Nanoliposomal irinotecan with fluorouracil and folinic acid in metastatic pancreatic cancer after previous gemcitabine-based therapy (NAPOLI-1): a global, randomised, open-label, phase 3 trial. Lancet. 2016;387(10,018):545–57.

Whitcomb DC, Frulloni L, Garg P, Greer JB, Schneider A, Yadav D, Shimosegawa T. Chronic pancreatitis: an international draft consensus proposal for a new mechanistic definition. Pancreatology. 2016;16(2):218–24.

Wittau M, Mayer B, Scheele J, Henne-Bruns D, Dellinger EP, Isenmann R. Systematic review and meta-analysis of antibiotic prophylaxis in severe acute pancreatitis. Scand J Gastroenterol. 2011;46(3):261–70.

Endoscopy and Upper Gastrointestinal Disorders

11

Marie Ooi and Nam Nguyen

11.1 Introduction

Most general surgeons, especially rural surgeons, include upper gastrointestinal endoscopy as part of their clinical practice, and many are competent at colonoscopy. When flexible upper endoscopy began about 50 years ago, almost all procedures were performed for diagnostic reasons. In contemporary practice, upper endoscopy is both diagnostic and therapeutic such that open or laparoscopic surgery of the upper gastrointestinal tract has become uncommon. One example is the management of upper gastrointestinal bleeding where the frequency of open surgery has markedly declined. Endoscopic therapy has also largely replaced surgical therapy in the management of esophageal varices, upper gastrointestinal strictures and the palliative therapy of several malignancies. This chapter will focus on the causes and endoscopic management of upper gastrointestinal bleeding and endoscopic therapy for benign and malignant disorders of the upper gastrointestinal tract, biliary tract and pancreas.

11.2 Causes of Upper Gastrointestinal Bleeding

Acute gastrointestinal bleeding is a common reason for presentation to emergency departments and continues to be associated with significant morbidity and mortality. The site of bleeding can usually be predicted by history with the broad

M. Ooi
Department of Gastroenterology and Hepatology, Royal Adelaide Hospital, Adelaide, SA, Australia
e-mail: marie.ooi@sa.gov.au

N. Nguyen (✉)
Department of Gastroenterology and Hepatology, Royal Adelaide Hospital, Adelaide, SA, Australia

Discipline of Medicine, University of Adelaide, Adelaide, SA, Australia
e-mail: quoc.nguyen@sa.gov.au

M. W. Wichmann et al. (eds.), *Gastroenterology For General Surgeons*,
https://doi.org/10.1007/978-3-319-92768-8_11

categories of bleeding from the upper or lower gastrointestinal tracts. These categories are important as they influence the evaluation and management of the patient. The incidence of upper gastrointestinal bleeding is approximately 40 to 150 cases per 100,000 per year in Western populations and is associated with significant medical costs. A common subclassification for upper gastrointestinal bleeding is division into nonvariceal and variceal bleeding as the latter often causes more severe bleeding, has distinctive therapy and is associated with a higher mortality.

In almost all surveys, the most common cause of upper gastrointestinal bleeding is peptic ulceration. This diagnosis applies in 30–40% of patients. The second most common cause is equally shared between hemorrhagic gastritis and esophageal varices. Although cirrhosis is the usual cause of varices, patients with cirrhosis can have alternative causes for bleeding such as peptic ulceration, gastroduodenal erosions, portal gastropathy and Mallory-Weiss tears. An additional issue, particularly in elderly patients, is prolongation of bleeding by a variety of anti-platelet drugs, warfarin and direct oral anticoagulants. This is discussed in more detail in Chapter 23. More common causes for upper gastrointestinal bleeding are briefly outlined below and illustrated in Fig. 11.1.

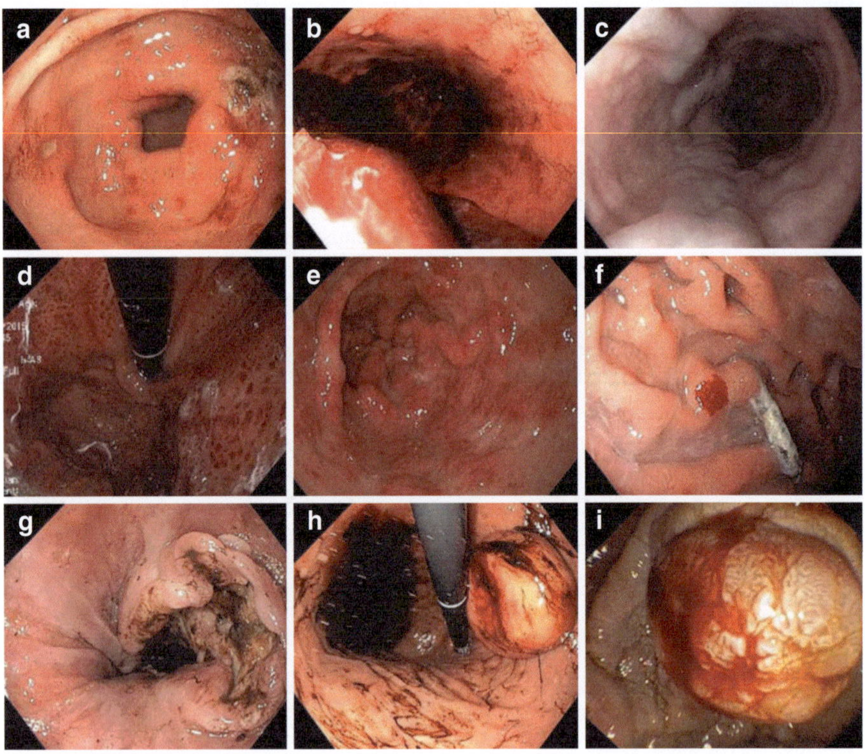

Fig. 11.1 Endoscopic appearance of (**a**) gastric ulceration with gastritis, (**b**) Mallory-Weiss tear, (**c**) esophageal varices, (**d**) portal gastropathy, (**e**) gastric antral vascular ectasia, (**f**) gastric angiodysplasia, (**g**) gastric cancer, (**h**) gastric stromal tumor and (**i**) tumor of the ampulla of Vater

Peptic ulcer disease. Peptic ulcers can be located in the stomach, duodenal cap or in both regions. The major risk factors are gastritis caused by *Helicobacter pylori* [*H. pylori*] and use of non-steroidal, anti-inflammatory drugs including aspirin. The prevalence of *H. pylori* in patients with duodenal and gastric ulcers is approximately 95% and 70%, respectively. In contrast, use of non-steroidal, anti-inflammatory drugs is more common in patients with gastric ulcers than in those with duodenal ulcers. Other risk factors for ulcers include smoking and genetic factors such as the ABH blood group non-secretor trait and genotypes of the Lewis blood group. A rare cause for severe peptic ulceration is gastrin-producing tumours associated with marked hypersecretion of gastric acid [gastrinoma or Zollinger-Ellison syndrome].

Esophageal varices. These are dilated submucosal veins, largely located in the lower one-third of the esophagus. The major cause is portal hypertension associated with cirrhosis, but other vascular causes occasionally apply. Bleeding due to varices is of increased importance because of life-threatening bleeding in some patients and a mortality rate of approximately 20%.

Hemorrhagic gastritis. The endoscopic appearance is that of multiple small bleeding lesions without overt ulceration. This is sometimes related to use of non-steroidal anti-inflammatory drugs and sometimes related to stress factors such as severe illness with admission to intensive care units.

Mallory-Weiss tear: This is a laceration of the mucous membrane, most commonly at the gastro-oesophageal junction that is usually related to repeated episodes of vomiting or dry retching. The typical history is vomiting of gastric contents followed by the vomiting of fresh red blood that gradually becomes darker. The tear is the result of an increase in intra-gastric and intra-abdominal pressure caused by repeated episodes of forceful vomiting.

Gastric antral vascular ectasia. This is also known as watermelon stomach because of the long erythematous streaks that are most prominent in the antrum and radiate into the pyloric region. These red streaks are caused by dilated small blood vessels in the submucosa. A minority have cirrhosis, but the pathogenesis in the remainder remains unclear. A presentation with iron-deficiency anaemia is more common than overt upper gastrointestinal bleeding.

Angiodysplasia. This is also called angioectasia or vascular ectasia in some publications. At endoscopy, there is a bright red area with either clearly demarcated margins or spidery small vessels radiating from a central area. Pathological changes include abnormally dilated, tortuous and thin-walled vessels involving small capillaries, veins and arteries. They are lined by endothelium with little or no smooth muscle and lack inflammatory or fibrotic changes. Although angiodysplasia can occur in the stomach, it is more common in the caecum, right colon and small bowel.

Upper gastrointestinal cancer. Cancer of the esophagus or stomach is a rare cause of acute upper gastrointestinal bleeding. However, acute bleeding can arise from the apex of a gastrointestinal stromal tumour or from other uncommon lesions such as a polypoid adenoma.

Other disorders. Rare causes of acute upper gastrointestinal bleeding include Dieulafoy lesions, Cameron's erosions and gastric or duodenal lymphomas as illustrated in Fig. 11.2. A Dieulafoy lesion is an anomalous submucosal artery usually

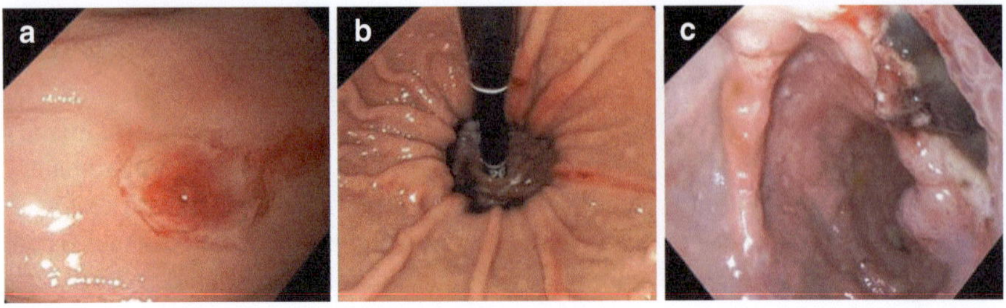

Fig. 11.2 Endoscopic images of (**a**) Dieulafoy lesion with active oozing, (**b**) a large hiatus hernia with Cameron erosions at the diaphragmatic border and (**c**) a T-cell lymphomatous ulcer in a patient with celiac disease

located in the proximal part of the stomach, often on the lesser curve. Bleeding can result in significant blood loss, sometimes in a periodic fashion where bleeding can cease temporarily and then recur. In the absence of bleeding, care needs to be taken at endoscopy in order to avoid missing a lesion that is usually suitable for endoscopic therapy. Cameron's erosions are linear erosions on gastric folds in the fundus of the stomach that are associated with a large hiatus hernia. These erosions may be related to gastric trauma or to restriction of the mucosal blood supply by the diaphragmatic border. With this disorder, iron deficiency anaemia is a more common presentation than acute bleeding. This also applies to gastrointestinal lymphomas which are sometimes associated with *Helicobacter pylori* [gastric mucosa-associated lymphoid tumor] or celiac disease [usually a small bowel T-cell lymphoma].

11.3 Endoscopic Management of Upper Gastrointestinal Bleeding

After clinical assessment and resuscitation, most patients are treated with high doses of a proton pump inhibitor to reduce gastric acid secretion. This decreases the risk of rebleeding and the need for endoscopic therapy. The next important step is endoscopic evaluation to identify the source of bleeding and to apply endoscopic interventions. Early endoscopy is recommended for most patients, usually within 24 h but more urgently in those with major bleeding. This practice also reduces the risk of rebleeding as well as decreasing blood transfusion requirements and the length of the hospital stay. In this section, non-variceal bleeding and variceal bleeding will be considered separately.

11.3.1 Non-variceal Bleeding

The risk of rebleeding, repeat endoscopic interventions, surgery and death from non-variceal bleeding can be predicted by the Forrest classification (Table 11.1). This important classification provides a guide as to the application of endoscopic

Table 11.1 Forrest classification of upper gastrointestinal ulcers

Endoscopic image	Forrest class	Lesion
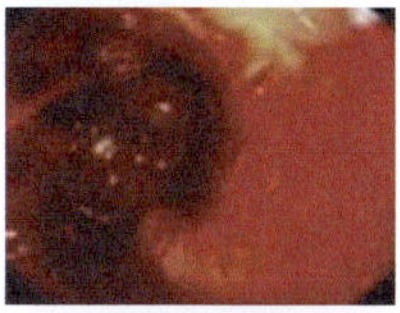	IA	Arterial spurting
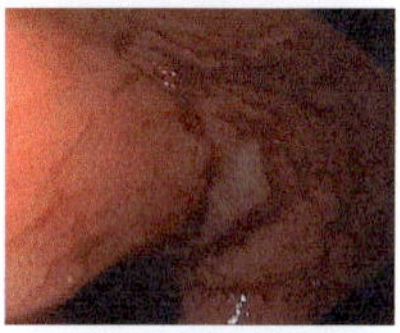	IB	Active oozing
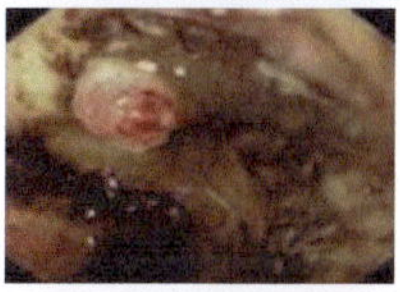	IIA	Ulcer with nonbleeding visible vessel
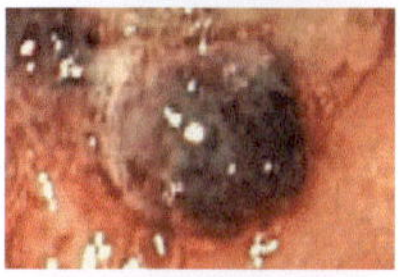	IIB	Ulcer with adherent clot on surface
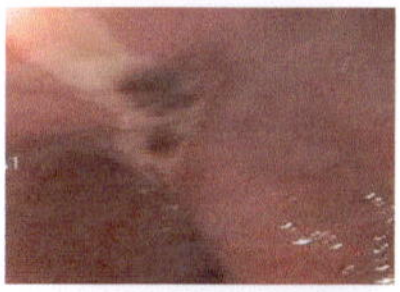	IIC	Ulcer with red flat spot
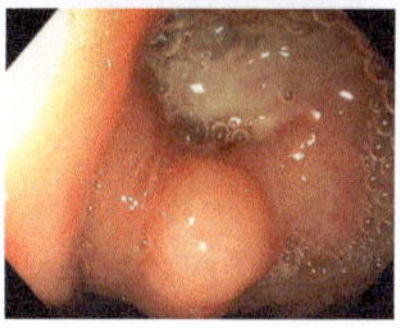	III	Ulcer with clean base

interventions for specific bleeding disorders. Current recommendations support endoscopic hemostatic therapy for patients with Forrest IA, IB, or IIA ulcers. For those ulcers with adherent clots (IIB), it is advisable to remove the overlying clots to accurately assess the underlying lesion as "blind endotherapy" over adherent clots does not reduce the risk of rebleeding. Ulcers with Forrest IIC and III subtypes do not require endotherapy and are best treated with acid suppression.

The submucosal injection of dilute adrenaline (epinephrine) should be within the practice of most general surgeons, and some will have access to thermal probes and endoscopic clips. These are illustrated in Figs. 11.3 and 11.4. The injection of dilute adrenaline (1:10,000 concentration) into the submucosal space adjacent to the bleeding vessel helps to achieve hemostasis by local vasoconstriction and tamponade. In some patients, the volume of adrenaline can reach 30–40 mL or more.

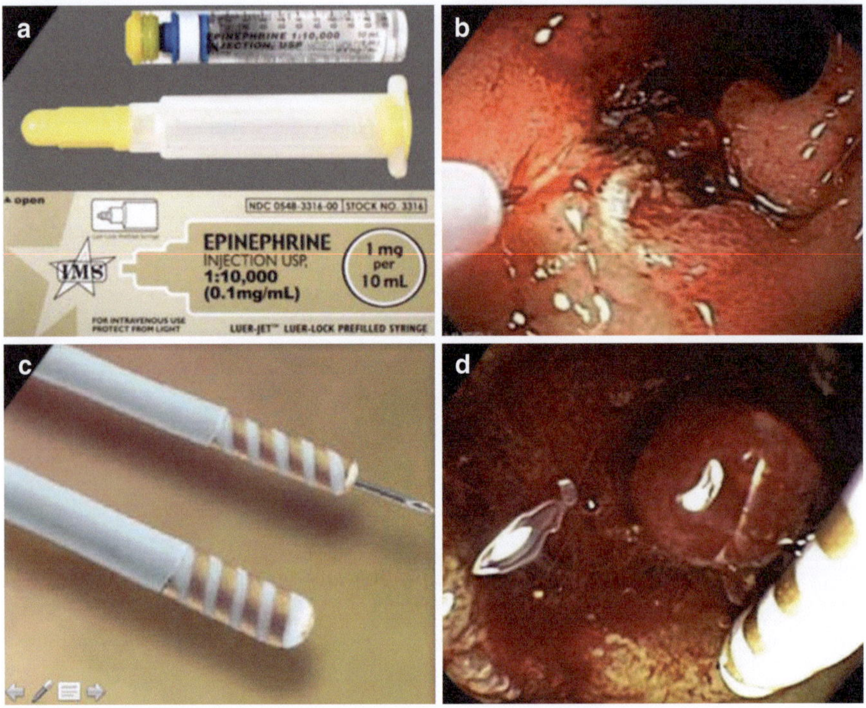

Fig. 11.3 Endoscopic therapy (**a**) diluted adrenaline, (**b**) use of an injector to administer the diluted adrenaline, (**c**) bipolar (gold) probe with an injector and (**d**) use of bipolar probe to inject and coagulate a lesion

As complications include hypertension, tachycardia and arrhythmias, it is important to monitor vital signs during the procedure. Although adrenaline injection alone is superior to non-endoscopic medical therapy, it is inferior to injection therapy followed by a thermal probe.

Current thermal probes can be either monopolar or bipolar. A bipolar probe, also known as the gold probe, is commonly used due to its "co-active" effect and is available in 7Fr and 10Fr. The gold probe is pressed firmly against the bleeding vessel to achieve hemostasis. However, potential adverse events include rebleeding due to avulsion of tissue adherent to the probe and, rarely, deeper tissue injury.

Another popular endoscopic therapy is the use of endoscopic clips. Currently, several models are available with various lengths, jaw widths and rotational capabilities. These clips are typically applied over bleeding sites or visible vessels and fall off spontaneously after days or weeks. One challenging area is deployment of the clips when bleeding is arising from an ulcer base that is hard and fibrotic. In this setting, shorter clips may be more effective than longer clips. Deployment can also be difficult when there is sharp angulation of the endoscope that may occur with lesions in the gastric fundus or posterior wall of the duodenum. A disadvantage of clips is that the clipped tissue is relatively superficial and that several clips are

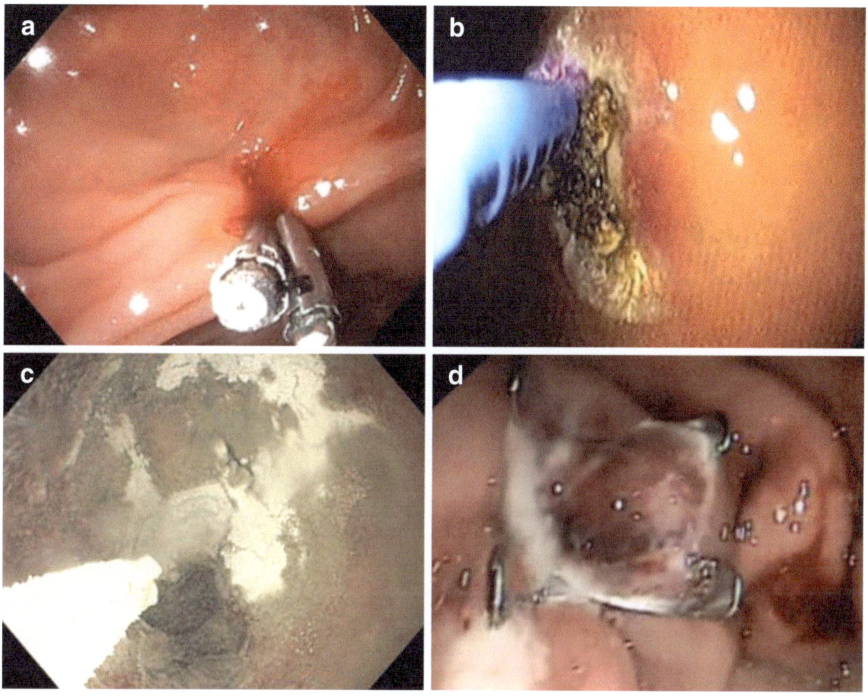

Fig. 11.4 Endoscopic images of endoscopic hemostatic intervention using (**a**) an endoscopic clip, (**b**) argon plasma coagulation, (**c**) a hemostatic spray and (**d**) "over-the-scope" clip

sometimes necessary to achieve haemostasis (thereby increasing the cost of the procedure).

Other endoscopic therapies are available but, at present, are only likely to be used in specialized or tertiary centres. One relatively simple product, currently in development, is a hemostatic powder spray that adheres to bleeding areas. The hemostatic effect is related to dehydration of bleeding tissue and the local application of clotting factors. Products of this nature could be widely used including bleeding from large areas such as those created by endoscopic mucosal resection. A second product, currently in use, is argon plasma coagulation. This is a non-contact, thermal method that uses a flexible catheter to deliver a monopolar electric current to bleeding tissue. However, the depth of the thermal coagulation is limited, and the procedure is largely restricted to superficial disorders such as gastric antral vascular ectasia and angiodysplasia. A much more complex procedure is an "over-the-scope clip" with the ability to effectively seal a large complex bleeding area or achieve full-thickness wall closure. These techniques are illustrated in Fig. 11.4.

A variety of accessories are also available to assist with the visualization of bleeding vessels and to enable endoscopic treatment to be delivered more accurately. These include endoscopic caps, waterjet options, endoscopes that bend in multiple directions and endoscopic overtubes. An endoscopic cap is a transparent

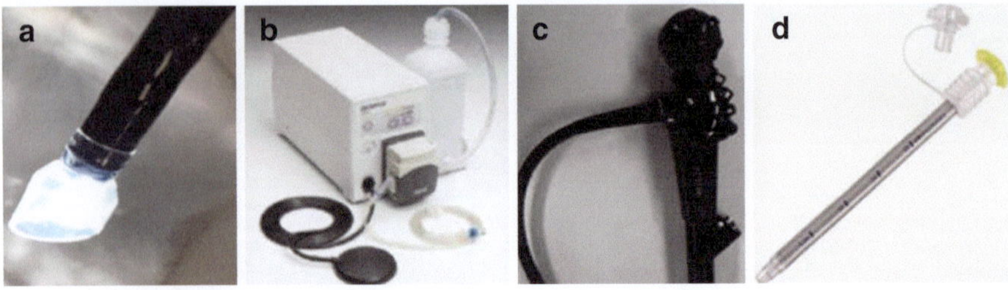

Fig. 11.5 Accessory devices: (**a**) cap-assisted endoscopy, (**b**) waterjet system, (**c**) multi-bend endoscope and (**d**) oesophageal overtube

cap mounted on the tip of an endoscope that may aid visualisation of the bleeding site and assist with the removal of larger blood clots. Studies have shown that use of a cap reduces the time to hemostasis. Endoscopes equipped with waterjets can also be helpful for removing clots and exposing the cause of major bleeding lesions. Multi-bending endoscope can facilitate access to difficult areas and, in addition, have two working channels that permit the simultaneous use of suction and therapeutic devices. Finally, overtubes can reduce the risk of aspiration pneumonia and facilitate endoscopy in patients who need repeated intubation because of extensive blood clots. These are illustrated in Fig. 11.5.

Although endoscopic therapy appears to achieve hemostasis in at least 90% of patients, a minority [10–20%] have recurrent bleeding. This is usually an indication for repeat endoscopy and endoscopic therapy. If this is unsuccessful, subsequent therapeutic options are limited to either emergency surgery or transarterial embolization.

11.3.2 Variceal Bleeding

Bleeding from esophageal varices is often a medical emergency and continues to be an important cause of mortality in patients with gastrointestinal bleeding. However, improved resuscitation measures and endoscopic therapy has reduced the mortality rate from approximately 40% to 20%. Mortality can also be viewed from the perspective of cirrhosis. Approximately 20% of patients with cirrhosis continue to die from bleeding varices. Apart from resuscitation, acute management should include prophylactic antibiotics, and there is some evidence of benefit from somatostatin analogues which reduce portal pressure by the promotion of splanchnic vasodilation. Rarely, it may be necessary to temporarily control major bleeding by balloon tamponade (usually a Minnesota tube).

Some general surgeons will feel competent to perform endoscopic variceal ligation. The purpose is to ligate varices at the distal end of the variceal columns so that the perforating veins which supply the mucosal venous plexus are thrombosed. Several commercial multiband devices are available with up to ten preloaded bands.

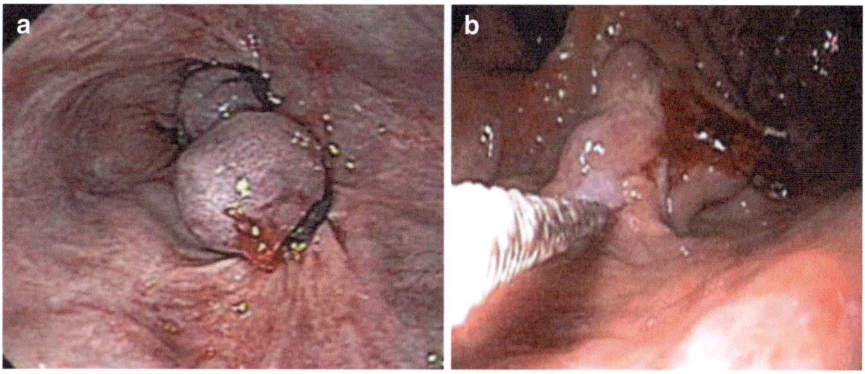

Fig. 11.6 (**a**) Esophageal varices after ligation and (**b**) injection of glue into gastric varices

All operate on the principle of placement of elastic bands on a varix after suction into a clear plastic cylinder attached to the tip of the endoscope. After the application of bands, the ligated tissue and the bands fall off within a few days (range 1–10 days). Eradication of varices may require up to four endoscopic sessions, but follow-up is necessary as varices recur.

The injection of cyanoacrylate at endoscopy has become the treatment of choice for bleeding varices in the fundus of the stomach (gastric varices) with a hemostasis rate of more than 95%. However, there is still a significant risk of rebleeding [20–35%] as well as other potential complications such as para-variceal injections, needle sticking in the varix, intraperitoneal injections and adherence of glue to the scope. Complications such as fever, mucosal necrosis, venous embolization and retro-gastric abscesses have also been reported.

The most commonly used agents are agents are n-butyl-2-cyanoacrylate (Histoacryl) and isobutyl-2-cyanoacrylate (Bucrylate). When injected into varices, the adhesive hardens within seconds forming a solid cast which is spontaneously extruded into the gastric lumen after several weeks. One option is radiological confirmation of the injection site using Lipiodol in a 1:1 ratio with the glue. A more recent development is the placement of coils in large gastric varices using endoscopic ultrasound followed by the endoscopic injection of glue. Banded oesophageal varices and the injection of gastric varices are illustrated in Fig. 11.6.

11.4 Endoscopic Management of Other Gastrointestinal Disorders

Over the past five decades, there has been a gradual expansion of the role of endoscopic therapy for a variety of gastrointestinal disorders. This began with the development of endoscopic sphincterotomy for bile duct stones in the 1970s and now includes therapy for gastrointestinal bleeding (as above) and various stents for biliary, pancreatic and gastrointestinal strictures. Importantly, advances in endoscope design have been accompanied by advances in the sophistication and capability of several accessories. For example, the first stents were composed of plastic, but subsequent developments led to the marketing of expanding metal stents and biodegradable stents. Metal stents, in particular, have improved stent patency with fewer stent-related complications and a subsequent improvement in quality of life. Biodegradable stents also have the potential to expand the indications for endoscopic stents into benign disorders such as benign esophageal and biliary strictures. The following section contains a brief overview of some of these developments.

11.4.1 Therapeutic Procedures Associated with Endoscopic Retrograde Cholangio-Pancreatography [ERCP]

Only a minority of general surgeons will have had the opportunity for training with ERCP. The major indication for the procedure is the removal of bile duct stones either before or after cholecystectomy. Pancreatic and biliary cancer is an unusual disease in rural centres but becomes a significant indication for endoscopic therapy in referral (tertiary) hospitals.

In contrast to other procedures, the technique of endoscopic sphincterotomy has only undergone minor modification since the first description in the 1970s. The principle is selective cannulation of the bile duct, retraction of a diathermy wire and use of an electric current to make an incision through the hood of the papilla. Bile duct stones can then be extracted using a wire basket or balloon catheter. Accessories now include use of guide wires to facilitate cannulation, more sophisticated diathermy units and a variety of baskets to crush or extract difficult stones. A debatable issue is the use of endoscopic ultrasound prior to sphincterotomy to confirm the presence of bile duct stones.

Pancreatic and biliary cancer is usually associated with a bile duct stricture causing jaundice. This frequently results in severe pruritus with a poor quality of life. In patients with inoperable tumors, the procedure of choice is usually a metal stent that extends from a position above the stricture into the duodenal lumen as shown in Fig. 11.7. The stent is inserted over a guide wire and expands to a diameter of approximately 1 cm. Expanding metal stents are composed of nitinol or elgiloy and can be uncovered, partly covered or fully covered. A fully covered stent reduces the risk of tumor ingrowth but increases the risk of stent migration. Removal of uncovered metal stents is difficult or impossible, and stent complications are usually treated by placement of a second stent within the first stent.

Plastic stents are still widely used for benign biliary and pancreatic disorders such as post-operative biliary strictures, post-operative bile leaks, sclerosing cholangitis, biliary strictures caused by chronic pancreatitis and pancreatic duct leaks,

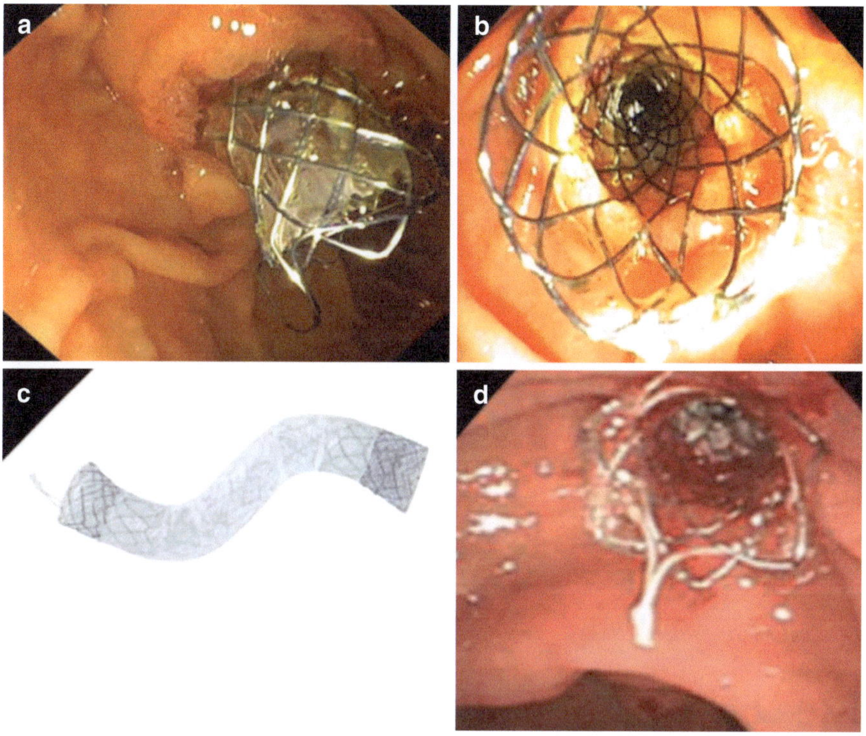

Fig. 11.7 Self-expanding metal stents: (**a**) covered metal stent, (**b**) uncovered metal stent, (**c**) Niti-S Taewoong stent (**d**) Niti-S Taewoong stent projecting into the duodenal lumen

and the prevention of pancreatitis after ERCP. As with metal stents, there are a variety of shapes, diameters, lengths and flaps or side holes. These stents also project into the duodenal lumen as shown in Fig. 11.8 and are readily removed by grasping the end of the stent with a loop catheter and withdrawing the stent through the endoscope. Plastic stents have smaller diameters than metal stents and have a higher frequency of complications such as cholangitis. This has led to the recommendation that new plastic stents be inserted prophylactically every 3 months if stenting needs to be continued for a prolonged period.

The major complications of stents relate to stent obstruction, cholangitis and stent migration. With plastic stents, the major reasons for obstruction are biofilm formation and biliary debris. For metal stents, obstruction can be due to tumor ingrowth, granulation tissue, biliary sludge or food debris. Obstruction is usually complicated by cholangitis and occasionally by a liver abscess. Stent migration is higher with plastic and covered metal stents, but the overall frequency of migration is usually low (<10%).

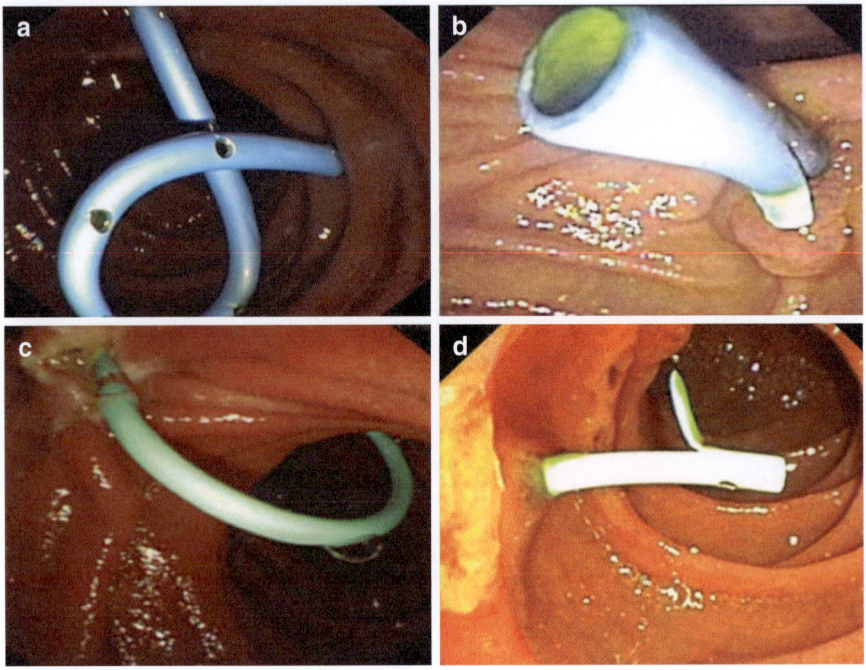

Fig. 11.8 Endoscopic appearance of plastic stents: (**a**) pigtail biliary stent (**b**) straight biliary stent, (**c**) pigtail pancreatic stent and (**d**) straight pancreatic stent

11.5 Luminal Stents

The initial indication for luminal stents was symptomatic malignant strictures of the gastrointestinal tract in patients predicted to have a limited life expectancy (usually 6 months or less). However, with the development of newer stents, particularly covered stents, indications have been expanded to include benign disorders such as esophageal strictures, post-operative leaks, iatrogenic perforations, tracheoesophageal fistulas and refractory bleeding from esophageal varices. Biodegradable stents are currently being trialled for benign strictures of the esophagus and may be useful for peptic strictures of the stomach and duodenum.

The placement of luminal stents usually involves passage of a guide wire through the stricture and passage of the stent over the guide wire into an appropriate position across the stricture. This is usually aided by fluoroscopy. The stent can then be gradually opened across the stricture. Covered stents have the advantage of potential endoscopic removal and a lower risk of tumor ingrowth but are associated with a higher risk of migration. The endoscopic appearance of opened luminal stents in a variety of locations is shown in Fig. 11.9.

The technical success and clinical success rates of stent placement have been over 90% and 80%, respectively. Failure is usually due to an inability to pass the

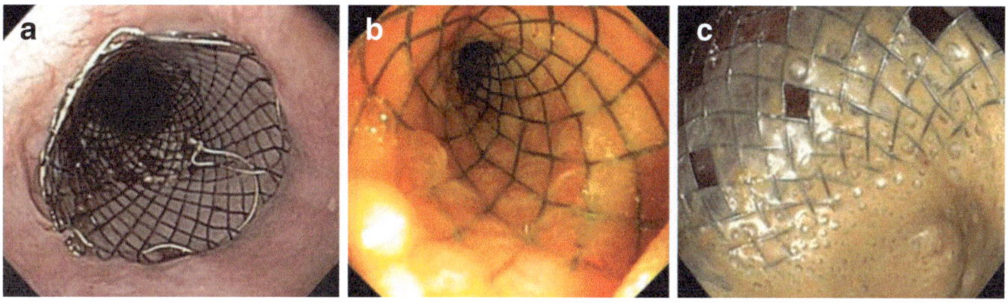

Fig. 11.9 (**a**) Esophageal stent, (**b**) gastric stent and (**c**) colonic stent

guide wire through the stricture or to major problems with looping and angulation. The median duration of stent patency is approximately 90%, 80% and 70% at 4 weeks, 3 months, and 6 months, respectively. Approximately 15% to 40% of patients require reintervention for recurrent symptoms. Apart from obstruction of the stent lumen, recurrent symptoms can also be caused by unidentified distal sites of malignant obstruction, diffuse peritoneal carcinomatosis with bowel encasement or functional outlet obstruction from neural (celiac axis) tumour involvement. Care needs to be taken with stents in the upper third of the oesophagus as a relatively proximal stent may cause an intolerable foreign body sensation.

11.6 Conclusion

The development of flexible endoscopy 50 years ago has led to a revolution in the management of upper gastrointestinal, biliary and pancreatic disorders. Whereas early endoscopic procedures were largely diagnostic, contemporary procedures are often therapeutic and involve a variety of techniques to address clinical problems such as gastrointestinal bleeding, bile duct stones, bile duct strictures, pancreatic disorders and benign and malignant strictures of the esophagus, stomach and duodenum. For general surgeons, competence in endoscopic procedures is likely to be highly variable, but most will have access to experienced endoscopists in tertiary centres who can undertake these procedures with high success rates and few complications.

Recommended Reading

American Society for Gastrointestinal Endoscopy Standard of Practice Committee. The role of endoscopy in the management of non-variceal acute upper gastrointestinal bleeding: guidelines for clinical application. Gastrointest Endosc. 1992;38:760–4.

Baron TH, Schöfl R, Puespoek A, Sakai Y. Expandable metal stent placement for gastric outlet obstruction. Endoscopy. 2001;33:623–8.

Baron TH. Expandable metal stents for the treatment of cancerous obstruction of the gastrointestinal tract. N Engl J Med. 2001;344:1681–7.

Chun HJ, Kim ES, Hyun JJ, Kwon YD, Keum B, Kim CD. Gastrointestinal and biliary stents. J Gastroenterol Hepatol. 2010;25:234–43.
Jeurnink SM, van Eijck CH, Steyerberg EW, Kuipers EJ, Siersema PD. Stent versus gastrojejunostomy for the palliation of gastric outlet obstruction: a systematic review. BMC Gastroenterol. 2007;7:18.
Kochar R, Shah N. Enteral stents: from esophagus to colon. Gastrointest Endosc. 2013;78:913–8.
Ramond MJ, Valla D, Mosnier JF, Degott C, Bernuau J, Rueff B, Benhamou JP. Successful endoscopic obturation of gastric varices with butyl cyanoacrylate. Hepatology. 1989;10:488–93.

Gastro-esophageal Reflux Disease 12

F. T. Kolligs and C. Kurz

The Montreal Classification provides a useful definition of GORD as heartburn symptoms or complications resulting from the reflux of gastric contents into the esophagus and up to the oral cavity, and lungs. The Montreal Classification further distinguishes between GORD with heartburn symptoms accompanied by endoscopic evidence of erosions (Erosive Reflux Disease, ERD) and GORD with heartburn symptoms but without endoscopic evidence of mucosal erosions (Non-Erosive Reflux Disease, NERD). It is important to distinguish NERD from functional heartburn. NERD is defined by typical reflux symptoms, absence of mucosal erosions, abnormal acid exposure on pH monitoring and responsiveness to proton pump inhibitors. In contrast, the Rome IV classification defines functional heartburn as the presence of retrosternal burning or pain for at least 3 months refractory to antisecretory therapy and the absence of GORD, histopathologic abnormalities, motility disorders and structural abnormalities.

Depending on the appearance of the esophageal mucosa on upper endoscopy three clinical settings of GORD need to be distinguished:

- *Erosive reflux disease (ERD)*—Erosive esophagitis is characterized by endoscopically visible lesions in the distal esophageal mucosa with or without troublesome symptoms of GORD.
- *Non-erosive reflux disease* (NERD)—Non-erosive reflux disease is characterized by the presence of symptoms of GORD without esophageal mucosal injury visible upon endoscopy.
- *Complications of GORD*—peptic stenosis, Barrett's esophagus, esophageal adenocarcinoma.

F. T. Kolligs (✉) · C. Kurz
Department of Internal Medicine and Gastroenterology, Helios Klinikum Berlin Buch, Berlin, Germany
e-mail: frank.kolligs@helios-gesundheit.de; christof.kurz@helios-gesundheit.de

M. W. Wichmann et al. (eds.), *Gastroenterology For General Surgeons*,
https://doi.org/10.1007/978-3-319-92768-8_12

12.1 Epidemiology/Pathogenesis/Risk Factors

The prevalence of GORD is 10–20% in Western countries; it is lower, for example, in China with 3–7% of the population affected. Roughly one third of patients with GORD have erosive lesions.

The development of GORD reflects an imbalance between aggressive (reflux events, acidity of reflux, esophageal hypersensitivity) and defensive factors (esophageal acid clearance, mucosal integrity). The antireflux barrier at the esophagogastric junction (EGJ) is anatomically and physiologically complex. Physiologically, both the diaphragm and the lower esophageal sphincter (LES) contribute to gastroesophageal sphincter competence and EGJ pressure. Three major mechanisms causing EGJ incompetence have been identified:

- Anatomic disruption of the EGJ, e.g. hiatus hernia
- Transient lower esophageal sphincter relaxations that are not associated with swallowing
- Incompetence of the LES function, e.g. due to medication, certain food contents, obesity and gravidity or other reasons for hypotensive LES function.

Medications negatively affecting LES function include calcium antagonists, beta mimetics and nitrates. The LES function is also negatively affected by the intake of chocolate, fat, alcohol and caffeine.

Esophageal clearance, mainly represented by propulsive peristalsis, is an important protective factor. Impaired propulsive peristalsis mostly occurs primarily, but can also occur secondary to collagenoses, e.g. sclerodermia. Rarely, secondary reflux disease can be caused by impaired gastric emptying due to gastroparesis or delayed gastric emptying.

12.2 Clinical Presentation

The characteristic symptoms of GORD are heartburn and regurgitation of acid. Other symptoms of GORD include dysphagia, chest pain, water brash (regurgitation of an excessive accumulation of saliva from the lower part of the esophagus), globus sensation and odynophagia. Extra-esophageal symptoms include chronic cough, hoarseness, wheezing and nausea. Important differential diagnoses are listed in Table 12.1. Complications can also arise in patients without typical esophageal symptoms. They can manifest within the esophagus (Barrett's esophagus, esophageal stricture, adenocarcinoma) or outside the esophagus (chronic laryngitis, asthma).

12.3 Diagnosis

The diagnosis of GORD can be based on clinical symptoms alone in patients with the typical symptoms of heartburn and regurgitation. In this situation, no diagnostic tests are necessary and it is recommended that a trial proton pump inhibitor therapy

Table 12.1 Differential diagnoses of gastro-esophageal reflux disease

Esophageal	Hypersensitive esophagus
	Functional heartburn
	Esophageal cancer
	Eosinophilic esophagitis
	Infectious esophagitis
	Pill esophagitis
	Motility disorders with impaired peristalsis
Extra-esophageal	Functional dyspepsia
	Depression
	Ischemic heart disease
	Gastric ulcer
	Gastric cancer

is initiated with a once daily standard dosing. Response to therapy confirms the diagnosis of GORD. It is important to mention that in patients presenting with chest pain as the only symptom and who are suspected of having GORD, cardiac causes of chest pain need to be excluded before initiating a proton pump inhibitor trial.

Gastroscopy—Gastroscopy is recommended when patients fail to respond to the initial proton pump inhibitor trial and in case of alarming symptoms: weight loss, dysphagia, odynophagia, unintentional weight loss and anemia. The recommendations regarding an early endoscopy also in patients with typical symptoms vary. While an early endoscopy is recommended by some, e.g. German guidelines, American guidelines recommend upper endoscopy only in case of alarm symptoms, non-response to empiric therapy with PPI, and in individuals at risk for Barrett's esophagus (see Table 12.4).

Biopsies are only required if Barrett's esophagus or carcinoma is suspected and when esophagitis has an atypical appearance. It is recommended that patients presenting with GORD should be tested and treated for *Helicobacter pylori* infection.

pH monitoring—Ambulatory pH monitoring can be performed with either a transnasally placed catheter or a wireless capsule that is endoscopically applied to the distal esophagus. 24 h pH monitoring is used to confirm the diagnosis of GORD in patients with persistent or continued symptoms under adequate therapy with PPI. pH electrode catheters are positioned 5 cm above the upper limit of the lower esophageal sphincter as defined by manometry. The wireless capsule is attached to the esophagus 6 cm proximal to the endoscopically defined squamocolumnar junction. Typically, tests with electrode catheters are conducted for 24 h and patients are advised to continue an unrestricted diet (Fig. 12.1). Studies with the capsule are conducted for 2–4 days, potentially varying the diet and therapeutic regimen between days.

Esophageal manometry—Esophageal manometry should be performed in case of suspected GORD with chest pain and/or dysphagia and a normal upper endoscopy to exclude an esophageal motility disorder. Manometry is also used to ensure correct placement of pH probes and to evaluate peristaltic function before antireflux surgery for GORD.

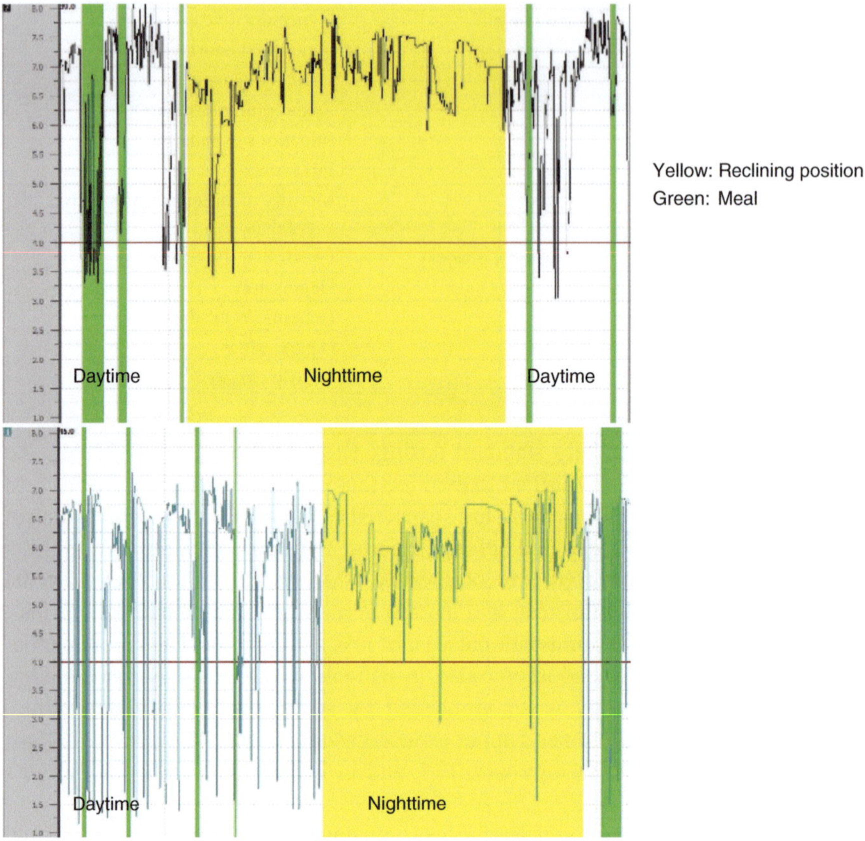

Fig. 12.1 24-hour pH monitoring. Normal (upper) and pathologic (lower) pH monitoring. Scale: pH. Yellow field: lying position. Green fields: Consumption of food

12.4 Endoscopic Classification

Two main endoscopic classifications are in use: Savary-Miller and Los Angeles, see Table 12.2 and Fig. 12.2.

The Savary-Miller classification is historically the most widely referenced grading of esophagitis. The Los Angeles classification is recommended by most current guidelines and grades esophagitis severity by the extent of mucosal abnormality, with complications recorded separately.

Table 12.2 Endoscopic classification of reflux esophagitis

Savary-Miller classification	Los Angeles classification
Grade I: One or more non-confluent reddish spots, with or without exudate	*Grade A*: One or more mucosal breaks each ≤5 mm in length *Grade B*: At least one mucosal break >5 mm long, but not continuous between the tops of adjacent mucosal folds
Grade II: Erosive and exudative lesions in the distal esophagus that may be confluent, but not circumferential	*Grade C*: At least one mucosal break that is continuous between the tops of adjacent mucosal folds, but which is not circumferential
Grade III: Circumferential erosions in the distal esophagus, covered by hemorrhagic and pseudomembranous exudate	*Grade D*: Mucosal break that involves at least three-fourths of the luminal circumference
Grade IV: Chronic complications such as deep ulcers, stenosis, scarring, or Barrett's metaplasia	–

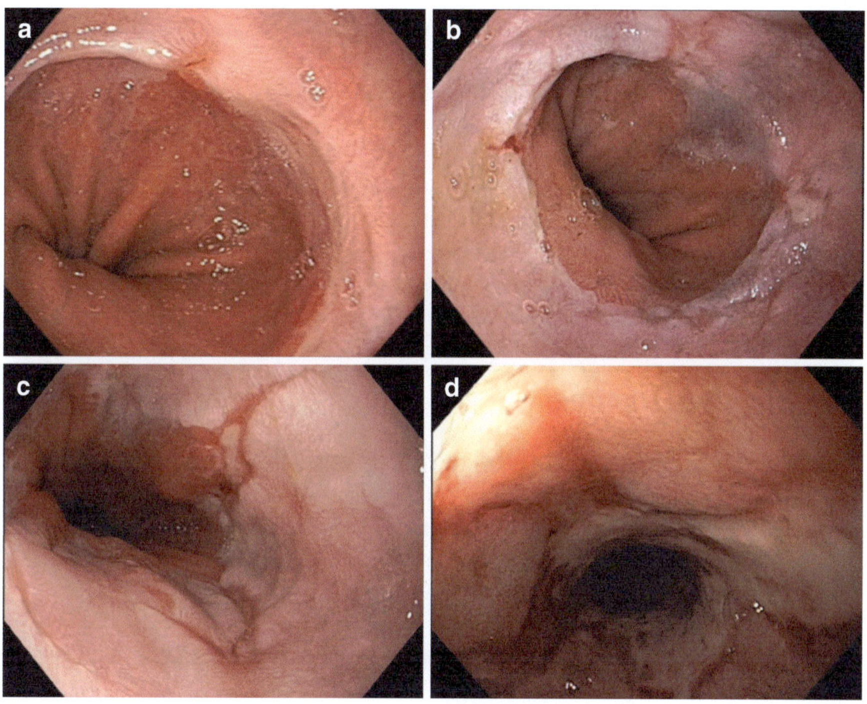

Fig. 12.2 Endoscopic pictures exemplifying the Los Angeles classification of erosive esophagitis, grades A–D

12.5 Treatment

Management of GORD includes life style, pharmacologic, endoscopic and surgical interventions.

Overview—The management of GORD is based on the frequency and severity of symptoms as well as the presence of erosive lesions.

In patients with mild and occasional symptoms (less than one episode per week) lifestyle and dietary modifications and a symptom-oriented medical approach with histamine-2 receptor antagonists, antacids and sodium alginate is often sufficient. If symptoms are not controlled by these measures or are more intense, a proton pump inhibitor should be initiated. When control of symptoms is achieved, treatment should be continued for at least 8 weeks.

In patients with more severe symptoms or erosive esophagitis a *step-down* therapy is recommended in order to achieve rapid symptom relief. Usually a treatment with a daily standard dose of a proton pump inhibitor (Table 12.3) is initiated for 8 weeks. Subsequently the dose is decreased. In case of full relief of symptoms acid suppression can be discontinued, in case of only mild or intermittent symptoms further dose-reduction, treatment on demand or switch to a histamine-2 receptor antagonist are possible options. Patients with severe erosive esophagitis require maintenance acid suppression with a proton pump inhibitor at standard dose due to a high risk of recurrence.

Lifestyle and diet—Recommended lifestyle and dietary modifications include

- Weight loss in obese patients.
- Elevation of the head of the bed when symptoms occur at night and especially in case of coughing, hoarseness and throat clearing.
- Avoiding meals 2–3 h before bedtime.
- Eliminating individual dietary triggers, e.g. caffeine, chocolate, fatty meals, sparkling beverages and peppermint.

12.6 Medical Treatment

Antacids—Antacids neutralize gastric pH. They have a role for the on-demand treatment of mild heartburn that occurs less frequently than once a week. They provide relief of symptoms within a few minutes, but the duration of their action is usually limited to 30–60 min. Currently available antacids are combinations of calcium carbonate, magnesium trisilicate and aluminium hydroxide.

Table 12.3 Equivalent standard dosing of proton pump inhibitors

Proton pump inhibitor	Standard dose
Omeprazole	40 mg
Esomeprazole	40 mg
Pantoprazole	40 mg
Rabeprazole	20 mg
Lansoprazole	30 mg

Sucralfate—Sucralfate adheres to and protects the mucosal surface. It can both protect from peptic injury and promote mucosal healing. Limitations are the short duration of action and low efficacy.

Histamine 2 receptor antagonists— Histamine-2 receptor antagonists decrease histamine stimulated acid secretion of the gastric parietal cell. Their onset of action is slower but their duration of action with 4 to 10 h is longer than that of antacids. Histamine-2 receptor antagonists are also more effective in terms of reducing frequency and severity of symptoms, but they have a limited efficacy in providing mucosal healing in patients with erosive esophagitis. A further limitation of their use is the development of a degree of tachyphylaxis within 2–6 weeks after start of regular intake. Therefore, they cannot be used as a maintenance therapy. Available histamine-2 receptor antagonists include cimetidine, ranitidine, nizatidine and famotidine.

Sodium alginate—Sodium alginate is an anionic polysaccharide derived from seaweed. When combined with water it forms a viscous gum and floats in the proximal stomach that is able to neutralize the postprandial acid pocket. Sodium alginate is used for the relief of mild postprandial reflux symptoms and as add-on therapy in patients with break-through symptoms under PPI therapy and patients with refractory GORD.

Proton pump inhibitors—Proton pump inhibitors (PPIs) bind to and irreversibly block the hydrogen-potassium ATPase pump of the parietal cell. PPIs are the most potent inhibitors of gastric acid secretion. They provide faster symptom relief than H2RAs and are the most potent drug to heal erosive esophagitis. Because the amount of proton pumps on parietal cells is highest after prolonged fast, PPIs are most effective when taken 30 min before the first meal of the day. The various PPIs are equally potent when used at equivalent dosing (Table 12.3). Typically, PPIs are started at a single standard dosing. In case of severe erosive esophagitis it may be necessary to start with a double standard dosing, each one tablet 30 minutes before breakfast and 30 min before dinner. In case of non-erosive disease or lower grade erosions (i.e. Savary Miller grade I or Los Angeles grade A or B) the PPI can be reduced to the half dose after 4 weeks. In case of higher grade erosions the dose should not be reduced before 6–8 weeks after initiation of therapy. When symptoms remain under control in patients with non-erosive disease or lower grade erosions the PPI can be withdrawn. In case of recurrence of symptoms a low dose continuous PPI therapy or a therapy on demand may be necessary. Patients with higher grade erosive esophagitis usually require continuous PPI medication.

12.7 Adverse Events Associated with Proton Pump Inhibitors

The most common adverse events of PPI use are headache, diarrhea and dyspepsia which occur in less than 2% of users. PPIs can cause hypomagnesemia at a median of 5.5 years after commencement of regular intake. Therefore patients at risk, e.g. those on diuretics, should be monitored for hypomagnesemia. PPI use has also been associated with a higher risk of cardiovascular events when used in conjunction with clopidogrel. However, these data are highly controversial. PPI use has also been associated with a possible higher risk of hip, wrist and spine fracture, but causality has not been proven so far. Furthermore, PPI use has also been associated with the development of pneumonia and *Clostridium difficile* colitis as well as other enteric infections. This may particularly apply to recurrent *Clostridium difficile* infection. PPI long-term use has also been associated with the development of atrophic gastritis, gastric polyp formation and gastric carcinoids.

12.8 Refractory Disease and Recurrent Symptoms

Up to 40% of patients treated with PPI fail to respond. The failure rate is higher in those with atypical than in those with typical symptoms. The first step in case of refractory GORD is to confirm adherence to therapy. Increasing a once daily dose to twice daily will improve symptoms in about 40% of patients. In partial responders with mostly nocturnal symptoms, the use of histamine-2 receptor antagonists at bedtime may be beneficial. As mentioned above, sodium alginate may be used as add-on to PPI therapy in patients with break-through symptoms. In patients with continued symptoms despite optimized therapy and confirmed compliance, a further medical workup is required. The first step is upper endoscopy to exclude non-GORD disease. Ambulatory pH monitoring may be helpful to objectivize acid reflux. If symptoms recur despite optimal PPI therapy or are insensitive to PPI at higher dose, patients should be evaluated for antireflux surgery.

12.9 Surgical and Endoscopic Management

Surgery is considered an option for the management of GORD in several clinical situations. Main indications are: persistent GORD symptoms or no resolution of esophageal erosions despite optimal medical therapy, non-compliance or lack of willingness to continue PPI use, medication side effects, the presence of large hiatal hernia, and high volume reflux. Surgical options include Nissen fundoplication, either laparoscopic or open, Belsey Mark IV, Hill gastropexy, and gastric bypass. A new FDA-approved approach is the LINX® reflux management system which works by augmenting the sphincter barrier via a system constructed of titanium beads. The system is introduced laparoscopically, does not alter gastric anatomy and is easily reversible. The device decreases esophageal acid exposure, improves reflux symptoms and quality of life, and allows cessation of PPIs in the majority of patients.

Preoperatively, upper endoscopy to assess gastric and esophageal mucosa and to rule out malignancy as well as manometry to rule out motility disorders is recommended. Patients benefitting most from surgery are those with typical GORD symptoms and/or regurgitation, and those responding well to PPI therapy. Patients with refractory dyspeptic symptoms such as nausea, vomiting and epigastric pain are less likely to achieve resolution of symptoms after surgery. Dysphagia and gas-bloat syndrome are common problems after fundoplication in 15–20% of patients. Many patients require further PPI therapy. Albeit at lower dose after surgery.

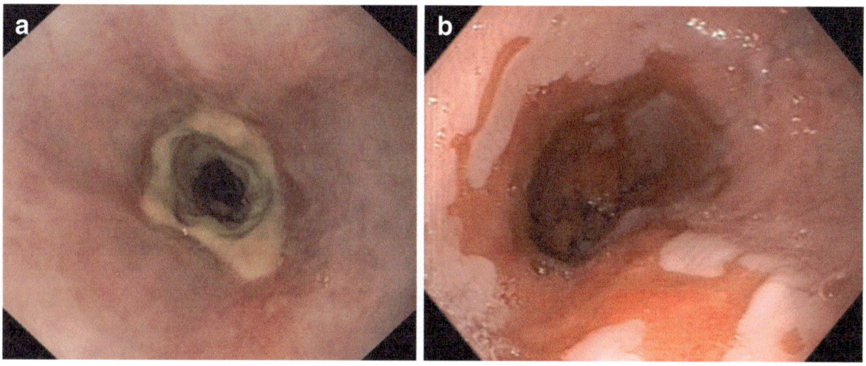

Fig. 12.3 Endoscopic pictures of a peptic stenosis of the esophagus (**a**) and of a histologically confirmed Barrett's esophagus (**b**)

Endoscopic methods are so far not considered a standard approach. In case of peptic stenosis (Fig. 12.3a) endoscopic treatment by dilation is usually sufficient. Repeat treatment sessions may be necessary. In severe cases surgery may be required.

12.10 Follow-Up of Patients with Severe Erosive Esophagitis

Patients with severe erosive esophagitis (Los Angeles classification grades C and D) on endoscopy should undergo control endoscopy after an 8 week course of PPI therapy to confirm healing and to rule out Barrett's esophagus.

12.11 Barrett's Esophagus

Barrett's esophagus is a precancerous condition associated with GORD (Fig. 12.3b). Esophageal adenocarcinoma in patients with Barrett's esophagus is thought to evolve through a sequence of genetic alterations that are associated with dysplastic changes of progressive severity (low to high grade).

Therefore, endoscopic screening for Barrett's esophagus is generally recommended for patients with multiple risk factors (Table 12.4). Patients with duration of GORD symptoms over 5 and more years should undergo upper endoscopy to rule out Barrett's esophagus.

Endoscopic surveillance of Barrett's esophagus includes the careful inspection of the epithelium with high-resolution white light endoscopy. Random-four quadrant biopsies should be obtained every 2 cm in patients without known dysplasia and every 1 cm in case of known or suspected dysplasia. Any visible abnormality should be removed with endoscopic mucosal resection. Advanced imaging techniques, e.g. chromoendoscopy (with acetic acid or indigo carmine) or virtual chromoendoscopy (e.g. NBI or FICE) can increase the diagnostic yield for dysplasia and cancer.

Table 12.4 Risk factors for Barrett's esophagus

Duration of GORD ≥5 years
Age ≥ 50 years
Male sex
White race
Hiatal hernia
Obesity
Nocturnal reflux
Tobacco use (current or past)
First-degree relative with Barrett's esophagus and/or adenocarcinoma

Endoscopic classification of Barrett's esophagus should follow the Prague C & M criteria to track the length of the Barrett segment over time. However, in the vast majority of patients the length of the Barrett's esophagus does not change over time. The key steps are: (1) identification of the gastro-esophageal junction (GEJ) at the top of the gastric mucosal folds; (2) definition of the extent of the circumferential columnar appearing mucosa above the GEJ in cm and (3) measuring the extent of tongue-like areas of columnar-appearing mucosa in cm above the GEJ.

Recommended Reading

Freedberg DE, Kim LS, Yang YX. The risks and benefits of long-term use of proton pump inhibitors: expert review and best practice advice from the American Gastroenterological Association. Gastroenterology. 2017;152:706.

Katz PO, Gerson LB, Vela MF. Guidelines for the diagnosis and management of gastroesophageal reflux disease. Am J Gastroenterol. 2013;108:308.

Ness-Jensen E, Hveem K, El-Serag H, Lagergren J. Lifestyle intervention in Gastroesophageal reflux disease. Clin Gastroenterol Hepatol. 2016;14:175.

Shaheen NJ, Falk GW, Iyer PG, et al. ACG clinical guideline: diagnosis and Management of Barrett's Esophagus. Am J Gastroenterol. 2016;111:30.

Sifrim D, Zerbib F. Diagnosis and management of patients with reflux symptoms refractory to proton pump inhibitors. Gut. 2012;61:1340.

Spechler SJ, Souza RF. Barrett's esophagus. N Engl J Med. 2014;371:836.

Surdea Blaga T, Dumitrascu D, Galmiche JP, Bruley des Varannes S. Functional heartburn: clinical characteristics and outcome. Eur J Gastroenterol Hepatol. 2013;25:282.

13 Surveillance and Premalignant Conditions

Matthias W. Wichmann and Timothy K. McCullough

13.1 Esophagus

13.1.1 Barrett's Esophagus

In patients with Barrett's esophagus, the squamous epithelium of the distal esophagus is replaced by metaplastic columnar epithelium. This condition develops as a consequence of chronic gastroesophageal reflux disease. The annual cancer incidence in patients with Barret's esophagus is estimated to be up to 0.4%, and the individual risk of developing esophageal cancer is increased 30-fold. Despite these significant findings, there is a lot of controversy regarding the surveillance and management of patients suffering from this condition because patients with Barrett's esophagus are usually elderly and much more likely to die from causes unrelated to esophageal cancer.

13.1.2 Management of Patients with Barrett's Esophagus

All patients with Barrett's esophagus should receive proton pump inhibitor treatment indefinitely independent of reflux symptoms. Aggressive antireflux treatment has been observed to prevent cancer and may result in regression of the specialized intestinal metaplasia. Whether or not antireflux surgery is more effective at preventing esophageal adenocarcinoma than medical therapy is unclear.

M. W. Wichmann (✉) · T. K. McCullough
Department of Surgery, Mount Gambier General Hospital, Mount Gambier, SA, Australia
e-mail: matthias.wichmann@sa.gov.au; timothy.mccullough@sa.gov.au

M. W. Wichmann et al. (eds.), *Gastroenterology For General Surgeons*,
https://doi.org/10.1007/978-3-319-92768-8_13

13.1.3 Surveillance

The goal of surveillance is to improve outcomes through early detection of dysplasia and/or malignant transformation. It is not clear whether surveillance is beneficial with regard to this goal. If surveillance has been agreed upon between the patient and his healthcare provider, an initial endoscopy should be performed with four-quadrant biopsies every 2 cm within the Barrett's segment. A second pathologist should confirm the diagnosis of dysplasia.

If the biopsies do not show any dysplasia, a repeat endoscopy should be performed after 3–5 years. If the biopsies are indefinite for dysplasia, antireflux treatment must be optimized, and repeat biopsies should be taken within 2–6 months (four-quadrant biopsies every 2 cm). In patients with dysplasia, endoscopic eradication should be performed as well as four-quadrant biopsies every 1 cm of the esophagus. Any mucosal irregularity should be removed endoscopically.

13.1.4 Management of Dysplasia

Dysplasia should be managed with endoscopic eradication (ablation or resection). Endoscopic ablation can be performed using radiofrequency ablation (RFA) or cryotherapy. RFA is very effective at removing all Barrett's epithelium with a low risk of complications. During endoscopic cryotherapy (nitrogen or carbon dioxide gas), the tissue is frozen for 40 s (2 × 20 s, 4 × 10 s). Follow-up after eradication depends on the initial degree of dysplasia as well as the success of the eradication treatment. Endoscopic resection includes mucosal resection (EMR) or submucosal dissection (ESD). These procedures provide tissue specimens that can be examined. In view of the significant morbidity and mortality (up to 12%) of esophagectomy for high-grade dysplasia, this form of treatment has been largely replaced by EMR and ESD and should be performed in highly specialized centers.

13.2 Stomach

13.2.1 Gastric Polyps

Gastric polyps are usually asymptomatic and are found incidentally during upper gastrointestinal endoscopy. A formal polypectomy should be performed for all polyps larger than 1 cm. If multiple polyps are identified, the largest polyp should be removed, and additional biopsies should be taken from the remaining polyps.

Routine gastric biopsies should include the antrum, angularis fold, body of stomach, and cardia.

Hyperplastic polyps are mostly associated with *Helicobacter pylori* (*H. pylori*) infection. They grow in response to a chronic inflammatory process within the stomach and contain dysplastic cells. The risk of malignancy is increased in polyps larger than 1 cm and in those with pedunculated growth. All hyperplastic polyps larger than 0.5 cm should be removed. Surveillance after removal of hyperplastic polyps should be performed at 6 months after resection and must be continued every 2 years in patient with increased risk for gastric cancer (atrophic gastritis, extensive intestinal metaplasia, family history).

Fundic gland polyps are common in countries with a low incidence of *H. pylori* infection. Fundic gland polyps are associated with polyposis syndromes, hypergastrinemia due to gastrinoma and long-term proton pump inhibitor medication. Fundic gland polyps larger than 1 cm, polyps with ulceration, or those located in the antrum should be removed to rule out dysplasia/neoplasia. Regular surveillance is not indicated for these polyps.

Gastric adenomas are the most common gastric neoplastic polyp (6–10% of gastric polyps) and are usually observed in patients with chronic atrophic gastritis. These lesions have a similar appearance as colonic adenomas and are usually less than 2 cm in size. In view of the increased risk of gastric cancer, all gastric adenomas must be resected. Surveillance endoscopy should be done 1 year after resection of gastric polyps.

Gastric neuroendocrine tumors (carcinoids) are subdivided into three types and are derived from enterochromaffin-like cells. Type I tumors (70–80%) are associated with prolonged hypergastrinemia (atrophic gastritis). Type II tumors (5–8%) result from a gastrin-secreting tumor (MEN-1 syndrome, Zollinger-Ellison syndrome). Type III tumors (20%) are sporadic and can be associated with atypical carcinoid syndrome. Types I and II are usually indolent, whereas two thirds of patients with type III tumors have locoregional or hepatic metastases at the time of resection. Types I and II tumors smaller than 2 cm should be resected endoscopically, whereas type III tumors require partial/total gastrectomy and lymph node dissection.

Surveillance endoscopy for tumor types I and II should be done at least annually.

13.2.2 Gastric Intestinal Metaplasia

This condition is considered a precancerous gastric lesion in the cancer cascade of chronic gastritis, atrophic gastritis, intestinal metaplasia, dysplasia, and adenocarcinoma. In gastric intestinal metaplasia, the surface, foveolar, and glandular epithelium is replaced by the intestinal epithelium. If small intestinal-type mucosa is found, this condition is classified as complete intestinal metaplasia. If colonic epithelium is identified, this condition is classified as incomplete intestinal metaplasia.

Risk factors for intestinal metaplasia are similar to those for gastric cancer and include *H. pylori* infection, high salt intake, smoking, alcohol, chronic bile reflux, and genetic factors. The risk of progression to gastric cancer is higher in patients with incomplete intestinal metaplasia.

To determine the subtype of metaplasia gastric biopsy mapping is performed. This mapping requires five nontargeted biopsies (lesser and greater curve of the antrum and corpus, incisura angularis). In patients at increased risk of gastric cancer (family history, non-Caucasian ethnicity), gastric biopsy mapping should be routinely performed.

Surveillance of patients with incomplete intestinal metaplasia or extensive intestinal metaplasia should be performed every 2 years.

13.2.3 Large Gastric Folds

Enlarged or giant mucosal folds in the stomach are associated with different proliferative, inflammatory, and infiltrative conditions. Large gastric folds are defined as greater than 1 cm in width and persistent after air insufflation into the stomach. In more than 50% of patients, the condition is benign. Gastric malignancy can be observed in approximately 10% of these patients.

Ménétrier's disease is a rare protein-losing hypertrophic gastropathy and is mostly seen in middle-aged men. The disease is usually progressive, and the pathogenesis is not well understood. The diagnosis is established on biopsy, and treatment includes eradication of gastric infections (CMV, *H. pylori*), proton pump inhibitor medication, octreotide (100–600 μg s.c./daily), cetuximab (monoclonal antibody to EGFR), and total gastrectomy.

Other conditions associated with large gastric folds are Zollinger-Ellison syndrome, ***H. pylori*** gastritis, and gastric neoplasia. Zollinger-Ellison syndrome results from gastric acid hypersecretion due to a gastrin-producing tumor. Gastric neoplasia associated with large gastric folds includes lymphoma, adenocarcinoma, and carcinoid tumors. All of these need to be excluded in patients with enlarged gastric folds.

13.2.4 Follow-Up After Gastric Cancer Treatment

Currently no globally accepted standard for the surveillance after curative treatment of gastric cancer has been published. The European Society for Medical Oncology (ESMO), European Society of Surgical Oncology (ESSO), and European Society for Radiotherapy and Oncology (ESTRO) have addressed this issue and suggest that regular follow-up may allow investigation and treatment of treatment-related symptoms and provide psychological support and early detection of recurrence. Until now there is no evidence that this approach improves survival outcomes. The aggressive nature of gastric cancer has so far prevented the concept of survivorship in these patients and is only now beginning to evolve.

13.3 Liver Lesions

The differential diagnosis of solid liver lesions is broad and can be challenging. Most lesions are solitary masses, but multiple lesions can be seen with hemangiomas, regenerative nodules, hepatocellular carcinoma, and metastatic disease.

Common **benign liver lesions** are:

- Hemangiomas: most common benign mesenchymal hepatic tumor; up to 80% of these are diagnosed between the ages of 30 and 50 years; most patients are female (female to male ratio 3:1); symptoms are usually observed in lesions bigger than 4 cm.
- Focal nodular hyperplasia (FNH): most commonly diagnosed in younger females (third/fourth decade); it appears to be a hyperplastic response to an anomalous artery; association of FNH with oral contraceptives has not been clearly established.
- Adenomas: most commonly seen in premenopausal women; most patients have used oral contraceptives for at least 2 years prior to diagnosis; small risk of neoplastic transformation.
- Idiopathic noncirrhotic portal hypertension: multiple foci of proliferating hepatocytes on the background of systemic autoimmune disease.
- Regenerative nodules: typically associated with liver cirrhosis.

Common **malignant liver lesions** are:

- Hepatocellular carcinoma (HCC): primary liver malignancy most often occurs in the setting of chronic liver disease (hepatitis B, cirrhosis of any cause); can cause hepatic failure in a patient with previously compensated cirrhosis.
- Cholangiocarcinoma (CCC): malignancy of the bile ducts; can involve intra- and extrahepatic ducts; main risk factors are primary sclerosing cholangitis and choledochal cysts.
- Metastatic disease: the most common malignant hepatic neoplasm in Western countries (North America and Europe).

13.3.1 Diagnosis and Management

Most patients with solid liver lesions are asymptomatic. The correct diagnosis regarding the etiology of the finding can usually be made based on the patient's history, physical examination, laboratory testing (liver function tests, serological studies, hemochromatosis, nonalcoholic fatty liver disease, tumor markers (CEA, CA19.9, alpha-fetoprotein)), and imaging (triple-phase CT scan, MRI, ultrasound).

Lesions smaller than 1 cm in patients who are not at increased risk for HCC are commonly benign. Some authors suggest to perform MRI (to exclude features of HCC) followed by two ultrasound investigations at 3 and 15 months. If the lesion is stable after three radiographic examinations, no further surveillance is indicated.

Fine needle aspiration (FNA) biopsy is controversial in patients with solid liver lesions. The biopsies are very often negative, and there is a significant risk of seeding of neoplastic cells in the peritoneal cavity or the needle tract. Surgical resection is therefore recommended for symptomatic lesions or if HCC cannot be excluded. In patients with suspected hepatic adenoma, surgical resection should be performed if the lesion is larger than 5 cm in diameter or if the lesion is symptomatic. The behavior of hepatic adenomas during pregnancy is unpredictable, and there is a risk of rupture. Radiofrequency ablation/resection of lesions larger than 2 cm in diameter is recommended prior to attempting pregnancy.

13.3.2 Biliary Cysts

Biliary cysts can occur throughout the biliary tree and are associated with significant complications. These complications include stricture, stone formation, cholangitis, rupture, biliary cirrhosis, and (depending on the cyst type) cancer. Six different types of biliary cysts have been described:

- **Type I** cysts (up to 85%): cystic or fusiform dilation of the common bile duct (CBD)
  - **IA**: CBD plus common hepatic duct and extrahepatic segments of left and right hepatic ducts
  - **IB**: focal, segmental dilation of an extrahepatic bile duct (often the distal CBD)
  - **IC**: smooth, fusiform dilation of all the extrahepatic bile ducts; associated with an abnormal pancreaticobiliary junction (APBJ)
  - **ID**: cystic dilation of CBD and cystic duct
- **Type II** cysts (2%): true diverticula of the extrahepatic bile ducts (narrow stalk); can arise from any portion of the extrahepatic bile duct
- **Type III** cysts (5%): limited to the intraduodenal portion of the CBD (choledochoceles)
  - **IIIA**: the bile duct and pancreatic duct enter the cyst.
  - **IIIB**: the diverticulum of intraduodenal CBD or intra-ampullary common duct.
- **Type IV** cysts (up to 35%): multiple cysts
  - **IVA**: intra- and extrahepatic dilations
  - **IVB**: no intrahepatic cysts
- **Type V** cysts (20%): dilations of the intrahepatic ducts; multiple dilations = Caroli disease
- **Type VI** cysts (rare): cystic duct only

The incidence of biliary cysts is low in Western populations (1:100,000) but can be as high as 1:1000 in some Asian countries (Japan) with a female to male ratio of 3:1. Abnormal pancreaticobiliary junction (APBJ) is defined as junction of the bile duct and pancreatic duct outside the duodenal wall with a long common ductal channel (up to 20 mm in length).

The classic clinical presentation of a biliary cyst includes the triad of abdominal pain, jaundice, and palpable mass. Other typical symptoms are nausea, vomiting, fever, pruritus, and weight loss as well as cholangitis, pancreatitis, and obstructive jaundice.

Biliary cysts carry an increased risk of cancer, particularly type I (up to 70% of malignancies) and type IV (up to 20% of malignancies) cysts. The risk of cholangiocarcinoma in biliary cysts is 20- to 30-fold increased over the general population, and the incidence of malignancy increases with age. The presence of an APBJ increases the risk of cancer, and in patient with an APBJ but no biliary cysts, a high incidence of gallbladder cancer has been observed. Prophylactic cholecystectomy should be performed in these patients.

Biliary cysts are often identified on ultrasound or computed tomography (CT) in patients being investigated for unclear abdominal pain or jaundice. Communication between the cysts and the biliary tree must be demonstrated to allow for differentiation between biliary cysts and other cystic lesions (pancreatic, mesenteric, hepatic). CT can detect all types of biliary cysts. Magnetic resonance cholangiopancreatography (MRCP) is the test of choice for diagnosing and evaluating biliary cysts because it does not expose the patient to ionizing radiation (like CT) and does not carry the risk of cholangitis or pancreatitis like ERCP (endoscopic retrograde cholangiopancreatography).

Patients with types I, II, and IV cysts usually undergo surgical resection due to the significant risk of malignant transformation. Types I and IV cysts should be completely resected, and reconstruction requires a Roux-en-Y hepaticojejunostomy. Type II cysts can be treated with cyst excision. Type III cysts only require treatment if they are symptomatic (sphincterotomy, endoscopic resection). Type V cysts require supportive treatment and management of complications (cholangitis, sepsis). Some patients with type V biliary cysts require liver transplantation. Post-excisional malignant disease is seen in up to 6% of patients, and regular follow-up is recommended (MRI, liver function tests).

13.4 Pancreas

Pancreatic cysts are detected in approximately 2% of cross-sectional studies (MRI, CT) performed for unrelated reasons. These cysts can be divided into inflammatory fluid collections, nonneoplastic pancreatic cysts and pancreatic cystic neoplasms (PCNs). PCNs account for more than half of pancreatic cysts, have significant malignant potential, and usually require resection.

Inflammatory fluid collections are not true epithelial cysts and are usually a complication of acute pancreatitis. These include acute peripancreatic fluid collections, pseudocysts, acute necrotic collections, and walled-off pancreatic necrosis.

Nonneoplastic pancreatic cysts (NNPC) are very rare and usually asymptomatic and do not require resection. They are usually identified after surgical resection of a lesion thought to be a PCN.

Pancreatic cystic neoplasms (PCNs) are important to be identified because some of these have malignant potential. Four subtypes of PCN have been described: serous cystic tumors, mucinous cystic neoplasms (MCN), intraductal papillary mucinous neoplasms (IPMN), solid pseudopapillary neoplasms (SPN). Each of these subtypes has benign and malignant forms.

Most **serous cystic tumors** are benign and can be followed conservatively unless symptomatic.

MCN have ovarian-like stroma and occur almost only in women. They are typically located in the tail or body and should be resected because of malignant potential.

IPMN are mucin-producing papillary neoplasms of the ductal system. IPMN can be main duct, branch duct, or mixed type. Management of IPMN involves surveillance and resection depending on risk of malignancy and patient factors.

IPMN are potentially malignant, typically more than 10 mm in size, and are composed of mucin-producing columnar cells. Branch-duct IPMN are at a low risk of malignancy (20% over 10 years), while main-duct IPMN have a higher risk (70%). Resection is typically recommended for IPMN with high-grade dysplasia (carcinoma in situ) on fine needle aspiration (FNA), progression to invasive carcinoma, and features concerning for malignancy or those at high risk for developing malignancy. Clear indications for surgery are main pancreatic duct diameter ≥ 10 mm, enhancing solid component in the IPMN, and obstructive jaundice. If no clear indication for surgery is identified, endoscopic FNA should be performed on IPMN ≥30 mm, enhancing cyst walls, non-enhancing nodules, associated pancreatitis, main-duct diameter 5–9 mm, and abrupt caliber change of the pancreatic duct. IPMN smaller than 10 mm in size should be followed up with imaging. Features on endoscopic ultrasound (EUS) suggestive of malignancy are main duct ≥7 mm in main-duct IPMN, irregular thick septum in a lesion ≥30 mm in branch-duct IPMN, and mural nodules larger than 10 mm for both forms of IPMN.

Surgery is the only treatment option in patients with high-grade dysplasia or after progression to invasive carcinoma. Resection should be attempted if there is no evidence of local vascular invasion or distant metastases. Chemotherapy after resection (even if non-curative) improves survival and should be offered.

Prognosis of IPMN-associated adenocarcinoma is better than that of pancreatic ductal adenocarcinoma.

IPMN are commonly classified according to the Tanaka or Fukuoka consensus guidelines.

Management of main-duct IPMN depends on degree of ductal dilatation: ≥10 mm resection, 5–9 mm FNA, and <5 mm follow-up MRI/CT after 2 years.

The risk of developing cancer in branch-duct IPMN is approximately 1%/year.

SPN are rare and typically occur in young women (<35 years). Resection is recommended due to malignant risk.

Cystic degeneration has been observed in most solid pancreatic tumors.

13.4.1 Pancreatic Cancer

Only 20% of patients with pancreatic cancer are candidates for curative surgery, and the prognosis is poor with less than 30% 5-year survival in node-negative disease and less than 10% 5-year survival in node-positive disease. Up to 10% of patients with pancreatic cancer have a family history of this disease. Inherited risk factors for pancreatic cancer are hereditary pancreatitis, familial pancreatic cancer, familial atypical multiple mole melanoma (FAMMM) syndrome, and Peutz-Jeghers syndrome. Non-inherited risk factors for pancreatic cancer are chronic pancreatitis (small increase from 1.3% to 1.8% of the population), diabetes mellitus (RR 2.08), IPMN, cigarette smoking (RR 1.5; accounts for 25% of all cases), and BMI ≥ 30 kg/m^2 (RR 1.72). Physical activity has a protective effect (RR 0.45). Data relating to the risk of certain diets and coffee or alcohol consumption on the risk of developing pancreatic cancer are inconclusive.

13.5 Large Bowel

13.5.1 Colon Polyps

A **hamartomatous polyp** consists of tissue that belongs in the area where the polyp is found but which grows in an unorganized fashion. Juvenile polyps belong to this group of polyps. These lesions are more commonly observed in children. The juvenile polyposis syndrome (autosomal dominant) is characterized by multiple juvenile polyps throughout the gastrointestinal tract and carries an increased risk of gastric and colorectal cancer. The Peutz-Jeghers polyp is a hamartomatous polyp which can grow and undergo malignant transformation. This polyp is associated with the Peutz-Jeghers syndrome (STK11 mutation), and these patients have increased risk of developing gastrointestinal and non-gastrointestinal cancers.

Serrated polyps are a group of polyps with variable malignant potential. This group consists of hyperplastic polyps, traditional serrated adenomas, and sessile serrated adenomas. The classification of these polyps is evolving. Hyperplastic polyps are the most common nonneoplastic polyps in the colon, and they are typically located in the distal sigmoid colon and rectum. They usually do not increase the risk of colorectal cancer. Large lesions especially when located in the ascending colon, however, must be resected completely. For patients with small lesions located in the rectosigmoid, surveillance should be scheduled after 10 years. Sessile serrated polyps/adenomas are more common in the proximal large bowel and are more likely to contain dysplastic cells. Dysplastic sessile serrated adenomas are considered to be precursors for microsatellite instability-high (MSI-H) colon cancers. Lesions larger than 10 mm and/or dysplasia should be considered as high-risk adenomas requiring a surveillance colonoscopy after a maximum of 36 months. The authors aim for a surveillance colonoscopy after 18 months. The serrated polyposis syndrome is characterized by multiple large and proximally located serrated polyps. The risk of colorectal cancer development is increased in these patients, and polyps larger than 10 mm need to be removed. Surveillance colonoscopy should be performed within 1–3 years. Colectomy should be considered in these patients if colorectal cancer is suspected, the polyposis is symptomatic (anemia), high-grade dysplasia develops, the polyp number significantly increases, and the patient cannot be followed up regularly or does not want regular colonoscopies. We also recommend surveillance colonoscopy for first-degree relatives of patients diagnosed with serrated polyposis syndrome.

Adenomatous polyps are the most common neoplastic polyp in the large bowel, and up to 50% of patients with one adenoma will have a second adenoma. At age 50 approximately 30% of patients have colonic adenomas. Risk factors for the development of adenomatous polyps are age, increased body mass index, and male gender. Approximately 5% of adenomas progress to cancer over a time period of 7–10 years. The risk of cancer development is higher in large polyps (>10 mm), villous adenomas, and polyps with high-grade dysplasia. The appearance of adenomas can be described as pedunculated, sessile, or flat. There are few depressed or excavated lesions as well (1%). Adenomas are tubular (80%), villous, or tubulovillous, and their cells are classified as low-grade or high-grade (intraepithelial carcinoma) dysplastic. All adenomas should be completely excised. If complete clearance of a high-risk adenoma is uncertain, a repeat colonoscopy should be performed within 3–6 months. Polyps with high-grade dysplasia are adequately treated with polypectomy if the resection margins are free of neoplastic tissue. After endoscopic clearance of a malignant polyp, a repeat colonoscopy should be performed after 3 months.

Polyps, which are poorly differentiated, show signs of lymphovascular invasion, are cancerous at the level of the resection margin (less than 2 mm margin), invade the lamina muscularis propria (T2), or arise from a flat polyp require colectomy. The likelihood of lymph node involvement in polyp cancers can be inferred by histological classifications (e.g., Haggitt and Kikuchi) and the depth of invasion in pedunculated and sessile polyps.

13.5.2 Surveillance After Resection of Colonic Polyps

Follow-up after resection of colonic polyps must consider risk of recurrence as well as risk of cancer development. Low-risk adenomas are one or two adenomas smaller than 10 mm. High-risk adenomas are either three or more in number or are larger than 10 mm or have villous histology or have high-grade dysplasia.

Surveillance after removal of high-risk adenoma should be done after 18 months to 3 years. Patients with high-risk adenomas remain in the high-risk group and should be followed up within the high-risk time frame even if a negative colonoscopy has been done. If complete resection of a high-risk polyp is uncertain, a repeat colonoscopy should be performed within 3–6 months. A malignant polyp should be followed up within 3 months.

The number of polyps removed at colonoscopy and the absolute number of polyps removed during all colonoscopies of an individual patient are the most significant risk factors for metachronous colorectal cancer.

Low-risk polyps should be followed up after 3–5 years. If a surveillance colonoscopy after removal of low-risk polyp is negative, a repeat colonoscopy should be done after a maximum of 10 years.

13.5.3 Surveillance After Colorectal Cancer Resection

Disease recurrence after resection of stage 2 (T3/T4, node negative) and stage 3 (any T, node positive) colorectal cancer can be observed in more than 40% of patients despite adequate adjuvant oncological treatment. The majority of tumor recurrences develop within the first 5 years after surgery. The early detection of metachronous and/or metastatic disease can potentially allow for live-saving surgery or an early start to palliative chemotherapy/radiotherapy. Published guidelines and surveillance protocols applied by treating physicians vary significantly, and there is no standardized follow-up program.

A survival benefit has been shown for patients participating in an intensive postoperative follow-up program. This program includes:

- Clinical reviews every 3 months for 2 years after surgery, followed by 6 monthly reviews until the end of year 5. We continue our follow-up program once a year until 10 years after resection.
- Tumor marker measurement (carcinoembryonic antigen, CEA) at every clinical review; it is recommended to use the same assay for each of these CEA measurements; the lead time of elevated CEA levels prior to detection of metastatic/recurrent disease has been observed to be as long as 6 months.
- Computed tomography (chest, abdomen, pelvis) yearly for 3 years after surgery (thereafter depending on other findings at the time of follow-up).
- Colonoscopy prior to and 1 year after surgery and every 3 years thereafter (intervals depend on colonoscopy findings); flexible sigmoidoscopy every 6 months for 3 years after resection of rectal cancer.

If a complete colonoscopy cannot be done at the time of surgery, this needs to be completed within 6 months of surgery to identify the potential existence of synchronous cancers (up to 5% of all patients). Metachronous cancers develop in up to 3% of patients within the first 5 years after surgery (half of these are found within the first 2 years after surgery and might have been missed at the time of initial diagnosis).

It appears that asymptomatic recurrent disease is more likely to undergo curative resection and the survival benefit for patients undergoing intensive follow-up after curative resection of colorectal cancer has been confirmed by meta-analysis of randomized trials.

The cost-effectiveness of intensive follow-up programs has been confirmed, and it has been shown that the adjusted cost per year of lives saved is US $5884 which is well below the accepted AU$ 50,000–100,000 per quality-adjusted life year gained.

Currently there is no clear recommendation to include patients after surgical treatment of stage 1 (T1 or T2, node negative) disease in the follow-up program. We routinely follow all patients including palliative resections with the same intensive follow-up program as outlined above. This approach to stage 4 disease is supported by other groups as well.

After the completion of an intensive follow-up program (5–10 years after surgery depending on the program), a clear understanding about who will be responsible for the surveillance during long-term survivorship needs to be reached between the patient, the clinician responsible for the intensive follow-up program (surgeon or medical oncologist), and the primary care provider (general practitioner).

13.5.4 Inflammatory Bowel Disease

Surveillance of patients with inflammatory bowel disease (IBD) aims to detect dysplasia early and to reduce mortality in patients who develop colorectal cancer. The risk of developing colorectal cancer is increased in patients suffering from IBD. The onset of disease is at an earlier mean age (50 years) when compared to patients with sporadic colorectal cancer (60 years).

13.5.5 Ulcerative Colitis (UC)

The risk for patients suffering from UC of developing colorectal cancer is increased with longer duration (longer than 20 years), higher activity, and larger extent (beyond the left colonic flexure) of the disease.

13.5.6 Crohn's Disease

The risk of developing colorectal cancer for patients with Crohn's disease of the colon appears to be similar to the risk of patients with UC.

Dysplasia can be found at sites distant from active inflammatory bowel disease (IBD) and synchronous tumors are more common in patient with IBD. Lesions detected on surveillance colonoscopy need to be described regarding their location (inside or outside of an area with colitis), morphology (polypoid or nonpolypoid), borders (distinct or indistinct), and evidence of submucosal invasion (ulceration, failure to lift).

Surveillance of patients with IBD should start at 5 years after initial diagnosis of colitis associated with IBD, and it is important to confirm mucosal healing after instituting treatment. In patients with extensive disease (more than one third of the bowel affected), surveillance should be performed every 3 years. Patients with a pouch (pouchoscopy) or a rectal stump after subtotal colectomy should be examined via endoscopy every 3 years. In patients with primary sclerosing cholangitis (PSC), screening should start with the diagnosis of PSC.

For surveillance, chromoendoscopy with the topical application of indigo carmine or methylene blue to enhance mucosal irregularities is recommended. Alternatively, high-definition white light colonoscopy with random and targeted biopsies can be used. With this approach to surveillance, four biopsies are taken every 10 cm from the caecum to the rectum, resulting in a minimum of 33 biopsies.

In patients with dysplastic polyps larger than 10 mm, surveillance colonoscopy is indicated at 6 and 12 months after the resection depending on the certainty of completeness of excision. Polyps smaller than 10 mm require surveillance at 12 months after resection.

The standard diagnostic procedure in long-lasting UC is to take four biopsies every 10 cm. Colitis-associated intraepithelial neoplasms may occur in flat mucosa of endoscopically normal appearance or may arise as dysplasia-associated lesion or mass (DALM), which may be indistinguishable from sporadic adenomas in healthy or non-colitis mucosa. For patients with DALM, (sub)total colectomy should be considered.

In patients with IBD, invisible dysplasia can be identified in random biopsies. This condition requires referral to a center offering high-definition chromoendoscopy.

Inflammatory pseudopolyps are islands of residual intact colonic mucosa and are a sign of prior severe inflammation and as such indicate the increased risk of colorectal cancer. Colonic strictures as a complication of IBD also indicate prior severe disease and require close surveillance due to the increased risk of colorectal cancer.

Chemoprevention of colorectal cancer in patients with IBD aims at control of disease activity and extent. No treatment has been shown to be superior in this setting. 5-aminosalicylates have a good safety profile, provide anti-inflammatory effects, and may have an anticarcinogenic effect. These agents (i.e., mesalamine) should be considered for chemoprevention in patients suffering from IBD.

13.5.7 Familial Adenomatous Polyposis (FAP)

FAP is an autosomal dominant disease caused by mutations in the Adenomatous Polyposis Coli gene. Classic FAP is characterized by presence of more than 100 colorectal polyps and carries a 100% risk of developing colorectal cancer. The attenuated form of FAP (AFAP) is characterized by fewer colorectal polyps with a later age of onset of disease and a 80% lifetime risk of developing colorectal cancer.

Screening or genetic testing for FAP is recommended in individuals:

- Who are first-degree relatives of patients with FAP with more than ten cumulative colorectal adenomas in combination with other features of FAP: duodenal adenoma, desmoid tumors, thyroid cancer, epidermal cysts, osteomas, and congenital hypertrophy of retinal pigment epithelium (CHRPE, present in 90% of the FAP population).

Screening should start at age 10 and should be repeated annually.

Indications for colectomy in these patients are:

- Colorectal cancer.
- The large number of adenomas makes endoscopic clearance impossible.
- High-grade dysplasia, multiple polyps larger than 6 mm.
- Significant increase in polyp number between investigations.
- Inability to perform adequate surveillance.

Surgical options for patients with FAP include total colectomy with ileorectal anastomosis (IRA), proctocolectomy with ileal pouch-anal anastomosis (IPAA), or proctocolectomy with end ileostomy. Elective colectomy can only be deferred to the late teens in patients with classic FAP who present with few (less than 10) or small polyps (less than 5 mm). The risk of colorectal cancer is not completely eliminated with proctocolectomy/colectomy, and the remnant large bowel must undergo endoscopy annually.

Additional screening for patients with FAP/AFAP must include:

- Endoscopic surveillance of the upper gastrointestinal tract every 3 years with the onset of colonic polyposis or at age 25, with all identified polyps removed.
- Annual thyroid ultrasound.

13.5.8 When to Transfer

If dysplasia is confirmed in a patient with Barrett's esophagus on four-quadrant biopsies, the patient should be referred for endoscopic eradication.

Adequate imaging must be carried out for diagnosis and surveillance of hepatic and pancreatic lesions. This includes MRI scanning and/or endoscopic ultrasound with or without, fine needle aspiration. If these diagnostic modalities are not available, patients should be referred to another center for these investigations to occur. Surgical treatment requires adequate intensive care support, the availability of radiological/endoscopic interventions, as well as surgical experience. Transfers should be arranged accordingly prior to elective surgery in patients suitable for surgical treatment.

Recommended Reading

https://radiopaedia.org/articles/fukuoka-consensus-guidelines-1.

Kastelein F, et al. Proton pump inhibitors reduce the risk of neoplastic progression in patients with Barrett's esophagus. Clin Gastroenterol Hepatol. 2013;11:382.

Neumann H, et al. Cancer risk in IBD: How to diagnose and how to manage DALM and ALM. World J Gastroenterol. 2011;17:3184–91.

Pita-Fernandez S, et al. Intensive follow-up strategies improve outcomes in nonmetastatic colorectal cancer patients after curative surgery: a systematic review and meta-analysis. Ann Oncol. 2015;26:644.

Renehan AG, O'Dwyer ST, Whynes DK. Cost effectiveness analysis of intensive versus conventional follow-up after curative resection for colorectal cancer. BMJ. 2004;328:81.

UpTo Date®: Barrett's esophagus: Surveillance and management.

UpTo Date®: Biliary cysts.

UpTo Date®: Classification of pancreatic cysts.

UpTo Date®: Epidemiology and nonfamilial risk factors for exocrine pancreatic cancer.

UpTo Date®: Familial adenomatous polyposis: Screening and management of patients and families.

UpTo Date®: Gastric intestinal metaplasia.

UpTo Date®: Gastric polyps.

UpTo Date®: Hepatic adenoma.

UpToDate®: Intraductal papillary mucinous neoplasm of the pancreas (IPPM): Evaluation and management

UpTo Date®: Large gastric folds: Hyperplastic and nonhyperplastic gastropathies.

UpTo Date®: Overview of colon polyps.

UpTo Date®: Solid liver lesions: Differential diagnosis and evaluation.

UpTo Date®: Surveillance after colorectal cancer resection.

UpTo Date®: Surveillance and management of dysplasia in patients with inflammatory bowel disease.

Waddel T, et al. Gastric cancer: ESMO-ESSO-ESTRO clinical practice guidelines for diagnosis, treatment and follow-up. EJSO. 2014;40:584–91.

Acute and Chronic Liver Failure

14

Garry R. Nind

Acute liver failure is defined as development of a severe, critical liver injury associated with hepatic encephalopathy and impaired hepatic synthetic function (INR > 1.5) in a patient not previously known to have liver disease. The latter part of this definition allows patients presenting with liver failure secondary to previously undiagnosed Wilson disease, autoimmune hepatitis and hepatitis B to be included in this definition even though they have an underlying liver disease and may even have cirrhosis. The time course that differentiates acute from chronic liver failure varies between guidelines, but if the liver disease has been present for less than 26 weeks, it is generally considered to be acute.

Chronic liver failure is also often referred to as decompensated cirrhosis. This is defined as the development of complications of cirrhosis such as variceal bleeding, ascites, encephalopathy, spontaneous bacterial peritonitis or the hepatorenal syndrome. Such patients usually have significantly impaired hepatic synthetic function and have a worse prognosis than those with compensated cirrhosis.

So why is it important for a surgeon to have an understanding of liver failure? Occasionally patients presenting with jaundice may have liver failure rather than biliary disease. Operating or performing procedures such as an endoscopic retrograde cholangiopancreatography [ERCP] on a patient with liver failure can result in significant morbidity and mortality.

G. R. Nind (✉)
Department of Gastroenterology and Hepatology, The Queen Elizabeth Hospital, Woodville South, SA, Australia
e-mail: garry.nind@sa.gov.au

M. W. Wichmann et al. (eds.), *Gastroenterology For General Surgeons*,
https://doi.org/10.1007/978-3-319-92768-8_14

14.1 Acute Liver Failure

Acute liver failure has a variety of causes with viruses and drugs being the most common worldwide. In the Western world, acetaminophen overdose is the most common cause. In Asia and Africa, it is still viral hepatitis.

The hepatotoxicity associated with acetaminophen is dose-dependent and rarely occurs when doses of less than 4 g/day are ingested, except in the setting of pre-existing liver disease. Most cases of overdose are related to attempted suicide, but occasional patients take multiple medications containing acetaminophen inadvertently or fail to take the drug as directed. Acetaminophen can also cause acute liver failure when taken in therapeutic doses, particularly in alcoholics or in patients taking certain medications such as anticonvulsant drugs which induce the cytochrome P450 system.

Idiosyncratic drug reactions or what is now commonly referred to as drug-induced liver injury (DILI) can cause liver failure in a dose-independent fashion, usually within 6 months of starting the drug. DILI is commonly caused by antibiotics and anticonvulsant drugs, but certain herbal treatments and dietary supplements can also be responsible.

Another cause that is being increasingly recognised is ischemic hepatitis. This is usually caused by systemic hypotension leading to hepatic hypoperfusion but may occasionally result from decreased perfusion of the liver alone. The common causes of systemic hypotension leading to hepatic hypoperfusion are sepsis, cardiac dysfunction and drugs, whereas isolated hepatic hypoperfusion can be seen with the Budd-Chiari syndrome and sinusoidal obstructive syndrome.

The development of acute liver failure from viral infections is uncommon in Western countries but may occur with hepatitis A, hepatitis B (with or without hepatitis D co-infection) and hepatitis E. Hepatitis C, herpes simplex viruses 1 and 2, and Epstein-Barr virus are rare causes of acute liver failure in immunocompetent individuals but need to be considered in immunosuppressed patients.

14.1.1 Clinical Manifestations of Acute Liver Failure

Patients with acute liver failure should have signs of hepatic encephalopathy and will often have jaundice, right upper quadrant pain and tender hepatomegaly. Early symptoms can be non-specific such as anorexia, nausea, vomiting, lethargy and fatigue. The features of encephalopathy range from subtle changes in behaviour to coma, and are outlined in the West Haven criteria (Fig. 14.1). The grade of encephalopathy is important because of the association with cerebral oedema and raised intracranial pressure. These complications are uncommon with encephalopathy grades 0–2 but occur in 25–35% of patients with grade 3 and in 75% of patients with grade 4. The signs of rising intracranial pressure are loss of pupillary responses due to brainstem herniation, and Cushing's triad of systemic hypertension, bradycardia and respiratory depression. It is important to differentiate acute liver failure from

West Haven criteria for classification of hepatic encephalopathy

- Grade 0 - No obvious changes, potentially mild decrease in intellectual ability and coordination
- Grade 1 - Trivial lack of awareness; euphoria or anxiety; shortened attention span; impaired performance of addition or subtraction
- Grade 2 - Lethargy or apathy; minimal disorientation for time or place; subtle personality change; inappropriate behaviour
- Grade 3 - Somnolence to semi-stupor, responsive to verbal stimuli; confusion; gross disorientation
- Grade 4 - Coma

Fig. 14.1 West Haven criteria for classification of hepatic encephalopathy

acute severe hepatitis with associated coagulopathy and a high serum bilirubin as the latter has a much better prognosis.

14.1.2 Laboratory Test and Imaging Abnormalities in Acute Liver Failure

In acute liver failure, the INR is $\geq$1.5, and the serum transaminases are commonly $\geq$1000 IU/mL with an elevated serum bilirubin. In relation to prognosis, the transaminases need to be viewed in the in the context of INR and serum bilirubin levels. If the transaminases fall and the INR and bilirubin improve, the liver failure is recovering. However, if the transaminases fall and the serum bilirubin and INR continue to rise, the liver failure is worsening as the falling transaminases signal a loss of functioning hepatic mass. Because of the importance of INR in determining the patient's prognosis, it is recommended that blood products such as fresh frozen plasma and cryoprecipitate only be administered if there is bleeding or the need for interventional procedures.

Approximately 30–70% of patients with acute liver failure have renal impairment. This appears to be a poor prognostic marker and may require treatment with hemodialysis. Hypoglycemia may also occur as the failing liver cannot make glucose from lactate via gluconeogenesis. This may lead to the development of a metabolic acidosis due to accumulation of lactate.

When a patient with suspected acute liver failure is admitted, appropriate imaging should be utilised to identify possibilities such as underlying cirrhosis and portal hypertension, Budd-Chiari syndrome and invasive malignancy. Abdominal ultrasound scans are frequently used as they do not involve the use of nephrotoxic contrast agents. However, if there is a suspicion that the patient may have Budd-Chiari syndrome or a malignancy and the ultrasound scan is inconclusive, an abdominal CT or MRI scan should be performed. If a cause cannot be determined by imaging or laboratory tests, a liver biopsy should be considered. This is usually performed by the transjugular approach because of concerns about bleeding.

The cause of an episode of acute liver failure can be determined in about 60% of cases. This is generally made by a combination of history, laboratory investigations and imaging studies. Liver biopsy is rarely needed but may guide initial management and provide prognostic information in some settings.

14.1.3 Management

The diagnosis of acute liver failure will almost always lead to referral to a tertiary hospital, ideally a liver transplant centre. Most will be managed in intensive care units, sometimes dedicated to acute and chronic liver disease. Particular issues include fluid balance, persistent hypotension, encephalopathy, renal impairment, gastrointestinal bleeding, infections, nutrition and the timing of liver transplantation. The major role of the general surgeon is the recognition of acute liver failure at an early stage and early referral to an appropriate liver unit.

An additional issue is the early use of *N*-acetyl cysteine in patients who have taken an overdose of acetaminophen. Cases of severe liver injury are largely abolished if *N*-acetyl cysteine is given within 12 h of acetaminophen ingestion, and, because of this, most hospitals have protocols for the administration of this drug in the emergency service and after admission as an inpatient. Whether *N*-acetyl cysteine is helpful in other causes of acute liver failure is debated. In one study, transplant-free survival in acute liver failure was somewhat higher in those randomised to *N*-acetyl cysteine [40%] than in those randomised to placebo [27%].

The detailed management of patients with acute liver failure is outside the scope of this chapter. However, one issue of relevance is fluid balance as many patients with acute liver failure are hypotensive, largely due to a decrease in systemic vascular resistance. The volume and choice of rehydration fluid will be influenced by levels of electrolytes, glucose, lactate and pH. Overhydration needs to be avoided as it may exacerbate cerebral edema. Even after fluid resuscitation, some patients are unable to maintain a mean arterial pressure of >75 mmHg. In this situation, vasopressor support is often initiated with noradrenaline to augment peripheral organ and splanchnic perfusion.

Another issue is the prophylactic use of antibiotics. Patients with liver failure in intensive care units are at high risk for the development of various infections including fungal infections. However, the prophylactic use of antibiotics is not recommended in guidelines from either the American Association for the Study of Liver Diseases (AASLD) or the European Association for the Study of the Liver (EASL). Rather, the recommendation is for regular surveillance cultures of blood and urine, as well as daily chest X-rays followed by treatment with antibiotics for active infections, positive surveillance cultures or unexplained clinical deterioration.

Oral nutrition should be encouraged in patients with grade I or II encephalopathy and is usually sufficient to meet caloric requirements. With grade III or IV encephalopathy, naso-enteric feeding may be adequate although some patients develop slow gastric emptying and may need a post-pyloric tube or, in rare cases, total parenteral nutrition. Because of the risk of bleeding from the upper gastrointestinal tract, most patients receive a proton-pump inhibitor despite a marginal increase in risk for *Clostridium difficile* colitis and pneumonia.

The management of encephalopathy and cerebral edema is a highly specialised area, largely restricted to dedicated transplant physicians. Patients who develop grade lll encephalopathy are usually intubated and ventilated to protect the airway. Intracranial pressure monitoring is helpful for documentation of intracranial pressure, but its use is now debated because of bleeding complications and a lack of evidence for an effect on patient outcomes. Therapeutic options for cerebral oedema include infusions of hypertonic saline or mannitol and hyperventilation.

Risks of acute kidney injury can be reduced by careful monitoring of fluid balance, maintenance of blood pressure, avoidance of nephrotoxic drugs and prompt treatment of infections. Kidney injury is more common with acetaminophen toxicity than with other causes of acute liver failure. Once kidney injury develops, it is usually progressive and is associated with a poor prognosis unless the patient receives a liver transplant.

14.1.4 Prognosis

King's criteria are often used to determine the prognosis in acute liver failure and to determine who should be considered for liver transplantation. These were developed at King's College London and are different for liver failure induced by acetaminophen to liver failure with other etiologies. For acetaminophen-induced acute liver failure, patients should be immediately referred for liver transplantation on arrival to hospital if:

- Arterial pH is <7.3 irrespective of grade of hepatic encephalopathy.
- Grade III or IV hepatic encephalopathy is present with INR of >6.5 or a serum creatinine of >300 µmol/L.

For other causes, any patient with an INR >6.5 should be referred to a liver transplant centre. Patients should also be referred if they have any three of the following:

- Age <10 or >40 years
- Unfavourable aetiology such as drug-induced liver injury, Wilson's disease or non-A and non-B viral hepatitis
- >7 days between the onset of jaundice and the development of encephalopathy
- INR > 3.5
- Serum bilirubin >300 µmol/L

The Model for End-Stage Liver Disease [MELD] score has also been used to predict survival in patients with acute liver failure and, if >32, has a similar predictive value for mortality as King's criteria. However, the ability of these criteria to predict mortality, particularly in non-acetaminophen overdose, is decreasing probably due to improvements in medical management. Currently, approximately 55% will survive without needing liver transplantation. For those who do undergo a transplant, the 1-year survival rate is 80%, with those who die usually doing so within the first 3 months post-transplant from neurologic complications or sepsis.

14.2 Chronic Liver Failure

Chronic liver failure is another term for decompensated cirrhosis. Cirrhosis represents the end stage of hepatic fibrosis with distortion of the normal hepatic lobular architecture and the formation of nodules. This was considered an irreversible process, but it is now known to be reversible in some patients if there is successful treatment of the underlying cause. The causes of cirrhosis are numerous and bring about hepatic fibrosis by causing either chronic hepatic inflammation or cholestasis. The most common causes of cirrhosis in the Western world are hepatitis C infection, alcohol abuse and non-alcoholic steatohepatitis (NASH). In contrast, viral hepatitis, particularly hepatitis B, is the most common cause of cirrhosis in Asia and Africa. Some patients have two or more factors causing them to develop cirrhosis such as hepatitis C and alcoholism. It is also relevant that not everyone who has alcoholism, viral hepatitis or NASH develops cirrhosis. This only occurs in 10–20% of alcoholics but has a higher frequency of up to 50% after prolonged infections with hepatitis C. The data for the risk of NASH progressing to cirrhosis is not currently clear.

The frequency of various causes for cirrhosis seems likely to change as increasing numbers of patients with hepatitis C are cured by new direct-acting antiviral drugs. However, the obesity epidemic in many Western countries such as the USA, UK and Australia raises the possibility of increasing numbers of patients with NASH such that this diagnosis will become the most common cause of cirrhosis in the future.

14.2.1 Clinical Features

The symptoms of compensated cirrhosis tend to be non-specific. With decompensated cirrhosis, symptoms are variable but include jaundice, pruritis, gastrointestinal bleeding, abdominal distension and confusion. Furthermore, patients with decompensated liver disease often develop sexual dysfunction. Women often stop ovulating and menstruating, and men can become impotent. These changes in men with cirrhosis are particularly associated with liver disease due to alcohol abuse or hemochromatosis.

Some of the physical signs of advanced liver disease can be evident with compensated cirrhosis. Common signs are spider naevi, palmar erythema and gynecomastia. With the development of portal hypertension and decompensation, signs include splenomegaly, ascites, a caput medusa and asterixis. Clubbing is more commonly seen with cholestatic liver diseases and the development of hepatopulmonary syndrome. The latter is due to intrapulmonary vascular shunts in the setting of advanced liver disease that cause dyspnea on standing. Hepatomegaly is unusual in cirrhosis as the liver tends to be small because of the fibrotic scarring. However, cirrhosis due to the cholestatic liver diseases, NASH and alcohol abuse can be associated with an enlarged liver.

Blood tests in decompensated liver disease usually reveal impaired hepatic synthetic function. This leads to elevation of the serum bilirubin and INR and lowering of the serum albumin. With the development of portal hypertension with splenomegaly, thrombocytopaenia and even pancytopaenia can occur because of splenic sequestration of blood cells. Renal function can also be impaired due to a variety of causes including adverse effects from medication, vascular changes associated with liver disease [hepatorenal syndrome] and disorders such as diabetes that are associated with NASH. As most patients with advanced liver disease have sarcopaenia, the serum urea and creatinine tend to be at the lower end of the normal range.

On abdominal ultrasound, CT or MRI, the presence of cirrhosis is suggested by the presence of an irregular liver margin, recanalization of the umbilical vein and/or a dilated portal vein. The latter finding indicates the development of portal hypertension which can be associated with radiologic evidence of splenomegaly, varices and ascites. If the diagnosis of cirrhosis is not clear from clinical examination, laboratory investigations and imaging, then either a liver biopsy or transient liver elastography can be performed. The latter is now in common use and provides a non-invasive way of assessing hepatic fibrosis. With this technique, waves of low frequency and amplitude are sent from a transducer placed on the skin in an intercostal space through the liver parenchyma. The speed at which these waves travel is higher in fibrotic or cirrhotic livers and is expressed as a higher kPa score. Although the test has some limitations, it has the advantages of simplicity and safety. Liver biopsy has now become infrequent because of the small risk of complications and the diagnostic accuracy of non-invasive investigations including various blood test and elastography.

The major complications of cirrhosis occur with the development of portal hypertension and include:

- Variceal hemorrhage
- Ascites and hepatic hydrothorax
- Spontaneous bacterial peritonitis
- Hepatic encephalopathy
- Hepatorenal syndrome

Portal hypertension develops when resistance to portal blood flow through the liver increases and results in an increase in portal collateral flow to get blood to the systemic circulation. The increased intrahepatic resistance to blood flow is due to structural changes in the liver and to dynamic vascular changes. The structural changes result from distortion of the hepatic circulation by fibrosis, cirrhotic nodule formation, vascular occlusion and angiogenesis. The dynamic changes result from contraction of myofibroblasts and activated stellate cells that surround the hepatic sinusoids in response to increased production of vasoconstrictor substances such as the endothelins and thromboxane A2 as well as reduced release of endothelial vasodilators such as nitric oxide. As the portal pressure increases, there is increased release of vasodilator substances such as nitric oxide in the splanchnic circulation, leading to arteriolar vasodilation and angiogenesis. In addition to allowing the portal pressure to increase further, these changes also can lead to systemic hypotension due to apparent underfilling of the systemic circulation. This results in the stimulation of endogenous vasoactive systems such as the renin-angiotensin-aldosterone system and sympathetic nervous system with increased absorption of sodium and water by the kidneys and increased cardiac output. Collateral blood vessels of clinical significance are usually located in the lower oesophagus, upper stomach and/or rectum and are commonly called varices.

The hepatic venous pressure gradient (HVPG) is the pressure gradient between the portal vein and inferior vena cava. The normal HVPG is 1–5 mmHg, but portal hypertension does not usually become clinically significant until the HVPG is ≥10 mmHg. Above 12 mmHg, there is an increased risk of variceal bleeding and other complications of portal hypertension such as ascites.

14.2.2 Complications of Decompensated Cirrhosis

14.2.2.1 Bleeding Varices

Here I will only deal with upper gastrointestinal variceal bleeding as rectal variceal bleeding is uncommon. Patients with upper gastrointestinal variceal hemorrhage present with hematemesis and/or melena. Overall, gastroesophageal varices are present in 50% of patients with cirrhosis. However, the more advanced the liver disease, the higher the risk of varices.

The outcome of an episode of variceal bleeding depends on whether the bleeding can be controlled and whether other major complications can be avoided. It is important to remember that not all upper GI bleeding in a patient with cirrhosis is due to varices. These patients may also have portal hypertensive gastropathy and are at increased risk for gastric antral vascular ectasia and peptic ulcers.

There are two phases of variceal bleeding: an acute phase and a late phase. Only about 50% of acute variceal bleeds cease spontaneously, and the rate is lower in patients with Child-Pugh C cirrhosis and in those with HVPG >20 mmHg or active infections. Because of the latter and the association with multi-organ failure, prophylactic antibiotics are recommended in patients with variceal bleeding. The risk of dying from variceal bleeding is 20–30%, and, for about 6 weeks post bleed, there is a high risk of recurrent bleeding. This risk is greatest in the first 48–72 h after the acute bleed and is higher in patients aged >60 years with large varices, an initial severe bleed or a bleed complicated by kidney injury. If the patient survives this 6-week period, the risk of having another variceal bleed and dying returns to that of a cirrhotic patient with the same degree of decompensation.

If a patient presents with a variceal bleed, they are categorised as having decompensated cirrhosis. However, survival depends on whether this is their first evidence of decompensation or if they already have had decompensation due to the development of such things as ascites or encephalopathy. For the former scenario, the 5-year mortality rate is 20%, but for the latter it is 80%. The three principles for the management of an acute variceal bleed are:

- Resuscitation
- Treatment of bleeding
- Prevention and treatment of complications

A variceal bleed is a medical emergency. The patient needs volume resuscitation to restore and maintain their circulating blood volume and hemodynamic stability. In cirrhosis, there is some evidence of benefit from a restrictive transfusion policy in patients with Child-Pugh A and B but not with Child-Pugh C. The restrictive policy defers transfusion until the haemoglobin level falls to 70 g/L or lower. At present, there is no evidence from randomized controlled trials to support correction of an elevated INR with fresh frozen plasma or recombinant factor VIIIa, or correction of a low platelet count with platelet transfusions.

Vasoactive drugs, either octreotide or terlipressin, should be started as soon as possible in a patient suspected of having a variceal bleed. These agents appear to be similarly effective with a lower 7-day all-cause mortality and a decrease in transfusion requirements. Endoscopy should be performed within 12 h of presentation to the emergency service, and, if varices appear to be the cause of the bleeding, they should be treated with variceal band ligation. Band ligation has been shown to have fewer complications and less rebleeding than sclerotherapy, although both are equivalent at initial control of bleeding. If the bleeding can be controlled by the above measures, the patient should remain on vasoactive drugs for up to 5 days, particularly if they have advanced liver disease.

If bleeding persists despite combined pharmacologic and endoscopic therapy, options include a second-look endoscopy for modest rebleeding and other options for major bleeding. The latter may include a Sengstaken-Blakemore, Linton or Minnesota tube, a covered esophageal stent or a transjugular intrahepatic portosystemic shunt [TIPS]. Experience with these techniques is likely to be limited, but some rural surgeons may feel competent to manage a Minnesota or similar tube. This involves passing the tube into the stomach, inflation of a large gastric balloon and maintenance of tension on the balloon for up to 24 h.

Following an episode of acute variceal hemorrhage, the aim should be to prevent further bleeding. In a patient who has not needed TIPS insertion, the combination of a non-selective β-blocker such as propranolol or nadolol, and band ligation is the preferred treatment option. This combination is better than band ligation alone and marginally better than a β-blocker alone.

Bleeding gastric varices are usually caused by portal hypertension, but a minority are related to portal or splenic vein thrombosis. Bleeding varices from portal hypertension are usually managed with the intravariceal injection of cyanoacrylate, but there is some risk of migration of glue into the lungs. As for esophageal varices, the combination of β-blockers and endoscopic therapy should be first-line therapy to prevent rebleeding. Varices associated with portal or splenic vein thromboses may require splenectomy or a complex radiological procedure called balloon-occluded retrograde transvenous occlusion that occludes splenorenal collaterals. The latter procedure is not widely available.

14.2.2.2 Ascites

Cirrhosis is the most common cause for ascites, accounting for approximately 85% of all cases. It is one of the consequences of portal hypertension and tends to develop after the formation of varices. In patients with compensated cirrhosis, 50% will develop this complication within 10 years.

Ascites develops because of a marked reduction in systemic vascular resistance, leading to a fall in mean arterial pressure and an increase in cardiac output. As a consequence of this and what appears to be a lack of circulating arterial blood volume, there is activation of the renin-angiotensin-aldosterone system and sympathetic nervous system as well as increased secretion of antidiuretic hormone. This leads to avid retention of sodium and water by the kidneys with the predominant movement of retained fluid to the splanchnic circulation. As portal pressure increases, changes in the balance of Starling's forces leads to an excess of ultrafiltration over reabsorption in the portal circulation and the development of ascites.

A patient who has developed ascites typically presents with abdominal distension, discomfort and shortness of breath. These symptoms usually develop gradually, and, on examination, the patient will demonstrate dullness of the flanks and, often, shifting dullness. They may also have pleural effusions, particularly on the right.

The presence of ascites, cirrhosis and portal hypertension can be confirmed by imaging. Abdominal CT and MRI scans can also largely exclude malignancy as the cause for the ascites. To confirm ascites is due to portal hypertension, a diagnostic ascitic tap should be performed and sent with a blood sample to determine the serum-to-ascites albumin gradient. A gradient of >11 g/L predicts that the ascites is due to portal hypertension in >97% of cases. A gradient of <11 g/L suggests that the ascites is due to malignancy, infection or some rarer cause.

The management of ascites includes a low-salt diet (<88 mmol of sodium per day) and oral diuretics. Fluid restriction is not required unless the patient has significant hyponatraemia that does not respond to cessation of diuretics. The initial diuretic regimen used by most hepatologists is the combination of spironolactone and furosemide. These are typically given in the ratio of spironolactone 100 mg/day: furosemide 40 mg/day and can be titrated up every 3–5 days to a maximum recommended dose of spironolactone of 400 mg/day and furosemide 160 mg/day. As spironolactone has a long half-life, it only needs to be given once daily, and giving both drugs together in the morning maximises patient adherence and drug effectiveness while minimising nocturia. The rate of fluid loss with the above regimen depends on the presence or absence of peripheral oedema. If peripheral edema is absent, fluid loss should be <0.75 kg per day as more rapid loss may cause the plasma volume to fall and precipitate acute kidney injury.

The initial treatment of tense ascites can include removal of fluid by paracentesis. Removal of less than 5 L of ascites does not appear to have hemodynamic or hormonal consequences and can be performed without the infusion of colloid. However, for volumes greater than 5 L, meta-analysis has shown a survival advantage when 6–8 g of albumin is administered for every 1 L of ascitic fluid removed.

About 10% of patients will develop refractory ascites, usually due to irreversible liver injury or to progress from diuretic-responsive ascites to diuretic-refractory ascites. It is important to exclude failure to adhere to dietary sodium restriction as the cause by checking urinary sodium excretion. This should be <78 mEq/day. If urinary sodium excretion is <30 mEq/day, diuretics should be ceased. It may also be helpful to cease drugs that decrease renal perfusion such as β-blockers, ACE inhibitors, angiotensin receptor blockers or non-steroidal anti-inflammatory drugs. If these measures do not help and the patient is not considered a candidate for liver transplantation, other available options are recurrent large volume paracenteses or the placement of a TIPS. The latter is only likely to be available in tertiary centres and is normally restricted to patients with a MELD score of <18 who have not had severe spontaneous encephalopathy and do not have cardiac failure or pulmonary hypertension.

14.2.2.3 Hepatic Hydrothorax

Hepatic hydrothorax is the development of a pleural effusion in a patient with ascites. Effusions develop because of the passage of ascitic fluid from the peritoneal to the pleural cavity through small defects in the tendinous portion of the diaphragm, defects that are more common in the right than the left hemi-diaphragm. The passage of the ascitic fluid is driven by the negative intrathoracic pressures that are generated during respiration. The treatment of hepatic hydrothorax is similar to that of ascites.

14.2.2.4 Spontaneous Bacterial Peritonitis

Spontaneous bacterial peritonitis is the development of an infection in ascitic fluid in the absence of evidence of another intra-abdominal source of infection. The typical presentation is with fever and abdominal pain, but other presentations include more severe ascites or decompensation of the liver disease. The diagnosis is established by the presence of an ascitic fluid neutrophil count of $\geq 250/\text{mm}^3$ and a positive ascitic fluid culture. However, if a cirrhotic patient is suspected of having spontaneous bacterial peritonitis, they should be started on empiric, broad-spectrum antibiotic therapy prior to the results of paracentesis. Often the patient will have culture-negative neutrocytic ascites where the ascitic fluid polymorph count is $>250\ \text{mm}^3$ but no organism is grown. Most of these patients actually have spontaneous bacterial peritonitis and should still be treated with broad-spectrum antibiotics.

Most cases of spontaneous bacterial peritonitis are due to *Escherichia coli* or *Klebsiella* species, but staphylococcal and streptococcal infections can occur. Therefore, broad-spectrum antibiotics need to be prescribed until the causative organism and antibiotic sensitivities are known. In the past, cefotaxime and ceftriaxone were the most commonly used antibiotics, but, with the increase in microbial resistance to third-generation cephalosporins, there is increasing use of antibiotics such as levofloxacin and piperacillin/tazobactam. Trials have shown that a 5-day course of antibiotics is usually effective for treatment unless the infecting organism is resistant to standard antibiotics or is associated with endocarditis.

Renal failure develops in 30–40% of patients who have spontaneous bacterial peritonitis and is associated with increased mortality. A meta-analysis has shown that infusion of concentrated albumin at 1.5 g/kg of body weight on day 1, then 1 g/kg of body weight on day 3, significantly decreases the incidence of renal impairment and lowers mortality. It should be used in those patients who have a serum creatinine of >88 μmol/L, a serum urea of >10.7 mmol/L and/or a bilirubin of >68 μmol.

The mortality from an episode of spontaneous bacterial peritonitis can be as high as 40%, partly because this complication is largely restricted to advanced liver disease. Furthermore, these patients have a 70% risk of recurrent disease within 12 months, a risk that can be reduced with prophylactic antibiotics, usually trimethoprim-sulphamethoxazole.

14.2.2.5 Hepatic Encephalopathy

Overt hepatic encephalopathy develops in 30–45% of patients with cirrhosis. It encompasses a spectrum of potentially reversible neuropsychiatric abnormalities ranging from mild confusion and altered behaviour (grade 1) to coma (grade 4). This results from the shunting of toxins normally metabolised or removed by the liver from the portal circulation to the systemic circulation, allowing them to reach the brain. Ammonia is the best characterised neurotoxin in hepatic encephalopathy, but other agents such as gamma-amino butyric acid have also been implicated.

The primary source of ammonia is the gastrointestinal tract, and it enters the circulation via the portal vein. A healthy liver normally clears almost all ammonia entering the portal vein and converts it back to glutamine. In advanced liver disease, the increase in blood ammonia levels largely reflects portosystemic shunting but is also partly caused by a decrease in extrahepatic removal of this agent by muscle due to the sarcopaenia.

Hepatic encephalopathy is characterised by both cognitive deficits and impaired neuromuscular function. The cognitive deficits range from subtle changes only revealed by psychometric testing (minimal encephalopathy) to impaired attention, reaction times and memory. The impairment of neuromuscular function can include bradykinesia, rigidity, myoclonus and asterixis. Disturbance of the sleep-wake cycle is also common.

The diagnosis is usually suspected in patients who have the above symptoms and decompensated liver disease. However, other neurological disorders may need to be considered. If the diagnosis is unclear, other tests such as arterial ammonia levels, psychometric tests and EEGs can be used to support the diagnosis. Once the diagnosis is made, precipitating factors such as gastrointestinal bleeding, infection, renal failure, hypokalaemia and constipation should be sought and managed.

Most of the currently available treatments for hepatic encephalopathy are based on managing elevated blood ammonia levels. After correcting any potential predisposing condition, the aim is to decrease ammonia production and absorption from the gut. Lactulose, a synthetic disaccharide, reduces ammonia absorption by decreasing the colonic transit time and reducing the colonic pH [thereby converting ammonia to ammonium ions that resist absorption]. The dose is normally titrated so that the patient is passing 2–3 loose stools per day and results in improvement in encephalopathy in 70–80% of patients.

Non-absorbable oral antibiotics can also be effective. Rifaximin, 550 mg bd, is now the antibiotic of choice and is added when a patient has recurrent bouts or worsening encephalopathy without a treatable cause and is already taking lactulose. Rifaximin appears to have similar efficacy to lactulose, but the combination of rifaximin and lactulose improves encephalopathy to a greater extent than lactulose alone.

14.2.2.6 Hepatorenal Syndrome

Acute kidney injury is common in acute and chronic liver failure. This can be caused by a variety of disorders including sepsis and prerenal injury. Hepatorenal syndrome only applies in a minority of patients, usually in the setting of decompensated cirrhosis with ascites but occasionally with severe alcoholic hepatitis, acute liver failure and metastatic malignancy. In cirrhosis, the risk of developing hepatorenal syndrome appears to be higher in those with hyponatremia and elevated serum renin levels.

The pathophysiology behind hepatorenal syndrome is complex. As the liver disease becomes more severe, there is increasing vasodilatation of the splanchnic blood vessels and a reduction in peripheral vascular resistance. This leads to a reduction in the effective circulating arterial blood volume and, consequently, to activation of the renin-angiotensin-aldosterone and sympathetic nervous systems. The kidney then retains more salt and water and expands the blood volume, but there is a decline in renal perfusion and deterioration of renal function.

Hepatorenal syndrome is characterised by a progressive rise in serum creatinine in the presence of an inactive urinary sediment, minimal or no proteinuria and low urinary sodium excretion (<10 mmol/L). There are two different types based on the rapidity of the decline in renal function:

- Type 1 where there is a twofold increase in the serum creatinine to >220 μmol/L in less than 2 weeks.
- Type 2 where the renal failure develops in greater than 2 weeks. This form generally develops in patients with refractory ascites.

Before making a diagnosis of hepatorenal syndrome, the patient should have an abdominal ultrasound looking at the kidneys and urinary tract and should have tests for urinary sediment and protein excretion. All potentially nephrotoxic drugs and diuretics should be stopped, and the circulating blood volume should be optimised by giving intravenous albumin 1 g/kg/day for 2 days. Any other factors that may have caused the deterioration in renal function, such as sepsis, should also be treated. If these measures do not help and there is no evidence of another cause for the renal injury, then the most likely diagnosis is hepatorenal syndrome.

Treatment is largely directed at improving liver function. This is difficult in many patients, but cessation of alcohol is helpful in alcoholic cirrhosis, and antiviral drugs may be useful in decompensated cirrhosis due to hepatitis B. In a patient who is not critically ill and does not need to be admitted to intensive care, albumin infusions can be combined with terlipressin. Terlipressin is an analogue of vasopressin and improves renal function by decreasing vasodilatation in the splanchnic vascular bed such that there is an increase in the effective circulating blood volume. This is effective in approximately 50% of these patients. If the patient is critically ill and in intensive care, albumin infusions can be combined with noradrenaline with similar outcomes for hepatorenal syndrome.

If these measures fail and the patient is not a candidate for liver transplantation, then selected patients could be considered for TIPS. Any patient who may be a candidate for liver transplantation should be referred to a liver transplant centre and, on occasions, may have hemodialysis while they await a transplant.

14.2.3 Assessing Surgical Risk in Advanced Liver Disease

The assessment of surgical risk in liver disease must include an evaluation of the severity of liver disease. Under most circumstances, this needs to be undertaken by a hepatologist/gastroenterologist or an experienced perioperative physician. Elective surgery should not be performed in patients with acute liver failure or alcoholic hepatitis. In cirrhotic patients, this risk depends on the severity of the underlying liver disease and the type of proposed surgery.

For elective surgical procedures, a number of retrospective studies have demonstrated that perioperative mortality and morbidity correlate with the patient's preoperative Child-Pugh score. However, it is important to note that there has been some decline in post-operative mortality rates in cirrhotic patients since the 2000s due to improvements in critical care management. A study of 100 patients undergoing abdominal surgery in 1984 demonstrated post-operative mortality rates of 10%, 31% and 76% in Child-Pugh classes A, B and C patients, respectively. In comparison, a similar study in 2011 revealed some reduction in mortality with rates of 10%, 17% and 63%.

The MELD score, which has been primarily used to select patients to undergo liver transplantation, has also been assessed for its ability to predict post-operative survival in cirrhotic patients. A study in 2007 from the Mayo Clinic revealed that the 30-day mortality for patients with cirrhosis undergoing gastrointestinal, orthopaedic or cardiothoracic surgery was only 6% if their MELD score was <8 but was >50% if their MELD was >20. This has led to the recommendation that cirrhotic patients with a MELD score of <10 can probably undergo elective surgery, but those with a MELD score of >15 should not. Patients needing semi-urgent or emergency surgery will need to be considered on an individual basis, but mortality rates may be higher than those for elective surgery.

Recommended Reading

D'Amico G, Pasta I, Morabito A, et al. Competing risks and prognostic stages of cirrhosis: a 25 year study. Aliment Pharmacol Ther. 2014;39:1180–93.

EASL clinical practice guidelines on the management of ascites, spontaneous bacterial peritonitis and hepatorenal syndrome in cirrhosis. J Hepatol. 2010;53:397–417.

EASL clinical practical guidelines on the management of acute [fulminant] liver failure. J Hepatol. 2017;66:1047–81.

Flamm SL, Yang YX, Singh S, Falck-Ytter YT, AGA Institute Clinical Guidelines Committee. American Gastroenterological Association Institute Guidelines for the Diagnosis and Management of Acute Liver Failure. Gastroenterology. 2017;152:644–7.

Garcia-Pagan JC, Gracia-Sancho J, Bosch J. Functional aspects on the pathophysiology of portal hypertension in cirrhosis. J Hepatol. 2012;57:458–61.

Gill RQ, Sterling RK. Acute liver failure. J Clin Gastroenterol. 2001;33:191–8.

Kamath PS, Wiesner RH, Malinchoc M, et al. A model to predict survival in patients with end-stage liver disease. Hepatology. 2001;33:464–70.

Lee WM. Etiologies of acute liver failure. Semin Liver Dis. 2008;28:142–52.

Seo YS, Park SY, Kim MY, et al. Lack of difference among terlipressin, somatostatin and octreotide in the control of acute gastroesophageal variceal haemorrhage. Hepatology. 2014;60:954–63.

Stravitz RT, Kramer DJ. Management of acute liver failure. Nat Rev Gastroenterol Hepatol. 2009:542–3.

Advanced Radiologic Imaging Techniques of the Gastrointestinal Tract

15

Frank Voyvodic, Melissa Jenkins, and Steven J. Knox

15.1 CT and MRI Enterography for Small Bowel Imaging

CT enterography (CTE) and MR enterography (MRE) are the current standards for radiologic imaging of the small intestine, especially for inflammatory disorders. Enterography findings have been shown to change management in a significant proportion of symptomatic patients independent of clinical, serologic and histologic findings.

Fluoroscopic barium contrast examination for small bowel disease has been superseded, and there is a limited residual role for fluoroscopy, e.g. for complex fistula road mapping in inflammatory bowel disease.

Enterography is widely available and easily performed at all sites providing CT and MRI services. Improved MRI technology means GIT imaging with MRI becomes a viable alternative to CT scanning depending on availability and expense. MRI may have a particular role in inflammatory bowel disease as multiple CT examinations can subject younger patients to significant cumulative radiation exposure.

15.1.1 Technique

Both CT and MR enterographies utilise a "negative" oral contrast agent to maximise visibility of adjacent mural contrast enhancement. An osmotically neutral

F. Voyvodic (✉)
Department of Radiology, Flinders University, Adelaide, SA, Australia

Benson Radiology, Adelaide, SA, Australia
e-mail: frank.Voyvodic@bensonradiology.com.au

M. Jenkins · S. J. Knox
Benson Radiology, Adelaide, SA, Australia

Department of Radiology, Royal Adelaide Hospital, Adelaide, SA, Australia
e-mail: sa.jenkins@bensonradiology.com.au; steven.knox@bensonradiology.som.au

M. W. Wichmann et al. (eds.), *Gastroenterology For General Surgeons*,
https://doi.org/10.1007/978-3-319-92768-8_15

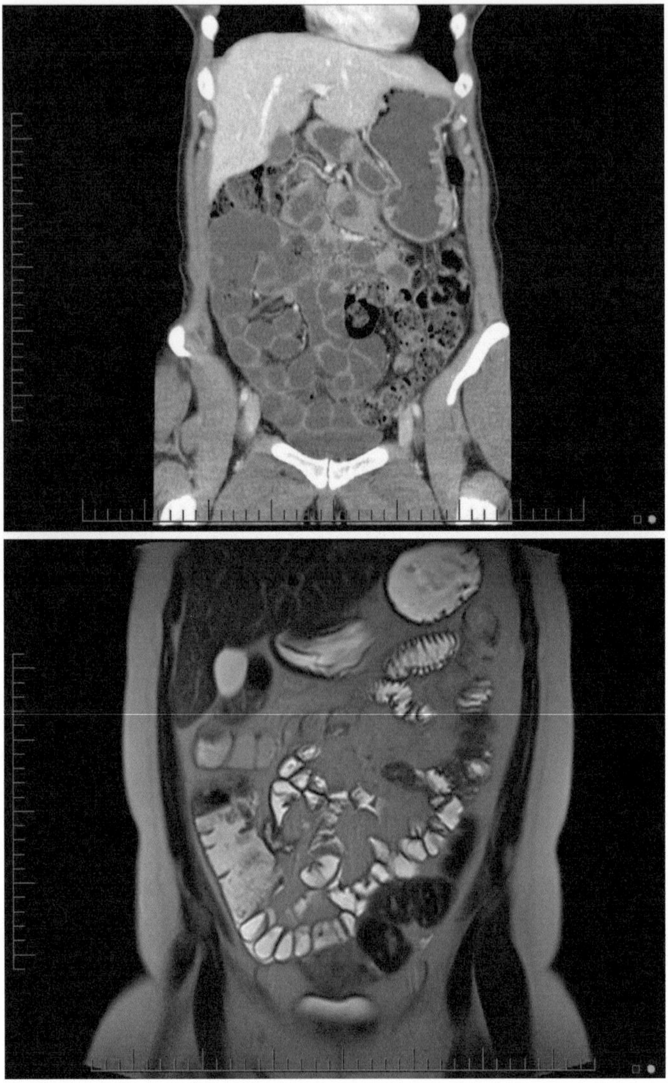

Fig. 15.1 Normal CT and MR enterogram (coronal orientation)

solution, as opposed to water alone, is used to prevent rapid reabsorption and therefore optimise distal small bowel distension (Fig. 15.1).

A large volume of fluid (1200 + mL) is slowly ingested orally over an extended period (60 + min). Note that enterography has replaced enteroclysis (which typically requires nasojejunal intubation) in routine usage.

Intravenous contrast is administered with scan timing in the "enteric phase" (approximately 40–45 s postinjection) to maximise bowel wall contrast enhancement. Note this is earlier than routine post IV contrast abdominal imaging which is performed in the portal venous phase of enhancement (70 s postinjection). Solid foods should be avoided for 4 h before the examination.

15.1.2 Role of CTE/MRE for Specific Indications

1. Crohn's disease (CD)—Assess extent, severity, and complications. High sensitivity for detection of enteric disease (>90%). Imaging is also used for assessment of response to therapy and bowel healing and to monitor progression of disease. Less sensitive than capsule endoscopy for early mucosal abnormalities. As CTE and MRE are utilised most commonly in CD diagnosis and assessment, this is discussed in more detail below.
2. Small bowel tumour detection, characterisation, and staging—Less sensitive than capsule endoscopy for small mucosal lesions.
3. Partial small bowel obstruction—Locate site and detect the cause.
4. Celiac disease—Assess complications especially lymphoma (subtle mucosal changes can be missed).
5. Ulcerative colitis—Exclude small bowel inflammation and extra-luminal complications. CTE and MRE have reduced sensitivity in colonic inflammation.
6. Occult GI bleeding—Unlike nuclear medicine studies, enterography does not have prolonged scanning capability to detect intermittent GI bleeding.

15.1.3 Imaging at Diagnosis of Crohn's Disease

Bowel inflammation, acute vs. chronic, location, length of involvement
Stricture detection
Penetrating disease (sinus, fistula, abscess)
Perianal sepsis
Malignancy
Extraintestinal manifestations
Alternate diagnoses

15.1.4 Bowel Inflammation

Acute bowel inflammation is characterised by mural thickening (3 mm+) in a distended segment of bowel associated with segmental mural hyperenhancement compared to the adjacent healthy bowel. Mural thickening can be graded as mild, moderate and severe depending on the degree of thickening (3–5 mm, 5–9 mm, $>=$ 10 mm). The hyperenhancement pattern can be uniform or stratified (inner wall hyperenhancement, i.e. target or halo sign) (Figs. 15.2 and 15.3). T2 signal hyperintensity and restricted diffusion are specific MRI features supporting active inflammation (Fig. 15.4). Perienteric edema is also a feature of acute mesenteric inflammation and correlates with elevation in serum inflammatory markers. Engorgement of the vasa recta of the affected bowel segment may be seen (comb sign) (Fig. 15.5). Visualisation of ulceration at CTE and MRE is a marker of more severe inflammation.

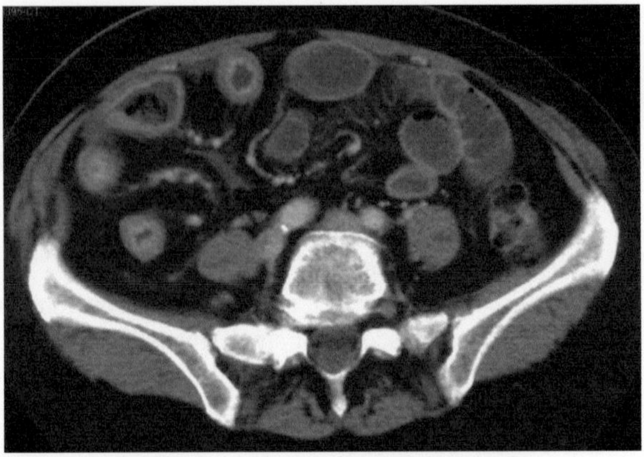

Fig. 15.2 CT enterogram—mural thickening and segmental hyperenhancement of the distal ileum in the right abdomen, compared to normal small bowel in the left abdomen. Note "target sign" with mural stratification

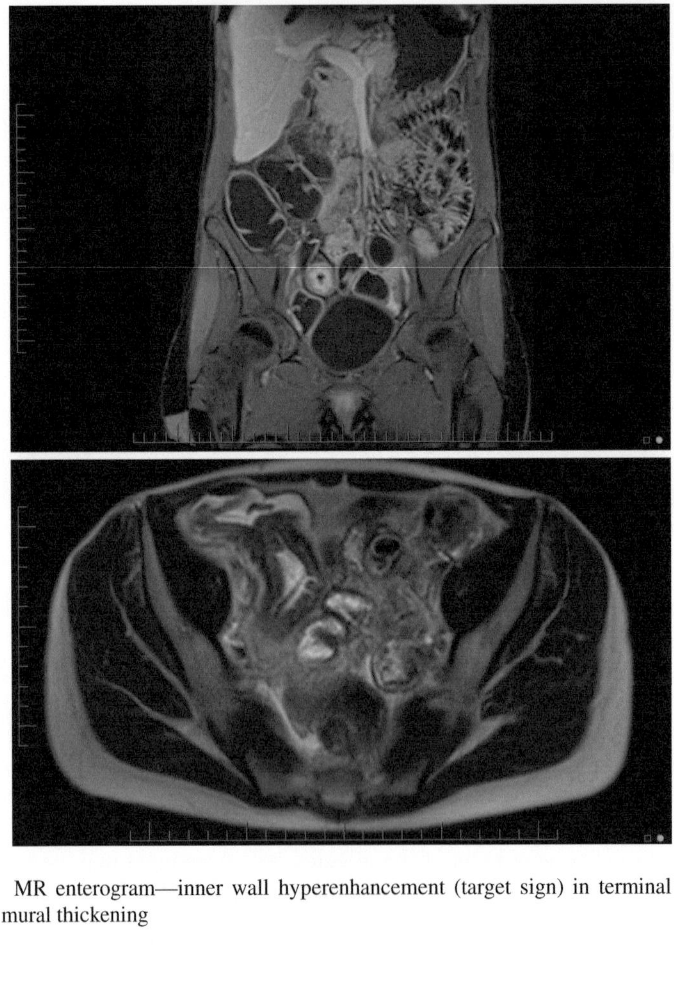

Fig. 15.3 MR enterogram—inner wall hyperenhancement (target sign) in terminal ileum and moderate mural thickening

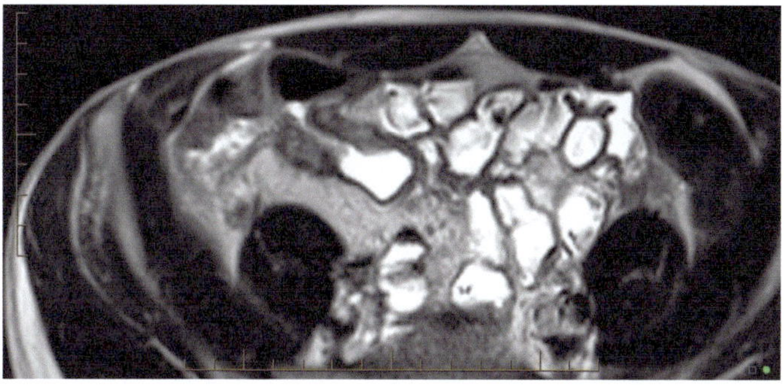

Fig. 15.4 T2 signal hyperintensity intestinal wall supports active inflammation

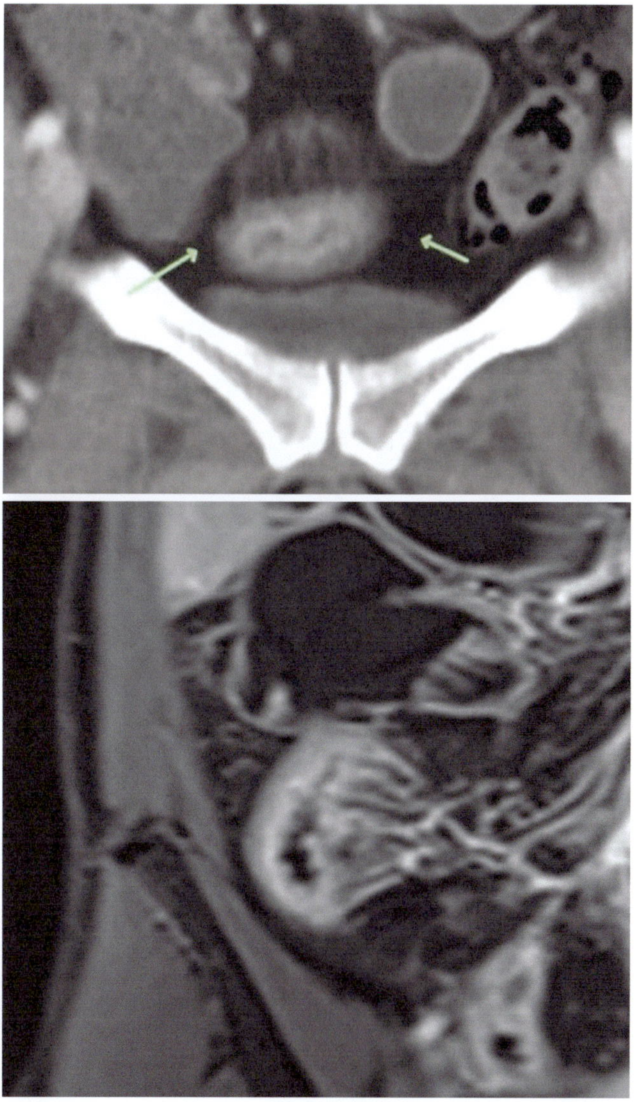

Fig. 15.5 CTE and MRE examples of engorged vasa recta associated with inflammation in a segment of small bowel (comb sign)

Note that wall thickening and hyperenhancement are not specific for Crohn's disease. Asymmetric wall thickening with inflammation typically sparing the mesenteric margin is pathognomonic for Crohn's disease.

When the sequelae of prior inflammation are present without active inflammation, the term "Crohn's disease with no imaging signs of active inflammation" is preferred to "chronic disease". Clinicians making decisions based on imaging findings should be aware that imaging criteria distinguishing between active and inactive disease do not always equate to histologic, endoscopic or clinically active or inactive disease.

Inactive bowel inflammation is also associated with focal bowel mural thickening and mural hyperenhancement, noting there is overlap with the imaging findings in active disease. Inactive disease does not typically show perienteric soft tissue stranding. Fibrofatty mesenteric proliferation or "creeping fat" is a feature of longstanding inflammation usually along the mesenteric border (Fig. 15.6). In longstanding inactive disease, the asymmetric fibrosis is associated with pseudosacculation formation (Fig. 15.7).

Reactive lymphadenopathy with short-axis diameter 10–15 mm is a common finding in active and inactive Crohn's disease.

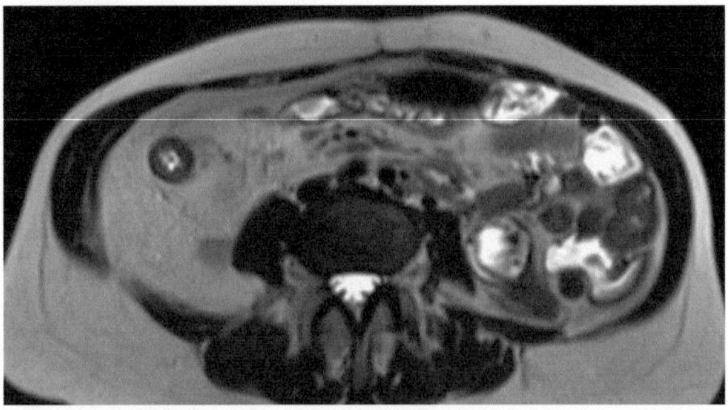

Fig. 15.6 Fibrofatty mesenteric proliferation or "creeping fat" is a feature of longstanding inactive disease

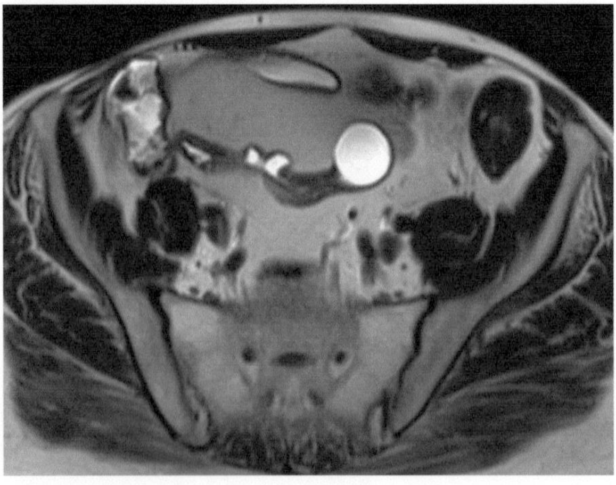

Fig. 15.7 Asymmetric mural fibrosis leading to pseudosacculations

Proximal small bowel disease is notable because of association with poorer prognosis, increased risk of surgery and hospitalisations.

15.1.5 Stricture Detection and Obstructing Disease

Stricturing disease is present in nearly 5% of CD patients. Strictures are diagnosed by the presence of luminal narrowing in an area of inflammatory disease with associated upstream bowel dilatation (>3 cm) (Fig. 15.8). Note that most Crohn's disease strictures have both inflammation and fibrosis with significant imaging overlap using standard enterographic techniques (Fig. 15.8).

15.1.6 Penetrating Disease

Extra-enteric inflammation is commonly detected in asymptomatic patients and found in approximately 15% of patients at the time of diagnosis of Crohn's disease. Its presence indicates active inflammation and is a poor prognostic sign for medical management. Penetrating disease can be characterised as simple or complex fistula, sinus tract, inflammatory mass or abscess depending upon lesion morphology (Figs. 15.9 and 15.10). CTE and MRE have similar and moderately high accuracy for detection of these entities (Fig. 15.11).

15.1.7 Perianal Sepsis

Imaging of the perianal region should be included in any CTE or MRE exam as 20–25% of cases of perianal sepsis present at or before the time of Crohn's disease diagnosis. Perianal fistulas in CD patients are usually more complicated with

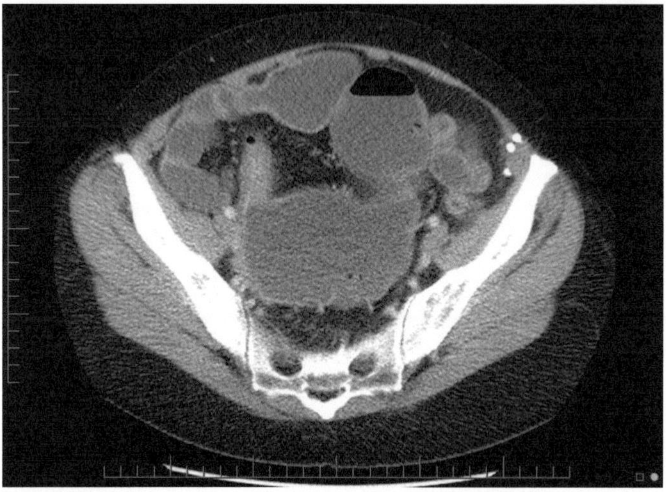

Fig. 15.8 Focal luminal narrowing with upstream dilatation consistent with stricture

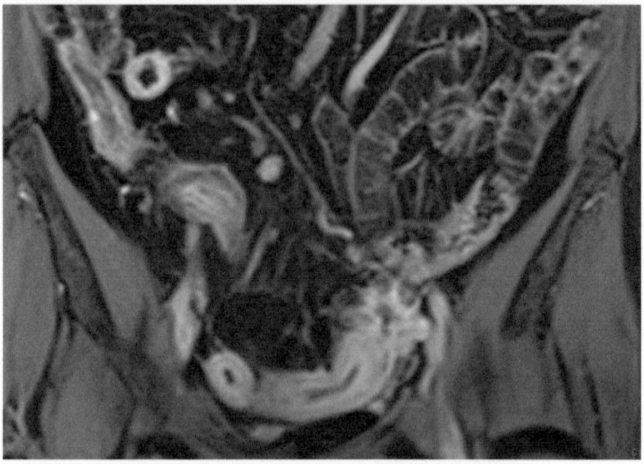

Fig. 15.9 Active terminal ileitis with enhancing perienteric abscess indicating penetrating disease

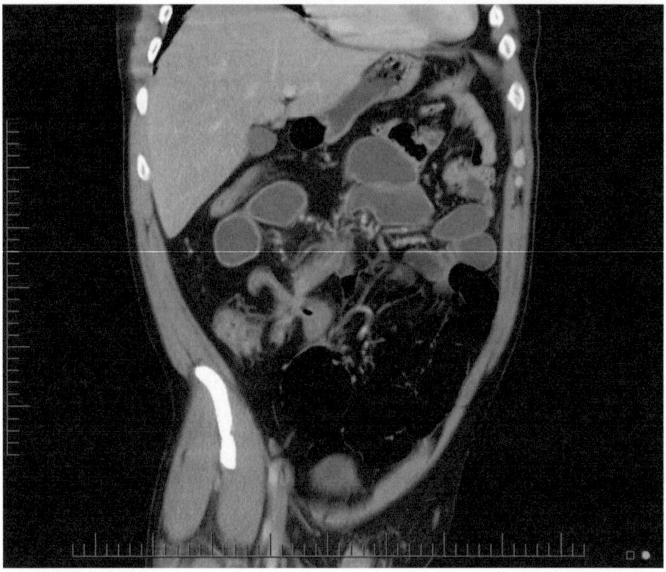

Fig. 15.10 Penetrating small bowel disease with complex entero-enteric fistula

increased frequency of secondary tract extension and abscess compared to the general population. Dedicated pelvic MRI is the most accurate imaging test for perianal disease detection and characterisation.

15.1.8 Malignancy

Patients diagnosed with Crohn's disease are known to be at increased risk of bowel cancer and lymphoma as well as many other cancers. Malignancy can be difficult to identify at imaging and can mimic a benign stricture. Consider the diagnosis of an

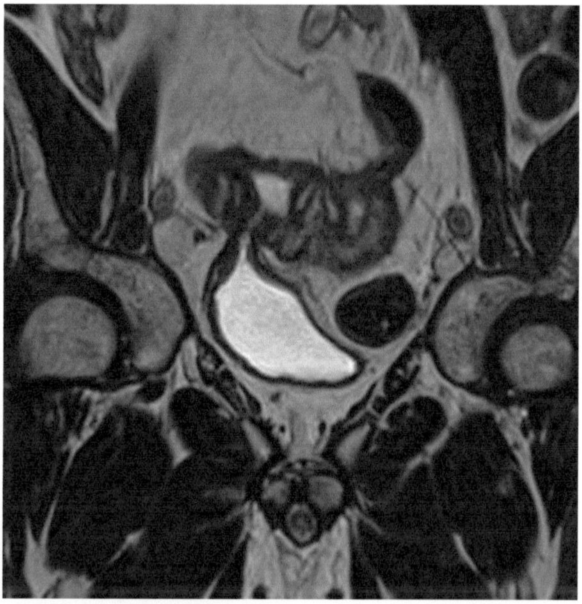

Fig. 15.11 MR enterography with loss of normal fat plane between the urinary bladder fundus and the antimesenteric margin of the sigmoid colon with underlying vesicocolic fistula

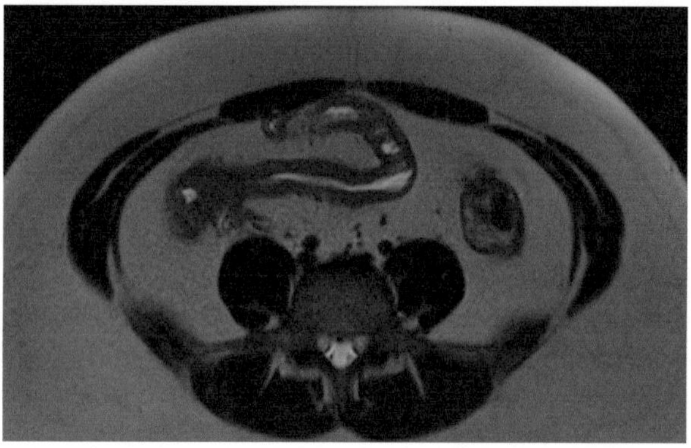

Fig. 15.12 Adenocarci noma arising in pre-existing Crohn's Disease

underlying bowel malignancy if the wall thickening is severe (>15 mm in diameter) (Fig. 15.12). A new obstructing lesion in the context of long-term inactive disease is also a red flag for increased risk of malignancy.

15.1.9 Alternative Diagnoses

Crohn's disease and intestinal tuberculosis (ITB) are both ulcerative diseases which can occur in any segment of the gastrointestinal tract. Differentiating these diseases can be difficult despite clinical evaluation, endoscopy and radiologic imaging. ITB should be excluded in all cases especially when the patient originates from an endemic country. Asymmetric non-circumferential wall involvement and

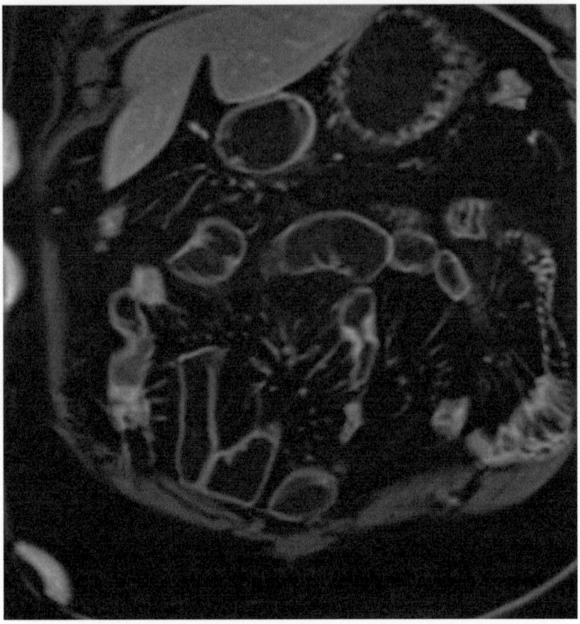

Fig. 15.13 Diaphragm-like strictures of NSAID enteropathy

skip lesions are more common in Crohn's disease, whereas contracture of the ileocecal valve and the presence of a fixed patulous ileocecal valve favour the diagnosis of ITB. Segmental vasa recta engorgement (comb sign), fistula and inflammatory masses are more likely to be found in Crohn's disease, whereas lymph nodes with central necrosis or calcification and ascites are more common in ITB patients. Other associated features of ITB include abdominal solid organ involvement in 15–20% and pulmonary TB in 15%.

Diaphragm-like strictures, i.e. circumferential, ringlike and very short, 5 to 10 mm in length, are the typical imaging features of NSAID enteropathy. Mild focal segmental wall thickening and mural hyperenhancement are recognised phenomena. Symmetric wall involvement, short stricture length and lack of predilection for the terminal ileum can help with differentiation from enteric Crohn's disease as well as the clinical context of chronic NSAID usage (Fig. 15.13).

15.1.10 Extraintestinal Disease Manifestations

These should be looked for in every CTE or MRE exam, and the most clinically important are sacroiliitis, primary sclerosing cholangitis and avascular necrosis, especially of the femoral heads (Fig. 15.14). Other findings may include nephrolithiasis, cholelithiasis and cutaneous disease including erythema nodosum, pyoderma gangrenosum and cutaneous vasculitis.

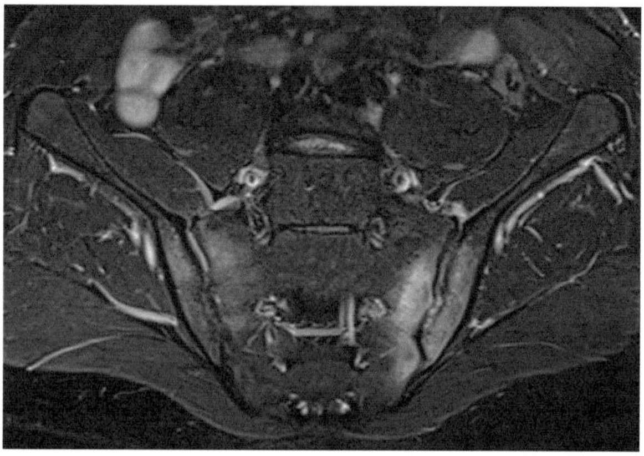

Fig. 15.14 Sacroiliitis on MRI

15.1.11 Imaging for Assessment of Disease Activity

Mucosal healing has been proposed as a treatment target for Crohn's disease and is associated with improved clinical outcomes (reduction in hospitalisation, surgeries and corticosteroid use).

Identifying radiologic transmural response by demonstrating the reduced length of segmental inflammation (or resolution) and no development of new inflammatory lesions may be a viable alternative to endoscopic assessment. This concept of radiologic response continues to gain momentum.

MRE may be preferred for follow-up imaging examination if available because it lacks radiation exposure and has validated sensitivity and specificity in children and adults.

Several radiologic scoring systems have been developed but are not in extensive clinical use. The most widely accepted is the MaRIA (magnetic resonance index of activity) scoring system which was developed and validated compared to endoscopic scoring systems.

15.2 Imaging of Perianal Sepsis

Accurate fistula characterisation helps determine appropriate management (medical vs. surgical). Failure to identify any secondary tracks or abscess can lead to recurrent sepsis. Inappropriate surgical fistulotomy can lead to loss of sphincter integrity and incontinence.

Fistulography with cannulation of the external opening of perianal fistula is of limited utility. External openings may be challenging to cannulate, all tracks may not opacify, and there is limited soft tissue resolution with plain radiography.

Endoanal ultrasound ± installation of hydrogen peroxide into fistula tracks is a useful but highly specialised technique with high sensitivity for identification of internal fistula opening but has limited availability especially in the rural context and requires specific US equipment and specialised training.

Standard transabdominal ultrasound techniques are not helpful in this condition. There is a recent interest in the role of transperineal ultrasound assessment using standard US transducers as a readily available, inexpensive and reliable modality for evaluation of perianal Crohn's disease.

CT scanning lacks soft tissue resolution and involves ionising radiation. There may be a limited role for CT fistulography when MRI is not available.

MR with surface coil imaging provides multiplanar imaging and excellent soft tissue resolution and involves no ionising radiation. A combination of fat-suppressed proton density or T2-weighted imaging is performed ± post IV gadolinium T1-weighted imaging. Short- and long-axis images are taken centred to the anal sphincter complex.

The inner and outer muscular layers are well identified on MRI, and with high-resolution T2-weighted imaging, it is possible to distinguish the deep, superficial and subcutaneous parts of the external anal sphincter (EAS) separately. The inter-sphincteric space, components of the levator ani muscle and the ischioanal and ischiorectal fossae are also evident (Fig. 15.15).

The role of MRI can be defined as follows:

1. Identify/exclude active perianal sepsis.
2. Help distinguish perianal fistula from pilonidal sinus and other conditions.
3. Anatomic classification of fistula path.
4. Identify the location of external and internal openings.
5. Identify secondary tracks and abscesses.
6. Exclude translevator and supralevator disease.
7. Identify rectal inflammation.
8. Grade disease activity.

The challenge for the radiologist is often adequately describing the information in the images in a form readily recognisable and of benefit to the referring clinician. Structured radiology reporting for MRI of perianal sepsis (as well as all other body applications) should be highly encouraged to ensure completeness of reports and facilitate communication to referrers.

15.2.1 Identify Active Perianal Sepsis

Active fistula track and abscesses will show high T2 (fluid) signal intensity (Fig. 15.16). Abscesses join fistula tracts and contain non-enhancing fluid or air. In inactive/chronic disease or complex postsurgical cases, there is a role for post IV contrast imaging to differentiate enhancing granulation tissue from fluid content. Inactive/chronic scarred tracks with fibrosis have reduced water content and low T2 signal. Seton sutures are usually clearly identified as linear signal "void" traversing fistula track and anal lumen (Fig. 15.17).

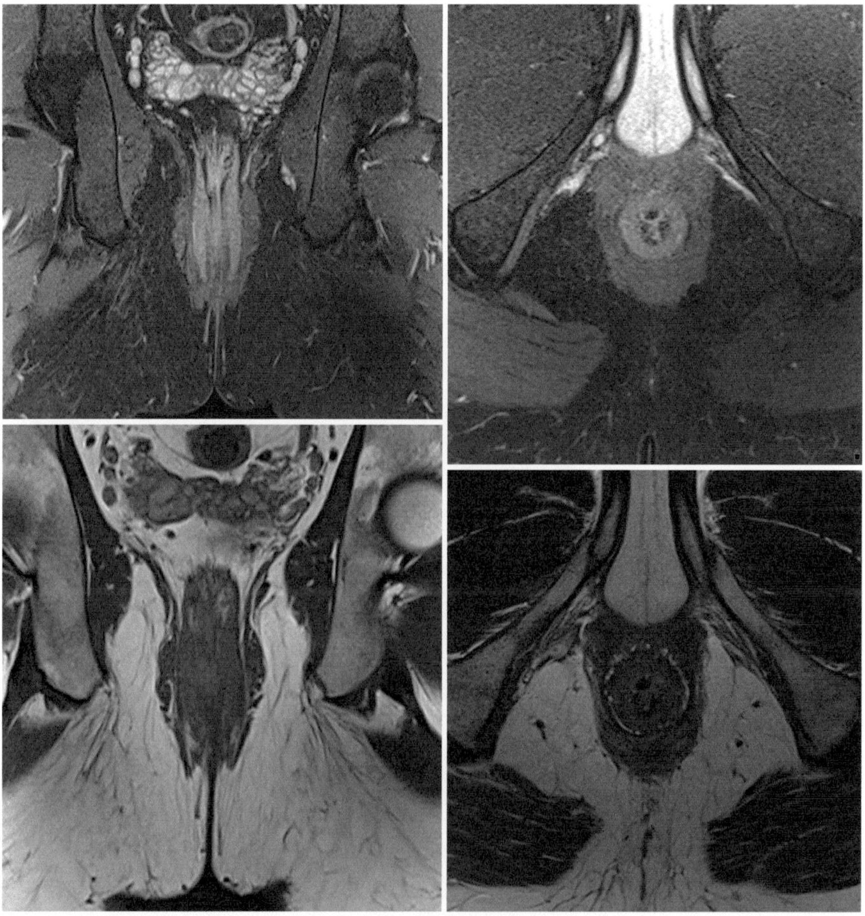

Fig. 15.15 Proton density fat suppression and T2-weighted coronal and axial images of normal anal sphincter muscle complex

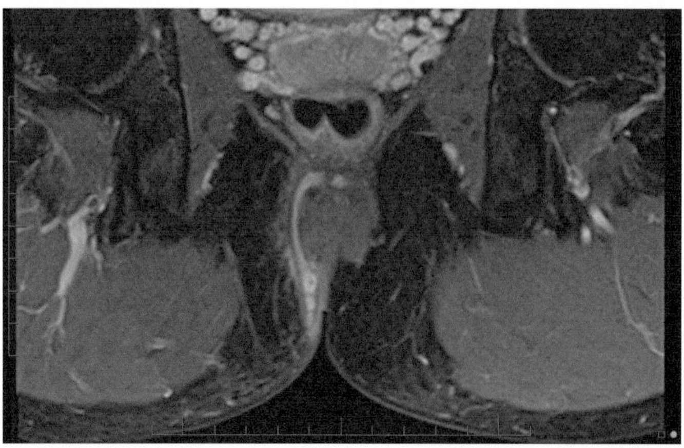

Fig. 15.16 Coronal MRI with active perianal sepsis—high T2 signal fluid within suprasphincteric fistula

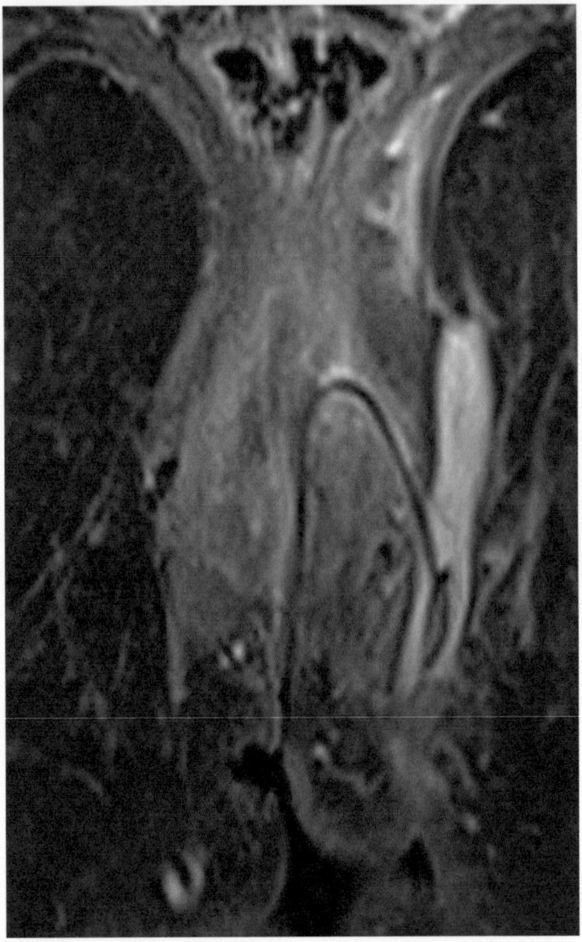

Fig. 15.17 Coronal MRI with linear low signal intensity seton suture within perianal fistula. Note undrained secondary track on left lateral margin

15.2.2 Anatomic Classification of Fistula Path

Anatomic and imaging-based classification schema encourages the use of consistent terminology in radiology reports and allows for improved communication between clinicians. There is no consensus for the classification of perianal fistula in Crohn's disease. Using the Parks classification, a fistula track can be described as intersphincteric, transphincteric, extrasphincteric or suprasphincteric in its course (Figs. 15.18, 15.19 and 15.20).

Unlike other types, an intersphincteric fistula will not be identified in either long or short axis outside of or crossing the external anal sphincter muscle (Fig. 15.18).

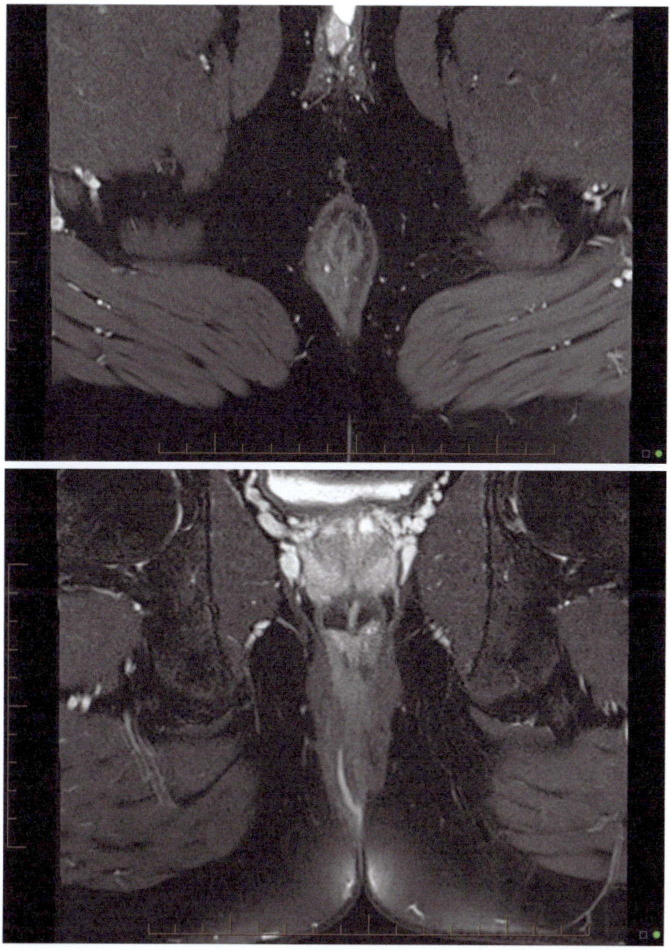

Fig. 15.18 Axial and coronal MR imaging of linear intersphincteric perianal fistula. Note the fistula track lies deep to the external anal sphincter muscle in both planes

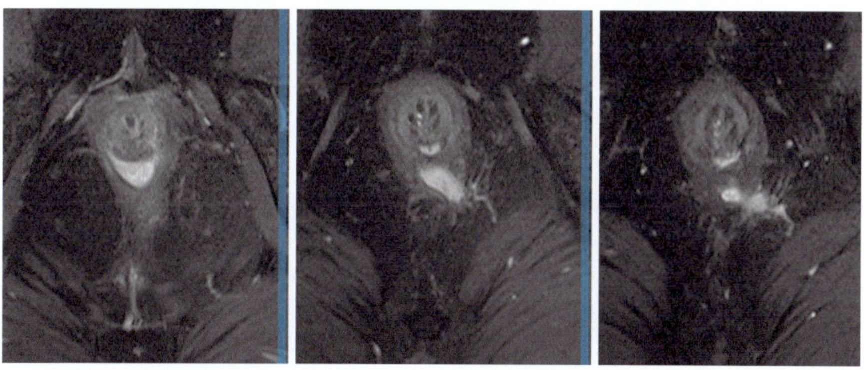

Fig. 15.19 Axial serial MR images of transphincteric perianal fistula with intersphincteric space abscess. Note the fistula track traverses at 5 o'clock

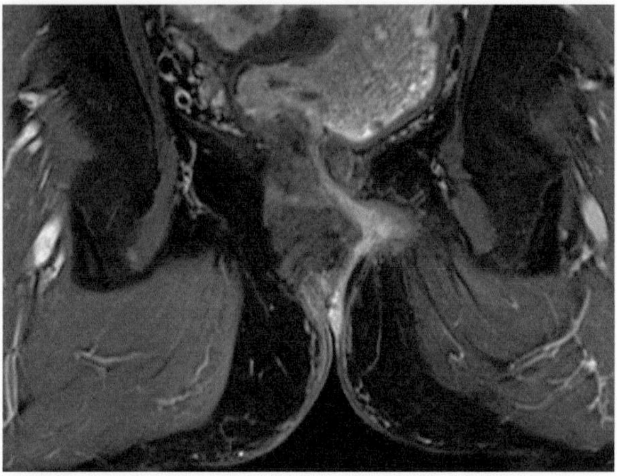

Fig. 15.20 Coronal MRI of suprasphincteric perianal fistula. Note cephalad extension and communication with low rectum above the levator ani muscles

15.2.3 Identification of Fistula Openings

The surgical localisation of external fistula openings utilises an anal "clock face" as seen in the lithotomy position. Note that MR imaging is acquired in the supine position with legs together, so some extrapolation is required to estimate the clock face position where the fistula tracks end in the skin. The distance to the ano-cutaneous junction can also be measured (Fig. 15.21).

Internal openings are not consistently seen with MRI of perianal fistulas. The term "predicted" internal opening may be used to signify that an internal opening is assumed to be at the clock face position and height that the fistula track crosses the external sphincter (Fig. 15.22). The dentate line on MRI is approximately 2 cm above ano-cutaneous junction but cannot be radiologically identified.

15.2.4 Secondary Tracks and Abscesses

Identification of these is crucial to guide surgical management and ensure optimal drainage. MRI has high accuracy for detection (Fig. 15.23).

15.2.5 Identify Rectal Inflammation

The simultaneous presence of proctitis will influence patient management as the chance of fistula healing is reduced leading to use of more aggressive medical management and avoidance of surgery. Dedicated MRI of the anorectum and perineum usually provides a sufficient field of view (25 × 25 cm) to image the rectum. Wall thickening, perimural oedema and enlarged mesorectal lymph nodes at MRI show a significant correlation to endoscopic findings and are reproducible in diagnosing proctitis.

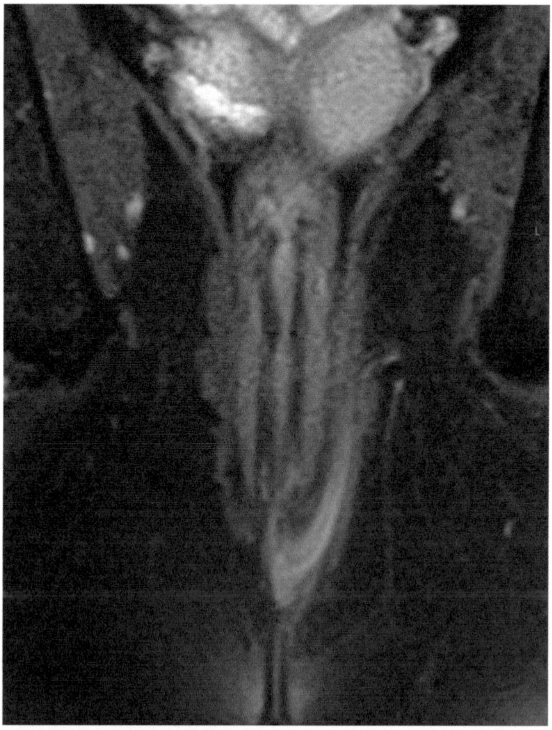

Fig. 15.21 Coronal MR image—external opening of fistula identified immediately adjacent to the ano-cutaneous junction at left lateral margin

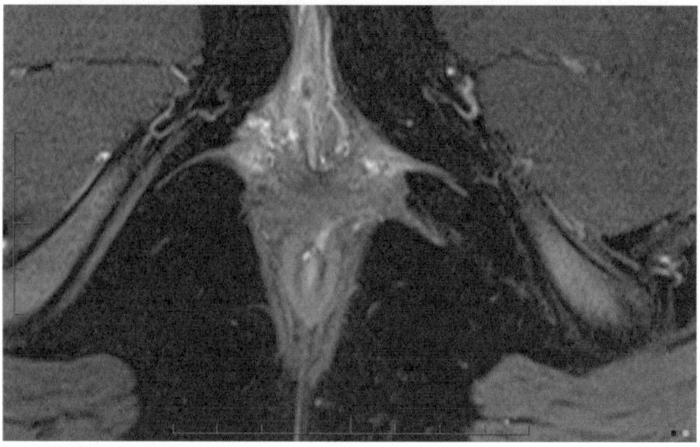

Fig. 15.22 Axial MR image of anterior transphincteric fistula crossing the EAS at 1 o'clock with predicted internal opening at this level

15.2.6 Grade Disease Activity

Radiologic assessment of healing disease can help in the follow-up of patients by evaluating the adequacy of therapy and the potential need for treatment modification. As fistulas heal, the high T2 signal becomes hypointense, and inactive healing/chronic fistula appear as non-enhancing low T1 and T2 signal intensity tracts lined by fibrous tissue. Some scoring systems for MRI are available as research tools, but these are not widely used or accepted into clinical surgical practice. The most widely validated is the Van Assche score which describes both the anatomic changes

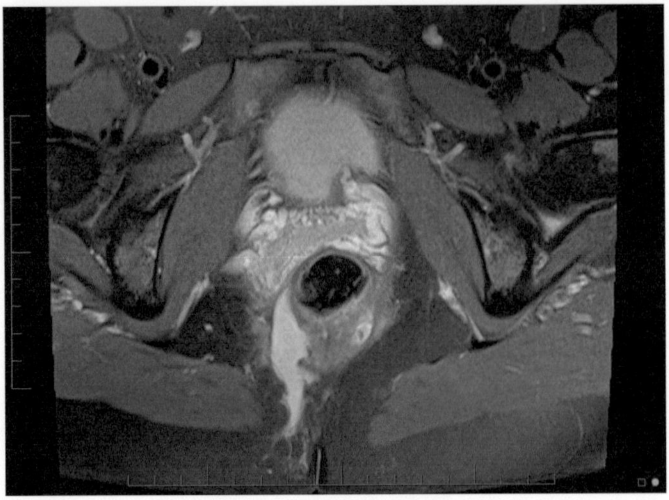

Fig. 15.23 Axial MR image—secondary track with abscess directed posteriorly in the right ischioanal fossa

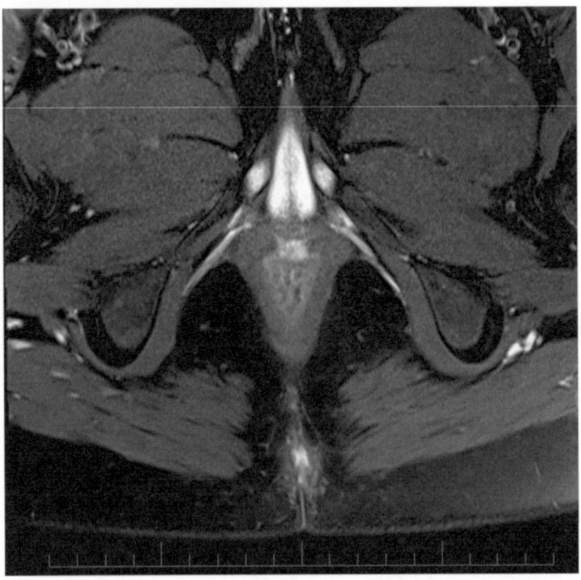

Fig. 15.24 Axial MR image—pilonidal sinus disease with small fluid collection and inflammatory change in midline natal cleft without communication to the anal sphincter muscle complex

and the inflammatory disease as seen on MRI (T2 signal, presence or absence of abscesses or proctitis). The clinical benefit of maintenance anti-TNF-alpha therapy has been correlated with significant improvement of the Van Assche score.

15.2.7 Natal Cleft Sepsis

Consider pilonidal sinus disease as an alternative diagnosis when sepsis is posterior and limited to the natal cleft (Fig. 15.24). The absence of intersphincteric sepsis or enteric opening allows reliable imaging distinction from perianal fistula.

Note that unlike perianal fistulas associated with Crohn's disease, detection and characterisation of anovaginal and rectovaginal fistulas are often difficult to identify because of the paucity of fat tissue for contrast and the absence of active inflammation and associated high T2 signal intensity.

15.3 CT Colonoscopy (CTC)

First performed in 1995, CT colonoscopy is a minimally invasive and safe technique for colonic visualisation and is the radiologic investigation of choice for colonic neoplasm. Virtual "fly-throughs" of the colon can be created simulating the view during the passage of an endoscope at optical colonoscopy. CTC typically uses a combination of 2D and 3D reviews of CT data sets acquired in two anatomic positions (usually supine and prone) following colonic cleansing preparation and gas insufflation (Fig. 15.25).

15.3.1 Technique

"Dry" or "wet" laxative preparations can be used for bowel preparation. The liquid residue is typically labelled or "tagged" with either orally ingested barium or iodine so that the liquid residue appears radio-opaque (white) enabling distinction between polyps and masses in fluid-filled segments (Figs. 15.26 and 15.27). There is potential for "same-day" endoscopy when a significant abnormality is found at CTC and also "same-day" CT when conventional colonoscopy is incomplete obviating the need for repeated bowel preparation.

All the latest generation, CT scanners permit fast breath-hold examinations and the ability to perform good-quality CTC with reduced radiation dose.

Thin flexible catheters are used (smaller than for barium enema), and the colon can be distended with either room air or CO_2 via automatic insufflator.

The patient is typically scanned in both the supine and prone positions to allow the redistribution of fluid and solid residue and optimise gaseous distension of colonic segments. Intravenous contrast is not routinely used unless staging a known colonic malignancy and low radiation dose technique is used.

Image data sets are assessed with specific CTC software systems (Figs. 15.28, 15.29 and 15.30). Reader operator training and experience are required, and subspecialty accreditation and ongoing competency are required by specialist colleges.

15.3.2 Accuracy

Barium enema has been replaced as the alternative imaging investigation of choice when colonoscopy is incomplete or the patient is considered unsuitable for colonoscopy. Fluoroscopic screening units are diminishing in number, and radiologist experience with barium GI procedures has also reduced over the last 10 years as cross-sectional GI imaging techniques increase in utility.

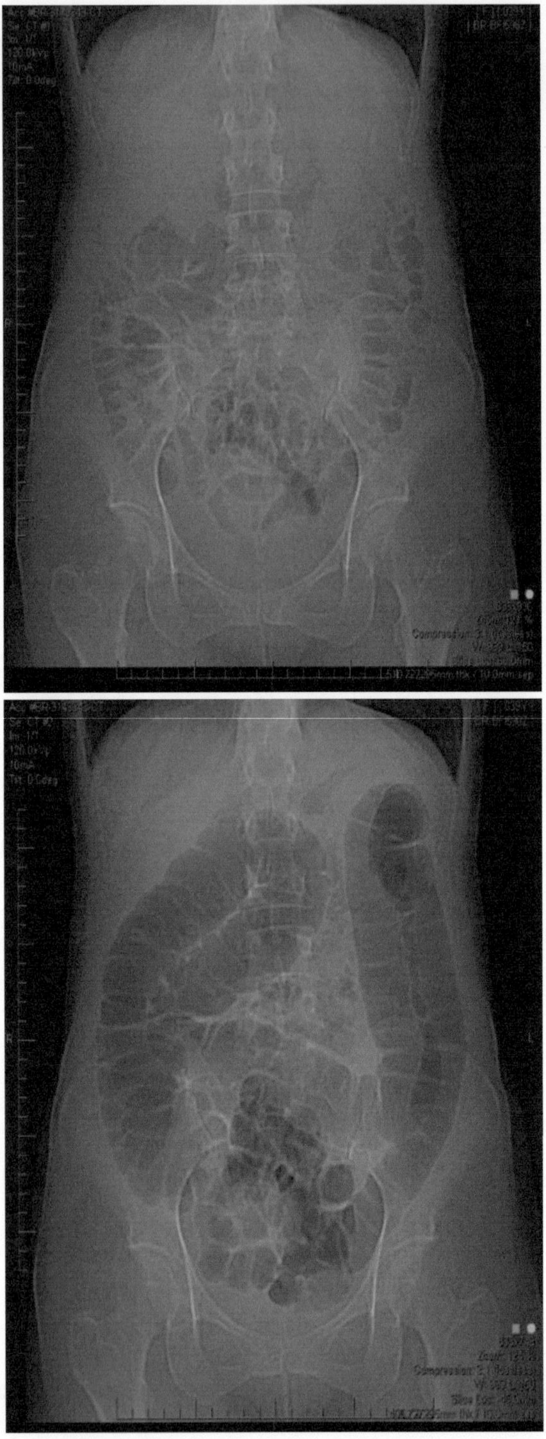

Fig. 15.25 Scout radiographs for CT colonoscopy pre- and post colon insufflation

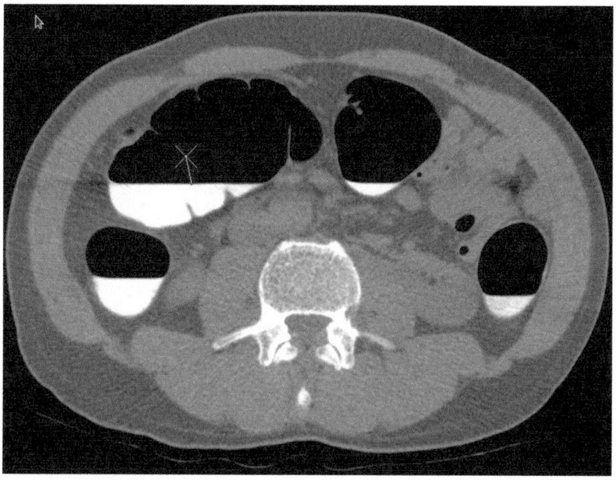

Fig. 15.26 Liquid colonic residue “tagged” with orally ingested positive oral contrast agent improving detection of focal abnormality in fluid-filled segments

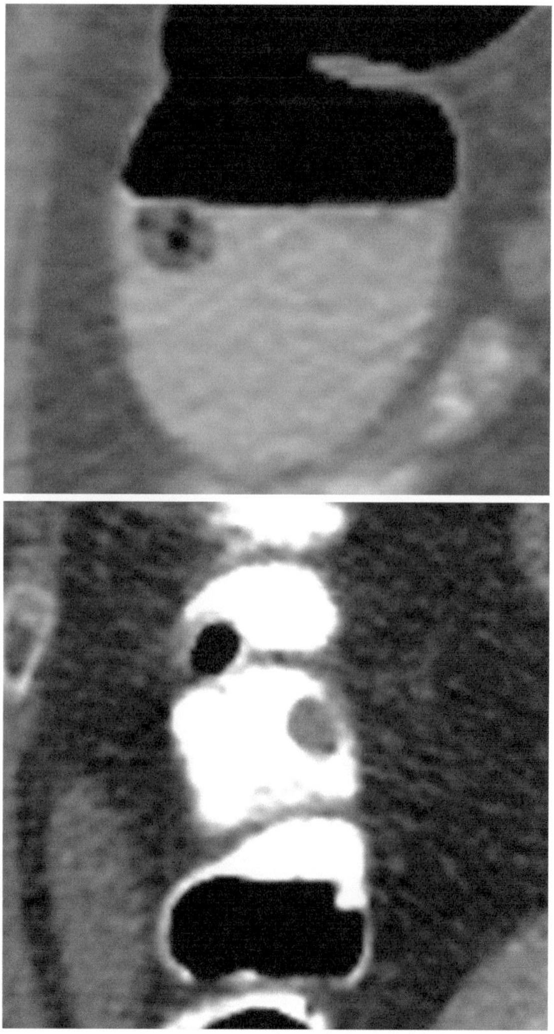

Fig. 15.27 CTC faecal residue (heterogeneous density with gas, mobile) versus polyp (homogenous soft tissue density, wall attachment)

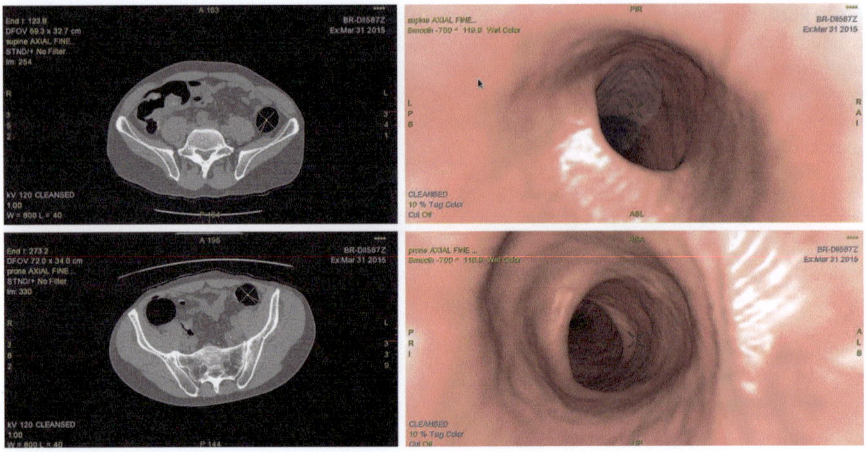

Fig. 15.28 2D (axial) and 3D ("fly-through") CT data sets for CTC

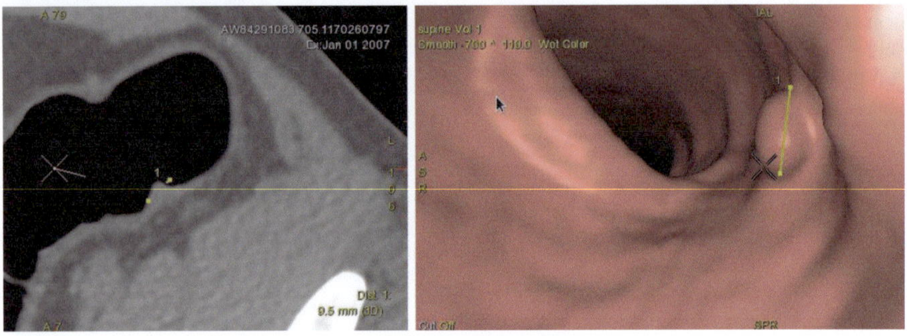

Fig. 15.29 10 mm diameter colonic polyp at CTC

Fig. 15.30 Annular carcinoma right colon at CTC

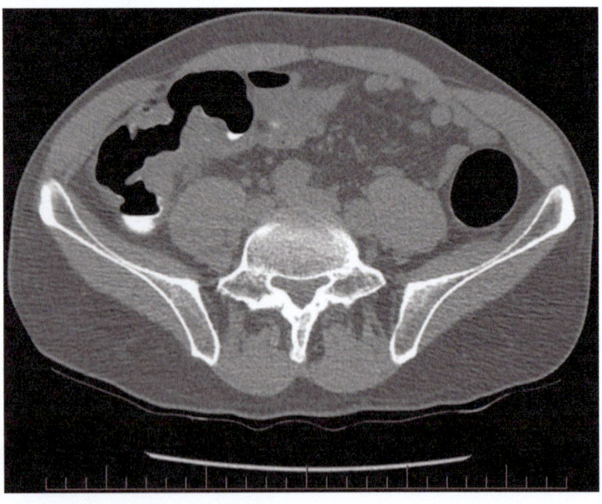

Compared with barium enema, CTC detects 30% more cancers and large polyps, and there is no significant difference in detection rates between CTC and conventional colonoscopy. Flat polyps and neoplasia can be challenging for both CTC and standard colonoscopy.

15.3.3 Safety

Colonic distension with CTC is associated with a small risk of perforation although no cases were reported in US series of over 11,700 exams in asymptomatic patients undergoing screening examinations.

Traditionally, most centres delay radiologic imaging of the colon after incomplete colonoscopy where a biopsy was performed due to the potential increased risk of perforation. However, mucosal biopsies and routine polypectomy do not involve the muscularis propria and are unlikely to result in perforation. More data is needed on the level of risk in those patients undergoing complex polypectomies or with a background of severe inflammatory bowel disease.

CT scanning is associated with the theoretical risk of cancer development associated with ionising radiation exposure although there is little evidence existing for risks below doses of 100 millisieverts (mSv). The median estimated effective dose in asymptomatic patients in a multicentre study from 24 European institutions indicated a dose from CTC of 5.7 mSv which compares to the background radiation in Australia of approximately 2–3 mSv. Repeat screening CTC examinations with cumulative radiation dose in younger patients have more potential cancer risk than scanning elderly patients given the potential latency period of cancer development.

15.3.4 Incidental Findings

One of the disadvantages of the increased resolution and utilisation of cross-sectional radiologic imaging technique is the high frequency of incidental findings with associated costs in terms of patient anxiety and further investigations. Government Medicare funding for CTC in Australia is restricted partly to minimise the cost burden of investigating incidental findings at CTC.

Over 40% of patients will have incidental findings reported at CTC. Most of these will not be clinically significant, but as CTC is usually performed without IV contrast and with a lower than standard radiation dose, the ability to definitively characterise some incidental findings is limited. Radiologist interpretations of these findings are therefore often inconsistent, and fear of litigation can lead to a tendency to recommend further imaging more often.

Efforts are well established for the development of expert consensus guidelines to define, report and manage incidental findings at radiologic imaging for multiple organ systems including CTC exams. The utilisation of such guidelines by radiologists leads to a reduction in imaging recommendations for incidental imaging findings.

15.3.5 Minimal Preparation CT Colon (MPCTC)

The risk of colorectal cancer (CRC) increases with age, and 40% of subjects will be aged 75 years or older at diagnosis. Standard colonic investigation by colonoscopy, barium enema or CTC requires full bowel preparation and colonic distension. Elderly or frail patients may not be able to tolerate standard bowel preparation due to reduced mobility and incontinence as well as general health issues.

MPCTC utilises a non-laxative technique without dietary restriction to non-invasively examine the colon and rectum. This technique involves drinking small volumes of water-soluble contrast medium 48–72 h before the examination. Typically, 50 mL of 2% Gastrografin© oral solution is given twice a day. A low-residue diet can be incorporated into the protocol but is not mandatory. An extended preparation (3 days) may be required for constipated patients especially without the use of dietary restriction.

Hyperdensity of the "tagged" fecal matter allows distinction between polyps and soft tissue masses in the colon which would otherwise be obscured (Fig. 15.31). Patients are scanned in the supine position, and some gas insufflation of the colon is helpful especially to improve rectosigmoid visualisation but is not essential. Prone positioning is often difficult in this group, and one or both decubitus positions may be a helpful adjunct to supine imaging. Post IV contrast examinations may be performed to optimise diagnostic information about significant non-colonic pathology which may be present in higher frequency in this elderly age group.

The diagnostic performance of this technique has been validated and shows high positive predictive value for detection of clinically significant polyps and malignancy (Fig. 15.32).

This well-tolerated technique is, therefore, a useful tool to identify or exclude significant polyps, masses and invasive malignancy in the elderly or frail without laxative bowel preparations.

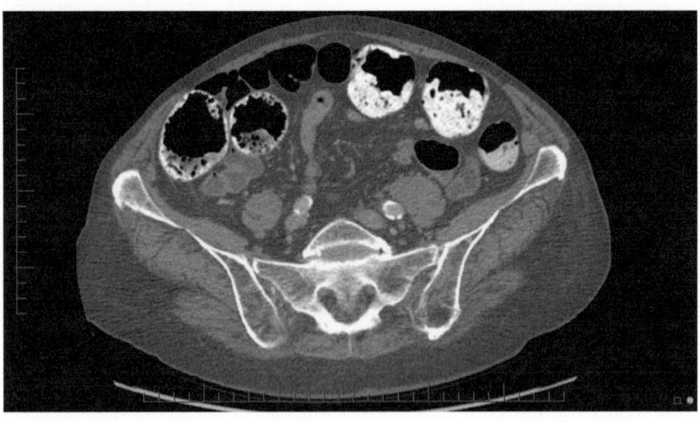

Fig. 15.31 Minimal preparation CTC—"tagging" of colonic feces to maximise the detection of focal lesions

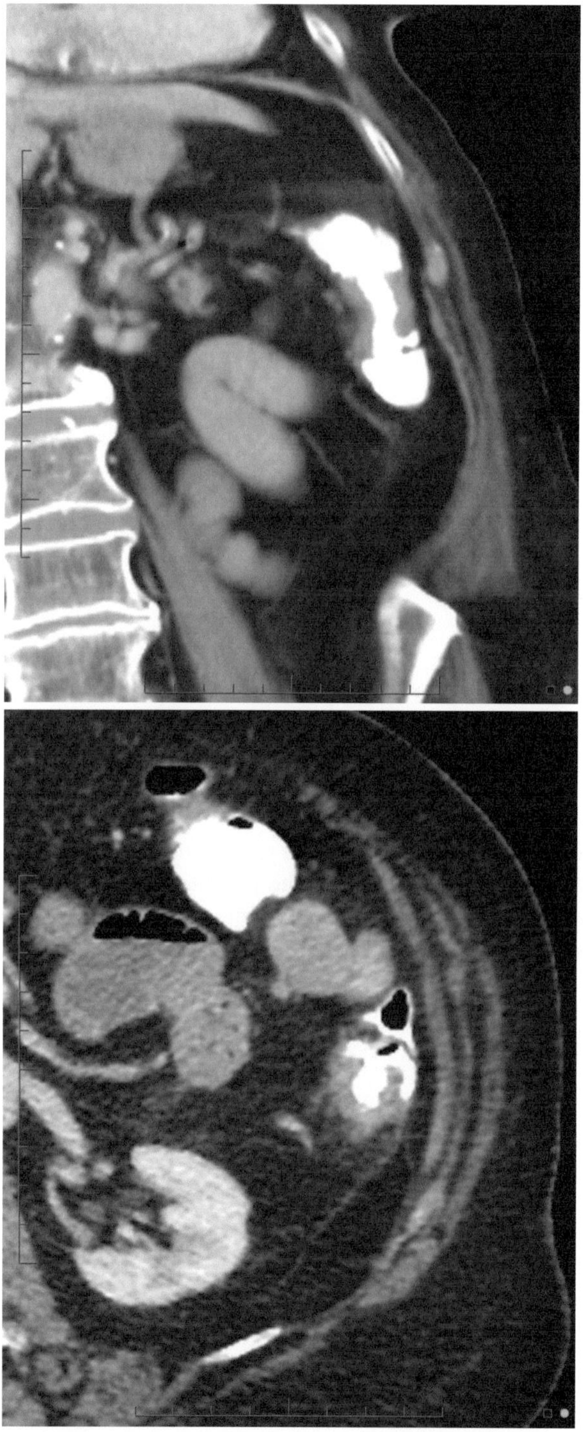

Fig. 15.32 Minimal preparation CTC demonstrates semi-annular carcinoma of descending colon (coronal and axial images)

15.4 MRI Staging for Rectal Cancer

15.4.1 Primary Staging

MR imaging plays an essential role in making management decisions in rectal cancer patients, particularly for the selection of those who would benefit from neoadjuvant therapy before surgery. Sagittal T2-weighted imaging provides long-axis view of the anorectum and is useful in the demonstration of a tumour marginal distance to the anal verge and the relationship to surrounding organs, the sacrum and the peritoneal reflection. Short-axis T2-weighted imaging is performed at the level of interest to assess the extramural extension of a tumour and the relationship to the mesorectal fascia (MRF).

The increased complexity of oncology radiology reporting leads to more diagnostic imaging parameters being included in oncologic guidelines, and accurate recording of all of the multiple vital features is required to guide clinical decision-making. Structured rather than free-text radiology reporting for body imaging especially oncologic applications is associated with improved referrer satisfaction, improves the completeness of radiology reports, facilitates interdisciplinary communication and also improves research data extraction.

15.4.2 Structured Reporting of Rectal Cancer MRI

15.4.2.1 Tumor Location and Characteristics

Longitudinal Tumor Location

The anal verge and the anorectal junction (upper margin of the puborectalis muscles) are used as reference structures. The distance from the lowest margin of a tumor to these structures is made using a composite measurement approximately along the luminal centre of the anorectum (Fig. 15.33).

The anterior rectal wall attachment of the peritoneal reflection is visible in most patients, and tumor relationship to this structure should also be described (below/astride/above). To adequately assess, the T2 sagittal and axial images should be reviewed.

Circumferential Tumor Location

Describing the extent and location of circumferential involvement (clock face descriptor) helps to identify the potential site of deepest invasion which typically exists near the central ulcerating component of a tumor (Fig. 15.34).

Tumor Length

The longitudinal tumor size (cranio-caudal extent along the long axis of the colorectum) influences the treatment planning in regard to surgical planning, potential radiation field and assessment of therapy-related responses.

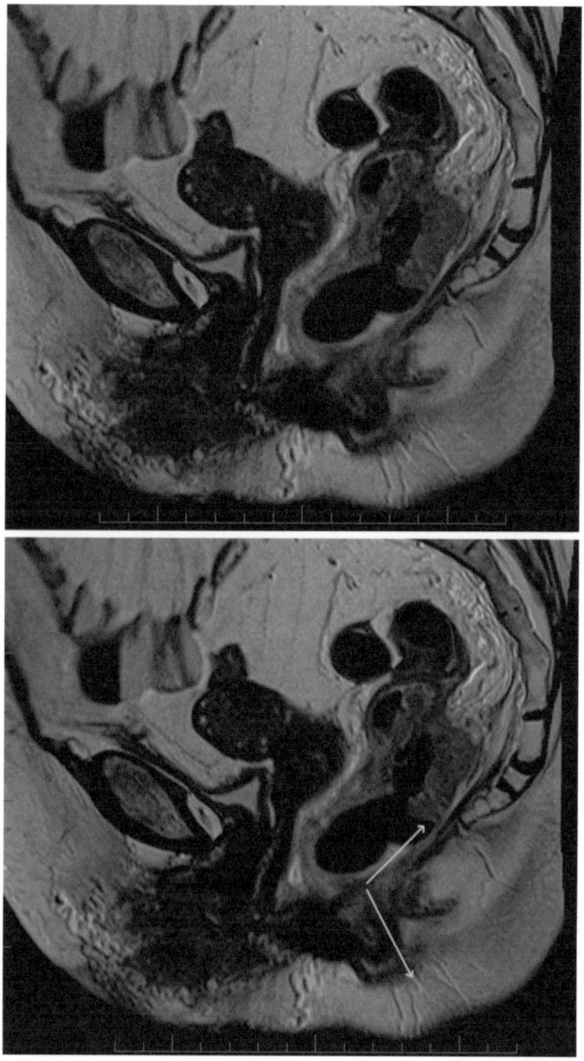

Fig. 15.33 Midline T2 sagittal MRI mid rectal cancer with measurement from lower margin tumor to ano-cutaneous junction (anal verge)

Tumor Composition

Mucin is prevalent in 15–20% of rectal cancer patients, and MRI is superior to biopsy in the preoperative detection (Fig. 15.35). This morphologic subtype is an independent marker for poor prognosis including poor response to preoperative CRT. Note that MRI after submucosal endoscopic resection procedures for cancerous polyps can lead to a false-positive diagnosis of infiltrating mucinous tumor due to the high T2 signal of the injectable colloid (Fig. 15.36).

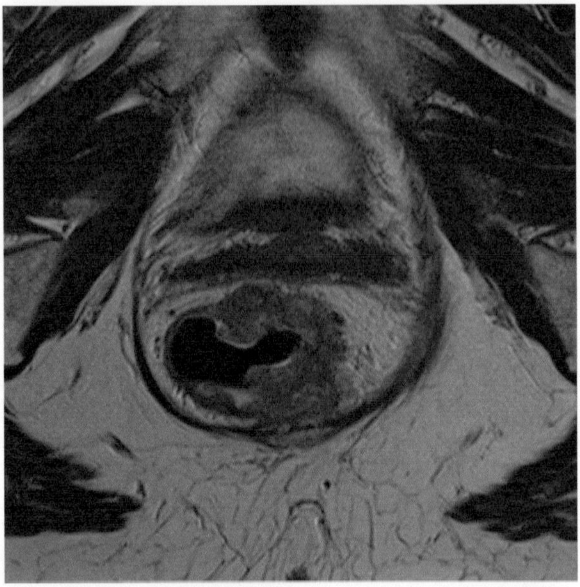

Fig. 15.34 T2 axial MRI semi-annular invasive carcinoma left lateral wall from 12 to 6 o'clock

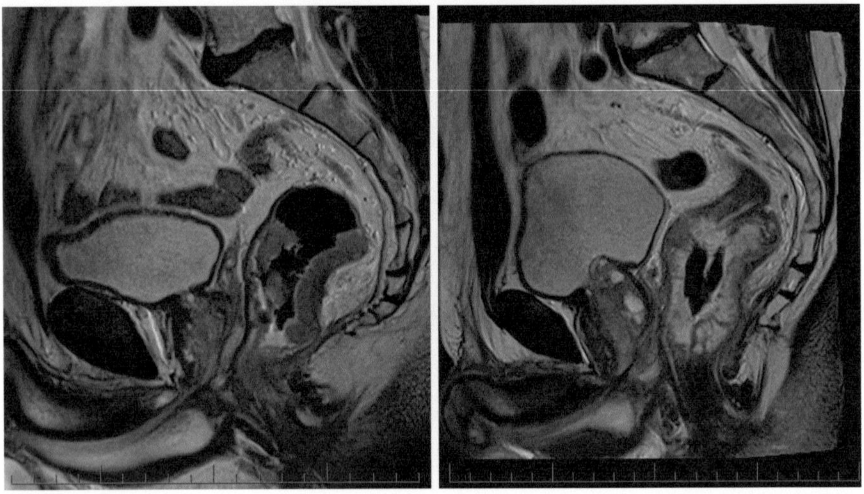

Fig. 15.35 Sagittal MR imaging non-mucinous and mucinous (high T2 signal) rectal cancers

15.4.2.2 Extramural Depth of Invasion and T Stage

The distinction between T1- and T2-stage rectal cancers is problematic on MRI. MRI has high accuracy in assessment of the depth of extramural invasion. Desmoplastic tumor response can give a spiculated appearance and lead to overstaging of T2 tumors, and fibrosis needs to be distinguished from the more nodular margin of tumor invasion (Fig. 15.37). Spiculation of the perirectal fat should be reported as a T2/early-T3 tumor.

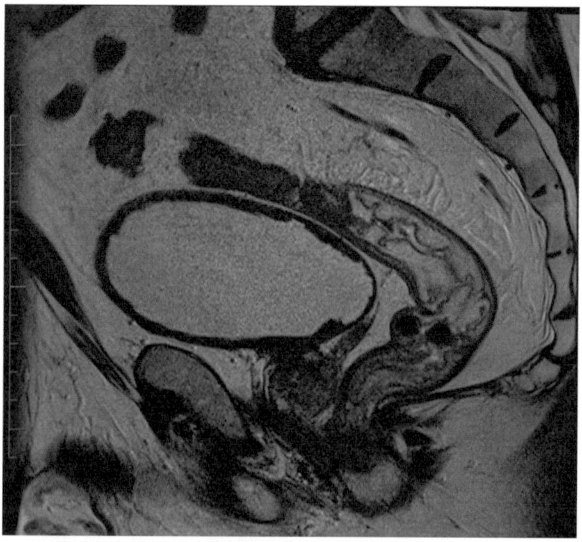

Fig. 15.36 Submucosal colloid injection at endoscopic rectal polyp resection mimicking mucinous tumor spread

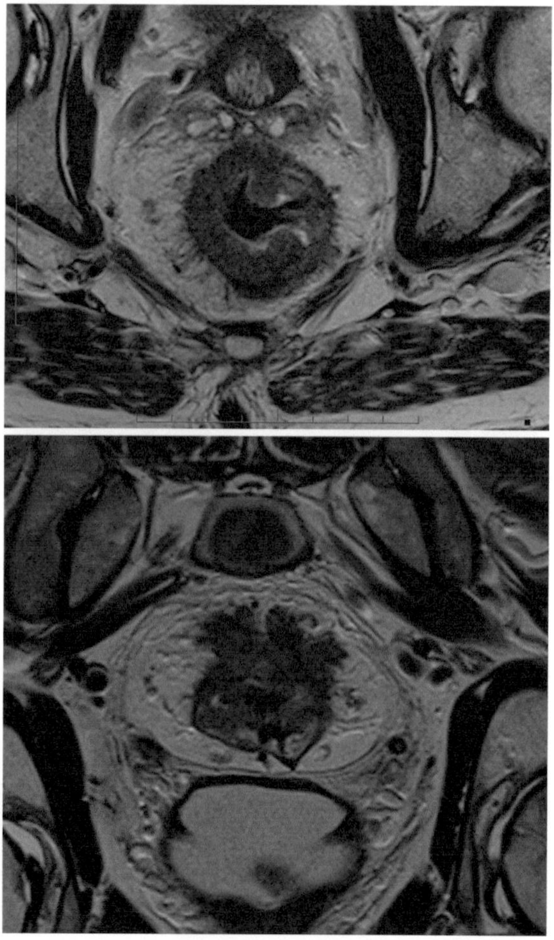

Fig. 15.37 Desmoplastic response with spiculated soft tissue stranding in mesorectal fat versus nodular tumor extension into the mesorectum

Recording the depth of extramural spread as T3 substage gives greater prognostic information by differentiating low-risk patients (<5 mm) against the poorer prognostic group with >5 mm depth of spread (Fig. 15.38). The measurement should include all types of tumor tissues that are contiguous with the primary tumor mass including extramural vascular invasion (EMVI).

Fig. 15.38 Axial MRI mid rectal cancers demonstrating depth of extramural tumor extension (<5 mm versus >5 mm)

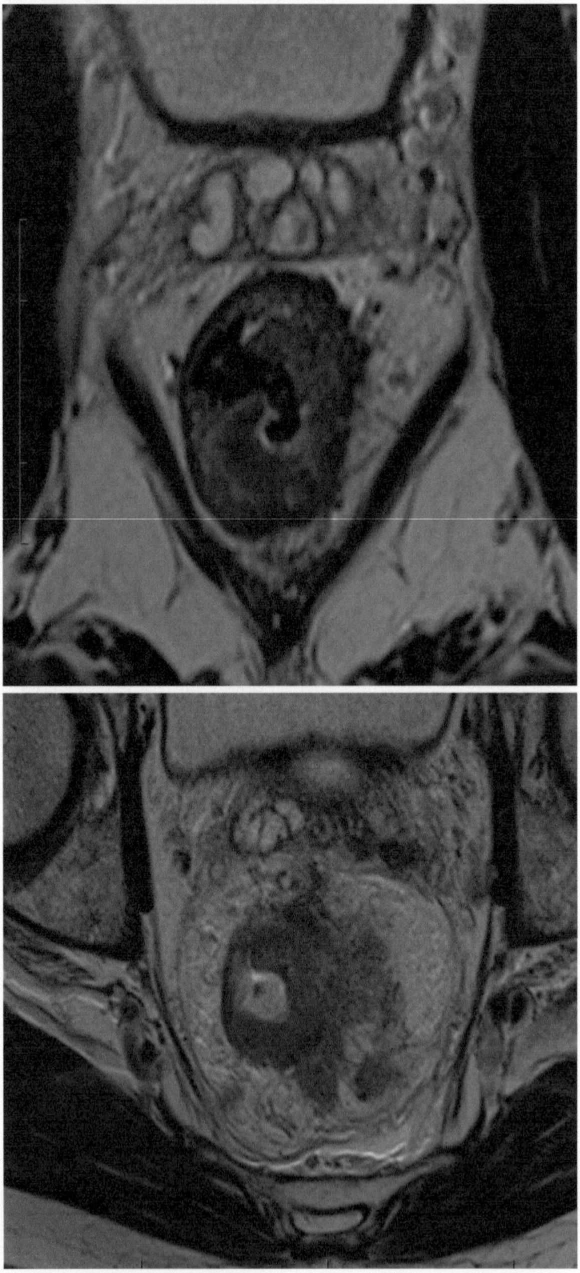

Definite invasion of adjacent organs is defined as loss of intervening fat plane and corresponding T2 signal abnormality within the organ, whereas possible invasion refers to the loss of the fat plane without a T2 signal change in the organ (Fig. 15.39). For T4b lesions, the involved structures should be specified.

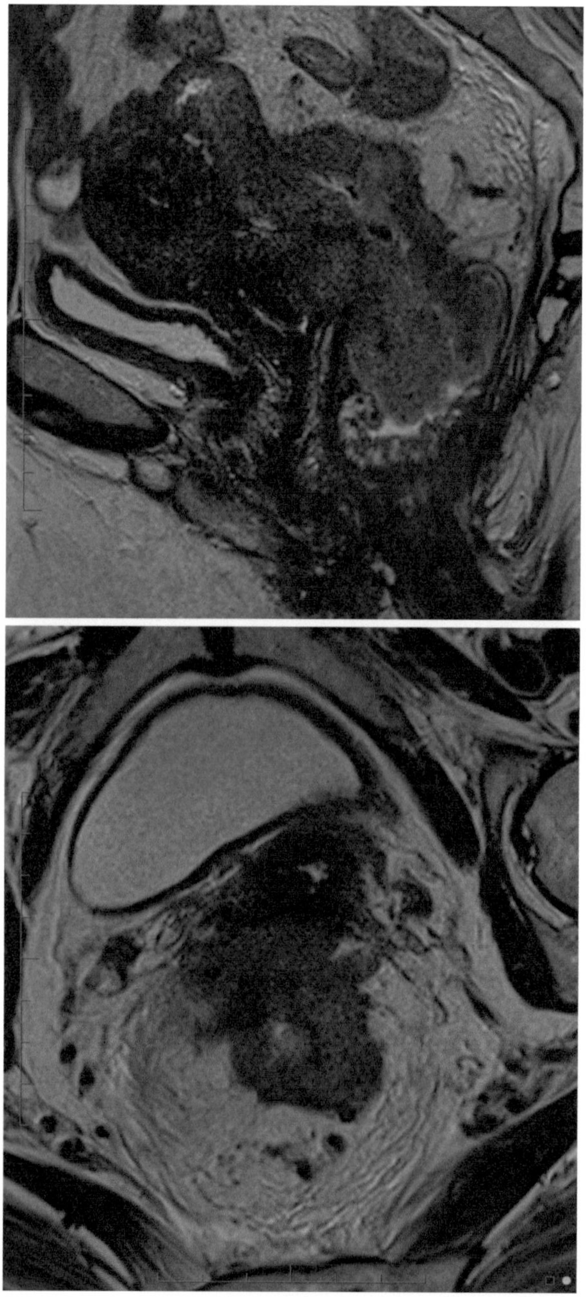

Fig. 15.39 Local locally invasive rectal cancer with involvement of the peritoneum, cervix and upper vagina

15.4.2.3 Relation of the Tumor to the Potential Circumferential Resection Margin (CRM)

The shortest tumor distance to the potential circumferential resection margin (CRM) (mesorectal fascia or levator muscles) should be stated (Fig. 15.40). The CRM is a pathologic term referring to the surgically dissected surface of a specimen and corresponds to the non-peritonealised aspect of the rectum. The CRM is only circumferential for rectal tumors below the anterior peritoneal reflection.

A distance on MRI of less than 1 mm to the mesorectal fascia has been shown to correlate with histopathologically confirmed positive CRM status. MRI +ve CRM status on baseline scans has been shown to be the most reliable prognostic factor for 5-year survival rates in MERCURY trial patients and is more important than T and N stage.

MR-identified lymph nodes involving mesorectal fascia are uncommonly a cause of CRM infiltration on final pathologic assessment. Involvement of the CRM by nodal disease only is uncommon. Caution should be used when recommending neoadjuvant therapy based solely on an MRI-detected lymph node close to the mesorectal fascia (MRF).

The distance to the MRF should be reported as "not applicable" for any tumor above the peritoneal reflection that involves peritonealised rectum (upper anterior and anterolateral tumors).

The MRF tapers below the pelvic sidewall attachments of the levator muscles, and for low rectal tumors, the distance to the levator muscles should be recorded.

Low rectal cancer outcomes remain worse than mid and upper rectal cancers with high positive pathological circumferential resection margin (pCRM) rates and high variation rates in permanent colostomies. Curative low rectal cancer restorative resection requires both the mesorectal fascia plane *and* the intersphincteric plane to be clear of a tumor.

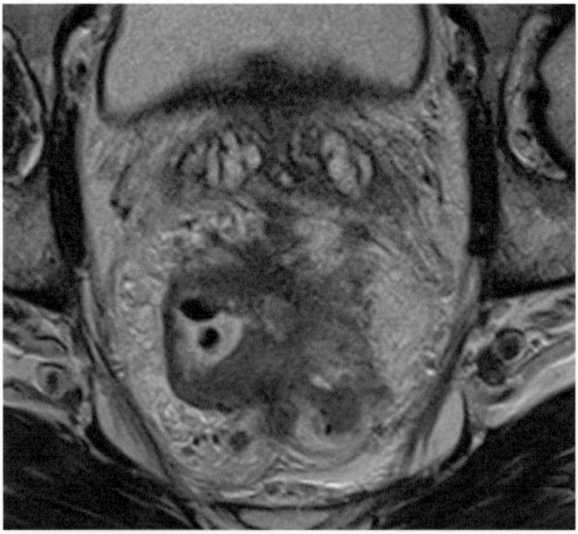

Fig. 15.40 T3d mid rectal cancer with multifocal contact with anterior mesorectal fascia (CRM positive)

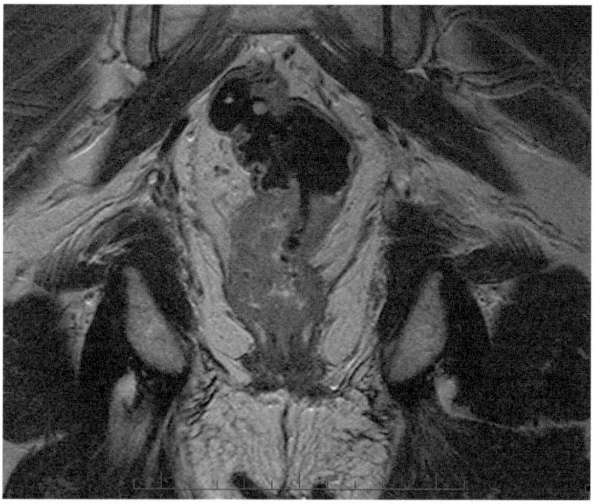

Fig. 15.41 Coronal T2 MRI low rectal cancer

For purposes of MRI reporting, low rectal cancer is classified into those with lower tumor margin above and those at or below the upper margin of the puborectalis muscle (Fig. 15.41).

Those above the puborectalis are reported similarly to upper and mid rectal tumors. Those below should be classified according to the extent of the sphincter and levator muscle involvement:

- Submucosal, no involvement of internal sphincter
- Confined to the internal sphincter, no intersphincteric fat involvement
- Intersphincteric fat involved
- Involves external sphincter and beyond

MRI staging can accurately assess the low rectal cancer surgical resection plane with improved clinical decision-making and outcomes.

15.4.2.4 Extramural Venous Invasion (EMVI)

MRI-detected EMVI is a strong predictor of poor prognosis, mainly related to the risk of liver metastases as well as local tumor recurrence.

EMVI is seen on MRI as intermediate tumour signal intensity within extramural vessels contiguous to the primary lesion (Fig. 15.42). Vessel expansion and contour irregularity by a tumor indicate increasing confidence for EMVI. MRI sensitivity is lower in small vessels (<=3 mm in diameter). Changes in MRI-detected EMVI status before and after preoperative CRT from positive to negative improve outcomes with increased disease-free survival.

15.4.2.5 Lymph Node Status

Size Criteria

Size criteria of 5 mm short-axis dimension are commonly used to assess nodal status, but there is no good evidence in the literature to support this with substantial overlap in size between benign and malignant lymph nodes. Most readers use size

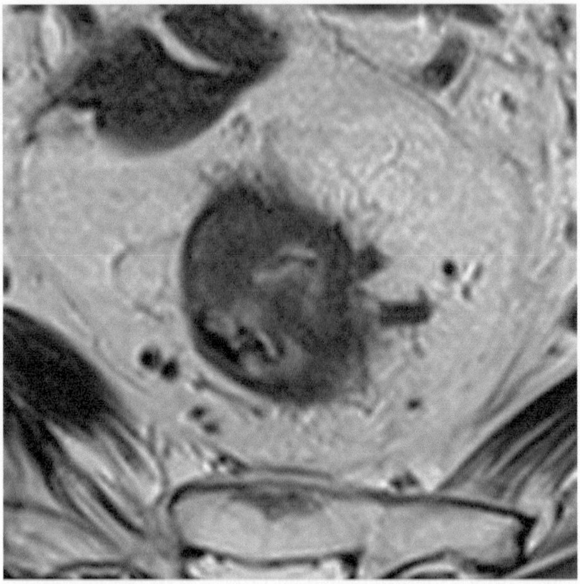

Fig. 15.42 Axial T2 MRI mid rectal cancer with multifocal EMVI left lateral margin

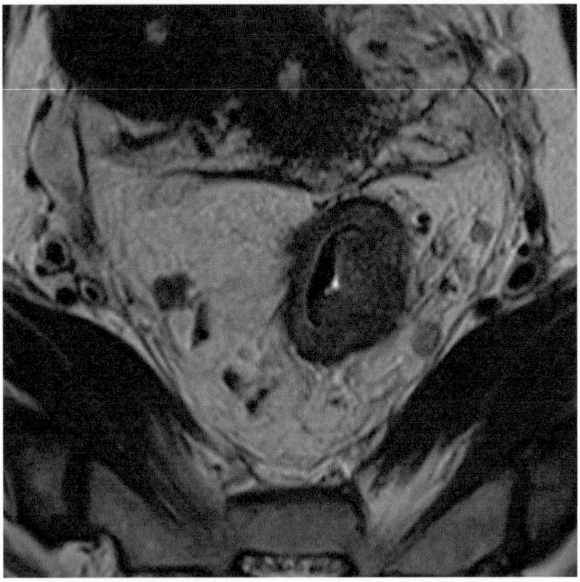

Fig. 15.43 Axial T2 MRI demonstrates variable mesorectal node appearance. Reactive node at 4 o'clock with smooth margins and T2 hyperintensity versus malignant node at 9 o'clock with heterogeneous signal intensity and irregular margins

criteria of 8 mm in the short axis, but there is reservation for recommending any particular size criteria because of the low accuracy of MRI N staging.

Border and Signal Characteristics

Published data suggest that morphological features such as heterogeneous signal intensity and irregular capsule borders are much more accurate predictors of metastatic spread within mesorectal nodes than size criteria alone (Fig. 15.43).

Distribution

Most involved mesorectal nodes are at the same level or proximal to a tumor.

Extramesorectal Nodes

If good-quality TME surgery is performed, mesorectal nodal status seems to be of no prognostic importance for local recurrence. In contrast, pelvic sidewall nodal involvement is associated with reduced disease-free survival. Any extramesorectal nodes with an irregular border, mixed-signal intensity and/or short-axis dimension >10 mm should be reported as "suspicious."

Some nodular structures in the mesorectum represent vascular deposits, a phenomenon that is difficult to assess on final histology as the absence of preserved nodular capsule precludes differentiating malignant lymph node with extracapsular invasion. Tumor deposits predict poorer prognosis.

MRI allows recognition of EMVI and discontinuous nodular deposits along infiltrated veins which probably represent venous deposits and can be classified according to the TNM seventh edition as N1c (extranodal tumor deposits) (Fig. 15.44).

15.4.3 MRI for Restaging Evaluation After Neoadjuvant Therapy

MRI is the imaging modality of choice for restaging rectal malignancy. High-resolution T2-weighted sequences are the primary sequence for morphologic assessment of tumor response.

The post CRT MRI exam is performed with the intent of ensuring negative margins, selecting those patients for less radical excision and to assess for the interval development of metastasis and extramesorectal lymphadenopathy.

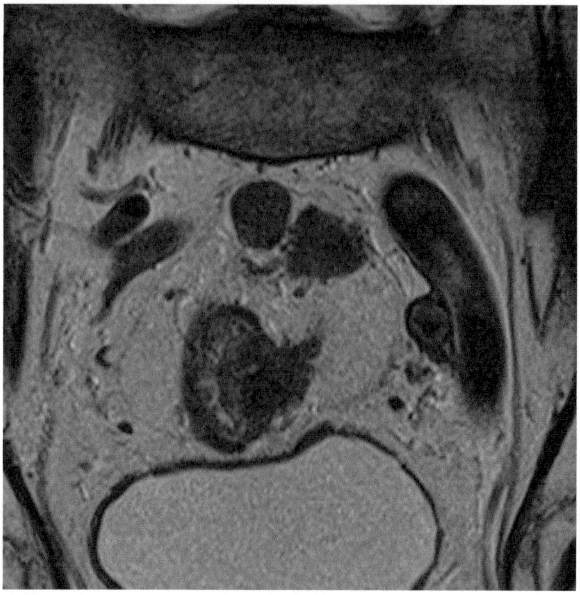

Fig. 15.44 Discontinuous nodular deposit of mesorectum at 1 o'clock along the path of extramural vascular invasion

The most widely used method to identify a complete pathologic response is the absence of endoscopic residual mucosal abnormality, but there is evidence that this underestimates the actual number of complete responders. MRI tumor regression grading systems based on the extent of visible fibrosis on MRI can identify more patients with pCR than clinical assessment with no significant compromise in false positive rate and has prognostic value in predicting long-term outcomes.

On post chemoradiotherapy (CRT) scans, T2-weighted MRI, areas of fibrosis have very low signal intensity, whereas areas of residual tumor have intermediate signal intensity (Figs. 15.45 and 15.46). The signal intensity of fibrosis is similar to that of the muscularis propria, and signal intensity of residual tumor is similar to that of baseline tumor. Evaluation of mucinous tumors on post-treatment MRI is challenging because these tumors remain hyperintense on T2WI, regardless of treatment response.

The MRI tumor regression grade (mrtRG) has predictive value for the distinction between good and poor responders to neoadjuvant therapy.

Because post-treatment fibrosis can sometimes be difficult to differentiate from a residual tumor on T2WI, there may be a role for the addition of functional diffusion-weighted imaging to improve restaging accuracy including for the identification of complete responders.

MRI-detected complete response is being used as a marker to select those patients who may be candidates for a watch and wait policy, rather than surgical intervention.

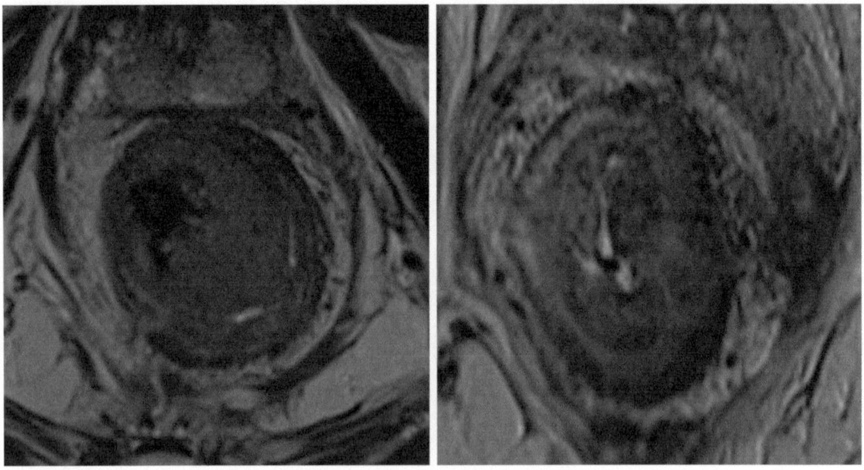

Fig. 15.45 Pre- and post chemoradiotherapy T2 axial scans show residual tumor of intermediate signal intensity post-treatment

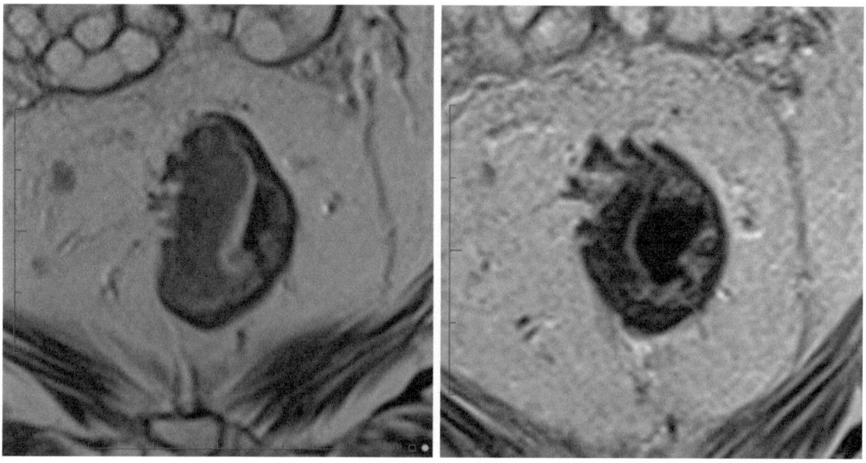

Fig. 15.46 Pre- and post chemoradiotherapy T2 axial scans show low T2 signal intensity wall thickening only on post-treatment scan indicating fibrosis

Recommended Reading

Bruning DH, Siddiki HA, Fletcher JG, et al. Benefit of computed tomography enterography in Crohn's disease: effects on patient management and physician level of confidence. Inflamm Bowel Dis. 2012;18:219–25.

Rimola J, Ordas I, Rodriguez S, et al. Magnetic resonance imaging for evaluation of Crohn's disease: validation of parameters of severity and quantitative index of activity. Inflamm Bowel Dis. 2011;17:1759–68.

Bruining DH, Zimmermann EM, Loftus EV Jr, et al. Consensus recommendations for evaluation, interpretation, and utilization of computed tomography and magnetic resonance enterography in patients with small bowel Crohn's disease. Radiology. 2018;286(3):776–99.

Cosnes J, Cattan S, Blain A, Beaugerie L, Carbonnel F, Parc R, Genre JP. Long-term evolution of disease behavior of Crohn's disease. Inflamm Bowel Dis. 2002;8(4):244–50.

Thia KT, Sandborn WJ, Harmsen WS, et al. Risk factors associated with progression to intestinal complications of Crohn's disease in a population-based cohort. Gastroenterology. 2010;139(4):1147–55.

Rimola J, Planell N, Rodriguez S, et al. Characterization of inflammation and fibrosis in Crohn's disease lesions by magnetic resonance imaging. Am J Gastroenterol. 2015;110:432–40.

Gomollon F, Dignass A, Annese V, et al. 3rd European Evidence-based Consensus on the Diagnosis and Management of Crohn's Disease 2016: Part 1: Diagnosis and Medical Management ECCO Guideline/Consensus Paper. J Crohn's Colitis. 2017;11(1):3–25.

Booya F, Akram S, Fletcher JG, et al. CT enterography and fistulising Crohn's disease: clinical benefits and radiographic findings. Abdom Imaging. 2009;34:467–75.

de Miguel CJ, del Salto LG, Rivas PF, et al. MR imaging of perianal fistulas: spectrum of imaging features. Radiographics. 2012;32:175–94.

Hemminki K, Li J, Sundquist K, et al. Cancer risks in Crohn disease patients. Ann Oncol. 2009;3:574–80.

Weber NK, Fletcher JG, Fidler JL, et al. Clinical characteristics and imaging features of small bowel adenocarcinomas in Crohn's disease. Abdom Imaging. 2015;40:1060–7.

Zhang T, Fan R, Wang Z, et al. Differential diagnosis between Crohn's disease and intestinal tuberculosis using integrated parameters including clinical manifestations, T-SPOT, endoscopy and CT enterography. Int J Clin Exp Med. 2015;8(10):17578–89.

Debi U, Ravisankar V, Prasad KK, Sinha SK, Sharma AK. Abdominal tuberculosis of the gastrointestinal tract: revisited. World J Gastroenterol. 2014;20(40):14831–40.

Frye JM, Hansel SL, Dolan SG, et al. NSAID enteropathy: appearance at CT and MR enterography in the age of multi-modality imaging and treatment. Abdom Imaging. 2015;40:1011–25.

Bouguen G, Levesque BG, Pola S, et al. Endoscopic assessment and treating to target increase the likelihood of mucosal healing in patients with Crohn's disease. Clin Gastroenterol Hepatol. 2014;12(6):978–85.

Deepak P, Fletcher JG, Fidlet JL, et al. Radiologic response is associated with better long-term outcomes and is a potential treatment target in patients with small bowel Crohn's disease. Am J Gastroenterol. 2016;111(7):997–1006.

Scardapane A, Ambrosi A, Salinaro E, et al. Assessment of disease activity in small bowel Crohn's disease: comparison between endoscopy and magnetic resonance enterography using MRIA and modified MRIA score. Gastroenterol Res Pract. 2015;2015:159641.

Bezzio C, Bryant RV, Manes G, et al. New horizons in the imaging of perianal Crohn's disease: transperineal ultrasonography. Expert Rev Gastroenterol Hepatol. 2017;11(6):523–30.

Ganeshan D, Duong PT, Probyn L, et al. Structured reporting in radiology. Acad Radiol. 2018;25(1):66–73.

Horsthuis K, Lavini C, Bipat S, et al. Perianal Crohn disease: evaluation of dynamic contrast-enhanced MR imaging as an indicator of disease activity. Radiology. 2009;251:380–7.

Gionchetti P, Dignass A, Danese S, et al. 3rd European Evidence-based Consensus on the Diagnosis and Management of Crohn's Disease 2016: Part 2: Surgical Management and Special Situations ECCO Guideline/Consensus Paper. J Crohns Colitis. 2017;11(2):135–49.

Erden A. MRI of anal canal: normal anatomy, imaging protocol, and perianal fistulas: part 1 abdominal. Radiology. 2018;43:1334–52.

Sheedy SP, Bruning DH, Dozols EJ, et al. MR imaging of perianal Crohn disease. Radiology. 2017;282(3):628–45.

Gecse K, Khanna R, Stoker J, et al. Fistulizing Crohn's disease: diagnosis and management. United European Gastroenterol J. 2013;1(3):206–13.

Nolthenius CJT, Bipat S, Mearadji B, et al. MRI characteristics of proctitis in Crohn's disease on perianal MRI. Abdom Radiol. 2016;41:1918–30.

Savoye-Collet C, Savoye G, Koning E, et al. Fistulizing perianal Crohn's disease: contrast-enhanced magnetic resonance imaging assessment at 1 year on maintenance anti-TNF-alpha therapy. Inflamm Bowel Dis. 2011;17(8):1751–8.

Taylor SA, Halligan S, Bartram CI. Pilonidal sinus disease: MR imaging distinction from fistula in ano. Radiology. 2003;226:662–7.

Atkin W, Dadswell E, Wooldrage K, et al. Computed tomographic colonography versus colonoscopy for investigation of patients with symptoms suggestive of colorectal cancer (SIGGAR): a multicentre randomised trial. Lancet. 2013;381:1194–202.

Halligan S, Wooldrage K, Dadswell E, et al. Computed tomographic colonography versus barium enema for diagnosis of colorectal cancer or large polyps in symptomatic patients (SIGGAR): a multicentre randomised trial. Lancet. 2013;381:1185–93.

Kim DH, Lubner MG, Cahoon AR, et al. Flat serrated polyps at CT colonography: relevance, appearance, and optimizing interpretation. Radiographics. 2018;38(1):60–74.

Pickhardt PJ. Incidence of colonic perforation at CT colonography; review of existing data and implications for screening of asymptomatic adults. Radiology. 2006;239:313–6.

Lara LF, Avalos D, Huynh H, et al. The safety of same-day CT colonography following incomplete colonoscopy with polypectomy. United European Gastroenterol J. 2015;3(4):358–63.

33. Hendee WR, O'Connor MK. Radiation risks of medical imaging: separating fact from fantasy. Radiology. 2012;264(2):312–21.

Liedenbaum MH, Venema HW, Stoker J. Radiation dose in CT colonography-trends in time and differences between daily practice and screening protocols. Eur Radiol. 2008;18:2222–30.

Lumbreras B, Donat L, Hernandez-Aguado I. Incidental findings in imaging diagnostic tests: a systematic review. Br J Radiol. 2010;83(988):276–89.

Meyer HJ, Pfeil A, Schramm D, et al. Renal incidental findings on computed tomography Frequency and distribution in a large non selected cohort. Medicine. 2017;96(26):1–5.

Berland LL. Incidental extracolonic findings on CT colonography: the impending deluge and its implications. J Am Coll Radiol. 2009;6(1):14–20.

Berland LL, Silverman SG, Megibow AJ, et al. ACR members' response to JACR white paper on the management of incidental abdominal CT findings. J Am Coll Radiol. 2014;11(1):30–5.

Johnson CM, Wei C, Ensor JE, et al. Meta-analyses of colorectal cancer risk factors. Cancer Causes Control. 2013;24(6):1207–22.

Amin MF, Hassanin AM. Diagnostic performance of CT colonography with limited cathartic preparation in colorectal cancer screening; comparison with conventional colonoscopy. Egypt J Radiol Nucl Med. 2015;46(3):591–8.

Liedenbaum MH, de Vries AH, Guow CI, et al. CT colonography with minimal bowel preparation: evaluation of tagging quality, patient acceptance and diagnostic accuracy in two iodine-based preparation schemes. Eur Radiol. 2010;20(2):367–76.

Zueco Z, Sampedro A, Corroto JD, et al. CT colonography without cathartic preparation: positive predictive value and patient experience in clinical practice. Eur Radiol. 2012;22(6):1195–204.

KSAR Study Group for Rectal Cancer. Essential Items for Structured Reporting of Rectal Cancer MRI: 2016 Consensus Recommendation from the Korean Society of Abdominal Radiology. Korean J Radiol. 2017;18(1):132–51.

Norenberg D, Sommer WH, Thasler W, et al. Structured reporting of rectal magnetic resonance imaging in suspected primary rectal cancer. Invest Radiol. 2017;52(4):232–9.

User's Guide for the Synoptic MRI Report for Pre-Operative Staging of Rectal Cancer. Cancer Care Ontario. 2015.

Yu SK, Chand M, Tait DM, et al. Magnetic resonance imaging defined mucinous rectal carcinoma is an independent imaging biomarker for poor prognosis and poor response to preoperative chemoradiotherapy. Eur J Cancer. 2014;50(5):920–7.

Barbaro B, Leccisott L, Vecchio FM, et al. The potential predictive value of MRI and PET-CT in mucinous and nonmucinous rectal cancer to identify patients at high risk of metastatic disease. Br J Radiol. 2017;90:20150836.

Beets-Tan RG, Lambregts DM, Maas M, et al. Magnetic resonance imaging for the clinical management of rectal cancer patients: recommendations from the 2012 European Society of Gastrointestinal and Abdominal Radiology (ESGAR) consensus meeting. Eur Radiol. 2013;23:2522–31.

Tong T, Sun Y, Cai S, et al. Extramural depth of rectal cancer tumor invasion at thin-section MRI: predicting treatment response to neoadjuvant chemoradiation. Oncotarget. 2015;6(30):30277–86.

Beets-Tan RG, Beets GL, Vliegen RF, et al. Accuracy of magnetic resonance imaging in prediction of tumour-free resection margin in rectal cancer surgery. Lancet. 2001;357:497–504.

Taylor FG, Quirle P, Heald RJ, et al. Preoperative magnetic resonance imaging assessment of circumferential resection margin predicts disease-free survival and local recurrence: 5-year follow-up results of the MERCURY study. J Clin Oncol. 2014;32(1):34–43.

Shihab OC, Quirke P, Heald RJ, et al. Magnetic resonance imaging-detected lymph nodes close to the mesorectal fascia are rarely a cause of margin involvement after total mesorectal excision. Br J Surg. 2010;97(9):1431–6.

Battersby NJ, How P, Moran B, et al. Prospective validation of a low rectal cancer magnetic resonance imaging staging system and development of a local recurrence risk stratification model: the MERCURY II study. Ann Surg. 2016;263(4):751–60.

Sohn B, Lim JS, Kim H, et al. MRI-detected extramural vascular invasion is an independent prognostic factor for synchronous metastasis in patients with rectal cancer. Eur Radiol. 2015;25:1347–55.

Jhaveri KS, Hosseini-Nik H, Thipphavong S, et al. MRI detection of extramural venous invasion in rectal cancer: correlation with histopathology using elastin stain. AJR Am J Roentgenol. 2016;206:747–55.

Chand M, Swift RI, Tekkis PP, et al. Extramural venous invasion is a potential imaging predictive biomarker of neoadjuvant treatment in rectal cancer. Br J Cancer. 2014;110(1):19–25.

Brown G, Richards CJ, Bourne MW, et al. Morphologic predictors of lymph node status in rectal cancer with use of high-spatial-resolution MR imaging with histopathologic comparison. Radiology. 2003;227:371–7.

Chand M, Moran BJ, Jones RG, et al. Lymph node status does not predict local recurrence in the total mesorectal excision era. Dis Colon Rectum. 2014;57(1):127–9.

Shihab OC, Taylor F, Bees N. Relevance of magnetic resonance imaging-detected pelvic sidewall lymph node involvement in rectal cancer. Br J Surg. 2011;98(12):1798–804.

Zhang LN, Xiao WW, Xi SY, et al. Tumor deposits: markers of poor prognosis in patients with locally advanced rectal cancer following neoadjuvant chemoradiotherapy. Oncotarget. 2016;7(5):6335–44.

Balyasnikova S, Brown G. Imaging advances in colorectal cancer. Curr Colorectal Cancer Rep. 2016;12:162–9.

Bhoday J, Smith F, Siddiqui M, et al. Magnetic resonance tumor regression grade and residual mucosal abnormality as predictors for pathological complete response in rectal cancer postneoadjuvant chemoradiotherapy. Dis Colon Rectum. 2016;59(10):925–33.

Kong JC, Guerra GR, Warrier SK, et al. Prognostic value of tumour regression grade in locally advanced rectal cancer: a systematic review and meta-analysis. Colorectal Dis. 2018;20(7):574–85. https://doi.org/10.1111/codi.14106.

Battersby NJ, Balyasnikova S, Brown G. Guiding post-treatment decisions in rectal cancer: mrTRG is a practical place to start. Oncology. 2014;28(8):667–77.

Fayaz M, Demian GA, Fathallal WM, et al. Significance of magnetic resonance imaging–assessed tumor response for locally advanced rectal cancer treated with preoperative long-course chemoradiation. J Glob Oncol. 2016;2(4):216–21.

Lee MA, Cho SH, Seo AN, et al. Modified 3-point MRI-based tumor regression grade incorporating DWI for locally advanced rectal cancer. AJR Am J Roentgenol. 2017;209(6):1247–55.

Patel UB, Taylor F, Blomqvist L, et al. Magnetic resonance imaging-detected tumor response for locally advanced rectal cancer predicts survival outcomes: MERCURY experience. J Clin Oncol. 2011;29:3753–60.

Moreno CC, Sullivan PS, Mittal PK. MRI evaluation of rectal cancer: staging and restaging. Curr Probl Diagn Radiol. 2017;46(3):234–41.

16 Nutrition and Parenteral Nutrition

Christopher K. Rayner and Marianne J. Chapman

16.1 Introduction

It is now recognized that surgery induces a catabolic response, such that two-thirds of patients will lose weight during their hospital admission. The risks of malnutrition in the surgical patient include susceptibility to infection, impaired wound healing, anastomotic leakage, pressure ulcers, prolonged hospital length of stay, increased readmission rates and higher costs, as well as increased mortality.

Provision of nutritional support to the surgical patient involves more than just supplying sufficient energy to maintain body mass. It can also improve outcomes by modulating immune responses and by ameliorating the harmful consequences of metabolic stress. This integration of nutritional therapy into the overall care of the surgical patient addresses a number of goals such as assessment of nutritional risk, avoidance of prolonged fasting, early feeding after surgery (where possible) and early mobilization to assist protein synthesis and preserve muscle function.

Evidence in support of nutritional interventions in hospitalized patients has been critically assessed in a number of meta-analyses and has been incorporated into guidelines published by national and international societies (see Recommended Reading). These form the basis for the information presented in the current chapter. However, the evidence is often of low quality and plagued by heterogeneity, variable disease severity and the absence of baseline nutritional data.

C. K. Rayner (✉)
Adelaide Medical School, The University of Adelaide, Adelaide, SA, Australia
e-mail: chris.rayner@adelaide.edu.au

M. J. Chapman
Intensive Care Unit, Royal Adelaide Hospital, Adelaide, SA, Australia
e-mail: marianne.chapman@sa.gov.au

M. W. Wichmann et al. (eds.), *Gastroenterology For General Surgeons*,
https://doi.org/10.1007/978-3-319-92768-8_16

This chapter will focus on evolving changes in nutritional practice in the perioperative setting, the assessment of nutritional risk, the indications and contraindications to enteral and parenteral feeding, composition of feeds, routes of delivery and monitoring of outcomes.

16.2 Changing Practices in Fasting and Resuming Feeding in the Surgical Patient

It is now recognized that the periods of perioperative fasting that were recommended in the past were often unnecessarily long. Issues with prolonged fasting include metabolic stress and impairment of mitochondrial function and insulin sensitivity.

The rate of gastric emptying is controlled by hormonal and neural feedback mechanisms that are dependent on the caloric and osmotic load of the stomach contents, the types of macronutrient ingested (fats empty more slowly than carbohydrate or protein) and whether the meal is solid or liquid. Gastric emptying is slowed by pain, some medications (e.g. opiates) and in some patients with disorders such as long-standing diabetes, Parkinson's disease, scleroderma and gastro-oesophageal reflux disease. In the absence of such risk factors, it is now recommended that patients fast from clear low-nutrient fluids for 2 h and from solids for 6 h prior to surgery. The provision of preoperative carbohydrate solutions, which has been advocated to reduce insulin resistance, has not been clearly shown to be better than giving water.

Similarly, in the past, patients were often ordered to delay resumption of oral intake after surgery until the return of normal gut motility. This could take 12–24 h for the small intestine, 24–48 h for the stomach, and 48–72 h for the colon. The return of bowel sounds is not a reliable marker of gut function and should not be the criterion for commencement of feeding. Early resumption of oral intake post-operatively (within 24 h) is now favoured in Enhanced Recovery After Surgery (ERAS) protocols that have been pioneered in colorectal surgery. The evidence is that early refeeding is safe and well-tolerated, especially after laparoscopic surgery, and is associated with enhanced recovery from ileus, lower risks of infection and a shorter hospital stay (without increasing the risk of anastomotic leakage). Furthermore, there is no need for a graded resumption of intake with progression from clear fluids to solids.

Despite the above, there are still some well-established contra-indications to early feeding. These include mechanical obstruction of the gastrointestinal tract, uncontrolled peritonitis, ischemic gut and some cases of high output fistulas. However, the presence of ileus, recent anastomosis, bowel wall edema, gastrointestinal bleeding and an open abdomen are no longer absolute contraindications to enteral feeding. Feeding can also be given in critically ill patients who are maintaining an adequate mean arterial blood pressure on catecholamine therapy.

16.3 Assessment of Nutritional Status and Nutritional Risk

Nutritional assessment of the surgical patient involves not just assessment of *nutritional status* but also *nutritional risk*. The latter recognizes that the underlying disease process, including surgery itself, evokes an inflammatory response and alters the utilization of available nutrients. Patients most at risk are those with severe underlying disease, poor baseline nutritional status and a low likelihood of resuming an oral intake within 5–7 days.

Clinical assessment of nutritional status involves both history and physical examination (Table 16.1). Important details include oral intake, duration of hospitalization, degree of weight loss, surgical history and coexisting infection or chronic disease. Indicators of severe malnutrition include loss of ≥5% body weight over 1 month, ≥7.5% over 3 months, ≥10% over 6 months or ≥20% over 1 year. Age itself (>70 years) is also a risk factor for malnutrition. In addition to weight and height, physical examination should evaluate loss of subcutaneous fat (particularly in the orbits, triceps folds and overlying the ribs), loss of muscle mass (especially the temporalis, chest, shoulder girdle, thigh and calf) and fluid accumulation (i.e. peripheral edema or ascites which may mask weight loss) as well as signs of specific nutritional deficiencies. Finally, grip strength can be tested. In obese patients, the assessor should be alert to the possibility of loss of fat-free mass even though body mass index (BMI) appears high.

Anthropometric measures such as the mid-arm muscle circumference, skin fold thickness or creatinine-height index are poorly reproducible and thus of limited value. Serum albumin is routinely measured in surgical patients; a concentration <30 g/L is a risk factor for complications of surgery, but albumin also falls with inflammation and may not increase again until the latter has resolved. Moreover, serum albumin is lowered by hepatic and renal disease. Pre-albumin and transferrin have been advocated as alternative measures given that they have shorter half-lives, but all acute phase reactants suffer from similar limitations.

Several tools have been developed to help evaluate nutritional status. These include the Mini-Nutritional Assessment (MNA), Simplified Nutritional Assessment

Table 16.1 Clinical assessment of nutritional status

History
• Energy intake as a proportion of requirements
• Weight loss (>5% in 1 month, 7.5% in 3 months, 10% in 6 months, or 20% in 1 year are indicators of severe malnutrition)
• Coexisting chronic disease or infection
• Surgical history
Physical examination
• Signs of specific nutritional deficiencies
• Loss of subcutaneous fat (orbits, triceps fold, overlying ribs)
• Loss of muscle mass (temporalis, chest, shoulder girdle, thigh, calf)
• Fluid accumulation (peripheral edema, ascites)
• Grip strength

Questionnaire (SNAQ), Subjective Global Assessment (SGA), Malnutrition Universal Screening Tool (MUST), and Nutritional Risk Index. These are suitable for patients on general wards, but they have not been validated in critical illness where indices that incorporate an assessment of nutritional risk become more important.

In critically unwell patients, either the Nutritional Risk Score-2002 (NRS-2002) or the Nutrition Risk in Intensive Care (NUTRIC) is appropriate for determining nutritional risk (Table 16.2). The NRS-2002 determines severity of impaired nutritional status (0–3 points) from weight loss, BMI, food intake and severity of disease (0–3 points) from broad diagnostic categories, with a total score >3 indicating risk and ≥5 indicating high risk. The NUTRIC score awards 0–3 points for Acute Physiology and Chronic Health Evaluation II (APACHE II) score, 0–2 points for each of age and organ failure assessment and 0–1 points for each of co-morbidities, days in the ICU and interleukin-6 (optional). Patients with ≥5 points are at high risk (≥6 if IL-6 is included). These indices have predictive value for determining which patients are most likely to benefit from intensive nutritional support. In a Chinese study, for example, patients with preoperative NRS-2002 scores ≥5 who met their nutritional targets had a 50% reduction in complications, including nosocomial infections, while in a Canadian study, patients receiving their target volume of nutrition had reduced mortality if the NUTRIC score was ≥6. Conversely, low scores (NRS-2002 ≤3, NUTRIC ≤5) suggest that a patient can tolerate 1 week in hospital without aggressive attempts to provide nutritional support.

16.4 Calculation of Nutritional Requirements

Indirect calorimetry is the most accurate means of determining the energy requirements of individual patients, but its availability is limited. Numerous equations have been developed as an alternative (e.g. Harris-Benedict), but these are less accurate than calorimetry, especially in those who are markedly over- or underweight. The obese are at particular risk of muscle loss, since their high insulin concentrations suppress lipid metabolism and result in increased muscle breakdown. The elderly are also at high risk as they have a reduced lean body mass and an increase in fat. In patients with edema, usual or dry body weight should be used in calculations of energy requirements.

For most patients, energy expenditure is in the range 25–30 kcal/kg/day. However, it remains uncertain whether providing this much energy is an important goal for short-term feeding (e.g. up to 1 week) in patients who were previously well nourished. For example, data from studies performed on critically ill patients suggest that the number of calories provided is not critical during a short stay in the ICU.

Given the benefits of stimulating the gut through enteral administration of nutrients, the concept of "trophic feeding" (providing around 400 kcal/day) or "permissive underfeeding or hypo-caloric feeding" (providing around 1000 kcal/day), while giving a full allowance of protein, has been suggested as a way of providing the benefits of enteral feeding on gut function while avoiding feeding intolerance. This strategy may be particularly suitable for obese patients and may be as good as providing full enteral nutrition over the first week.

Table 16.2 Nutritional risk assessment

(A) NRS-2002					
Impaired nutritional status					
Absent					0 points
Mild					
• Weight loss >5% in 3 months					
• Intake <50–75% of needs in past week					1 point
Moderate					
• Weight loss >5% in 2 months					
• Intake 25–50% of needs in past week					
• BMI 18.5–20.5 with impaired condition					2 points
Severe					
• Weight loss >5% in 1 month or 15% in 3 months					
• Intake <25% of needs in past week					
• BMI < 18.5 with impaired condition					3 points
Severity of disease					
Absent					0 points
Mild					
• Hip fracture					
• Acute complications of chronic disease (cirrhosis, COPD)					
• Chronic disease (diabetes, oncology, haemodialysis)					1 point
Moderate					
• Major abdominal surgery					
• Stroke					
• Severe pneumonia					
• Hematological malignancy					2 points
Severe					
• Head injury					
• Bone marrow transplant					
• ICU (APACHE II >10)					3 points
Interpretation of total score					
>3 points: at risk					
≥5 points: high risk					
(B) NUTRIC					
	0 points	*1 point*	*2 points*	*3 points*	
Age	<50 years	50–74 years	≥75 years	–	
APACHE II score	<15	15–19	20–27	≥28	
Simplified Organ Failure Assessment (SOFA) score	<6	6–9	≥10	–	
Number of co-morbidities	0–1	≥2	–	–	
Days in hospital prior to ICU	0	≥1	–	–	
IL-6 (optional)	<400 pg/mL	≥400 pg/mL			
Interpretation of total score					
≥5 points (≥6 points if IL-6 included): high risk					

It is now known that protein is the most important macronutrient. Although recommendations are not based on robust evidence, guidelines indicate that 1.2–2.0 g protein/kg/day should be provided, with higher amounts in patients with burns, trauma, or large wounds. Serum protein markers (albumin, pre-albumin, transferrin and C-reactive protein) have not been validated for monitoring the adequacy of protein administration and typically lag behind improvements in nutritional status.

Attention to nutritional support in at-risk patients should be considered early, even in the preoperative period. The concept of "pre-habilitation" refers to a multimodal approach that provides nutritional supplements and exercise programs (including the respiratory muscles) in advance of surgery in order to reduce postoperative complications. Such programs have been shown to shorten length of stay after cardiac and abdominal surgery and to improve outcomes after liver resection.

Similarly, ongoing monitoring of nutritional status after discharge from hospital continues to be important, particularly in high-risk patients such as those who have had esophagectomy or gastrectomy. In such patients, supplemental overnight feeds via a jejunostomy are associated with weight gain and improved preservation of muscle and fat mass.

16.5 Approach to Feeding in the Critically Ill Surgical Patient

When compared to withholding feeding, commencing enteral nutritional early (within 24–36 h) in critically unwell patients is associated with a reduction in infectious complications and lower mortality. Many of these trials have included patients with severe acute pancreatitis and abdominal trauma and those who have undergone major gastrointestinal surgery.

Feeding into the gut has a number of advantages over parenteral nutrition (Table 16.3). These include the maintenance of mucosal integrity and absorptive capacity by mechanisms such as stimulation of gut hormones and secretion of bile salts. Critically ill patients deprived of enteral nutrition manifest changes in gut permeability within hours which predispose to bacterial translocation with consequent inflammation and multi-organ failure. The metabolic response to feeding is also better controlled when nutrients are delivered enterally due to modulation by gut hormones including the incretins. Enteral nutrition helps to maintain a healthy microbiome within the gut lumen which, in turn, regulates immune responses not only in the gut but also at distant sites such as the lungs, liver and kidneys. Furthermore, patients receiving enteral nutrition are less prone to infectious complications, have fewer anastomotic leaks after gastrointestinal resections and have shorter hospital stays. Another important issue is costs since enteral feeding is less expensive than parenteral nutrition.

Table 16.3 Advantages of enteral over parenteral feeding

• Maintenance of gut integrity and absorptive capacity
• Improved metabolic response through gut hormone secretion
• Immune modulation
• Maintenance of microbiome
• Cost

The importance of enteral nutrition has also been highlighted by outcomes in patients who fail to achieve their caloric targets. Observational studies indicate that the magnitude of this caloric deficit is associated with increases in organ failure, length of hospital stay and infectious and other complications. This can be addressed, at least in part, by nurse-driven protocols that allow for missed feeds (e.g. when fasting for a procedure) to be administered at flexible times.

For most patients, a standard polymeric formula is suitable for enteral feeding. This provides 1.0–1.5 kcal/mL and may include fermentable soluble fibre such as fructo-oligosaccharides or inulin. Antioxidants (e.g. vitamins E and C) and trace minerals (selenium, zinc and copper) appear to reduce mortality slightly in clinical trials, but the optimal dose and formulation of each remain unclear. Glutamine may be of benefit in patients with burns but is contraindicated in those with multi-organ failure. At present, there is insufficient evidence to recommend routine provision of probiotics. In one study, small intestinal administration of a probiotic was associated with increased mortality in patients with pancreatitis.

A wide array of specialized feeds is available, but, in general, there is limited evidence to support their use. More concentrated feeds (1.5 kcal vs. 1.0 kcal/mL) may help to achieve goals for nutrient delivery. "Immune-modulating" formulas containing arginine and fish oil have been associated with a reduction in infections and length of hospital stay but not mortality. However, studies in this area have considerable heterogeneity of trial design. When used, these feeds should commence 5–7 days preoperatively and continue in the post-operative phase.

16.6 Gastrointestinal Tolerance of Enteral Feeding in Critical Illness

It is well-established that gastrointestinal motility is frequently disordered in critically unwell patients. Gastric emptying is often delayed and has been associated with raised cholecystokinin and peptide YY concentrations. Small intestinal transit is highly variable and has been associated with impaired absorption of glucose and fat (absorption of protein has been less well studied). It is therefore not surprising that up to 50% of mechanically ventilated patients manifest features of gastrointestinal intolerance to feeding including absent or diminished bowel sounds, vomiting, high gastric residual volumes, intestinal dilatation or diarrhoea. The more of these features that are present, the longer the stay in ICU. These issues have led to the recommendation that the rate of delivery of enteral feeding be increased in increments over 2–3 days until the target volume is reached.

16.7 Monitoring and Complications of Enteral Feeding

Enteral nutrition should be monitored for adequacy of meeting prescribed requirements for both total energy and protein. Studies in critically ill patients indicate that, on average, only 60–80% of energy needs are prescribed and only 80% of what is prescribed is actually delivered. Thus the typical patient only receives 50% of their needs. Volume-based rather than rate-based goals should be set, with protocols that allow nurses to make up any lag in volume in the event of interruptions to feeding.

Tolerance of feeds should be monitored by daily assessment of volume status, abdominal distension, bowel sounds and passage of flatus and stool. In patients with a baseline BMI <20 kg/m^2 or a history of weight loss or prolonged impairment of oral intake, clinicians should be alert to the risk of the refeeding syndrome. Such patients should undergo slow initiation of feeds over 3–4 days, whether by the enteral or parenteral route, with careful monitoring for low plasma concentrations of potassium, phosphate and magnesium.

Aspiration of feeds is another risk of enteral nutrition, particularly in the setting of motor dysfunction of the gut. Other risk factors for aspiration include inability to protect the airway, supine positioning, mechanical ventilation, poor oral hygiene, reduced levels of consciousness or neurologic deficits, age over 70 years, low nurse/patient ratios and bolus rather than continuous feeding.

Routine measurement of the gastric residual volume is controversial. The technique is poorly standardized and time-consuming and may block the feeding tube. Furthermore, it carries the risk of contributing to underfeeding and has not been shown to improve outcomes. Nevertheless, one study showed that all patients with a gastric residual volume >250 mL were found to have delayed gastric emptying when measured by scintigraphy. Therefore, if this measurement is used, volumes >250 mL should prompt measures to improve nutrient delivery to the small intestine, either by the administration of prokinetic drugs or the placement of a small intestinal feeding tube. Feeds should only be ceased if volumes are ≥500 mL.

The first choices for prokinetic drugs are erythromycin, metoclopramide or both in combination. There is good evidence that feeding through post-pyloric or jejunal tubes reduces the aspiration risk, although the contribution from upper respiratory tract colonization and aspiration of oropharyngeal secretions means that this risk is not eliminated. Other measures including elevation of the bed head, continuous rather than bolus feeds and chlorhexidine mouthwashes are supported only by low levels of evidence.

Diarrhoa is commonly reported in association with enteral feeding, but its incidence is widely variable (between 2% and 95%), at least in part because its definition, whether by stool frequency, weight or altered consistency, is not standardized. In the first instance, a specific cause should be sought. This includes careful review of potential contributing medications (Table 16.4) and exclusion of infection. *Clostridium difficile* is responsible for up to 20% of cases of diarrhoa in the critically ill because of contributing factors such as use of antibiotics and proton pump inhibitors, advanced age and institutional care. If no specific cause is identified, general measures include the addition of soluble fibre (inulin, fructo-oligosaccharides or guar gum), with or without insoluble fibre. Feeds do not usually need to be interrupted. Changing to a small peptide and mixed chain triglyceride formula has been advocated but is not supported by available clinical trial evidence.

Hyperglycemia is commonly encountered in critically ill patients with a frequency of up to 50% of patients in ICU. This “critical illness hyperglycemia” is defined as a blood glucose concentration of ≥7 mmol/L when fasting or >11.1 mmol/L

Table 16.4 Medications that may contribute to diarrhoa

• Antibiotics
• Proton-pump inhibitors
• Prokinetics
• Metformin
• Nonsteroidal anti-inflammatory drugs
• Colchicine
• Antineoplastic drugs
• Selective serotonin reuptake inhibitors
• Cholinesterase inhibitors
• Prostaglandins
• Sorbitol-containing preparations
• Magnesium salts
• Laxatives

when fed, in the absence of pre-existing diabetes. An initial report in surgical ICU patients indicated a lower mortality if blood glucose was tightly controlled, but a subsequent multi-centre trial showed that overly tight control of blood glucose (4.5–6.0 mmol/L) resulted in increased mortality from hypoglycemia and that the preferred option was moderate control (keeping the blood glucose <10 mmol/L).

16.8 Feeding in Specific Surgical Conditions

16.8.1 Acute Pancreatitis

The approach to nutritional support varies depending on whether acute pancreatitis is classed as mild or moderate/severe. In mild pancreatitis, an oral diet can be provided without specific nutritional intervention. In moderate to severe disease, enteral nutrition should be provided via a tube, commencing at "trophic" rates and increasing progressively to target. Feeds can usually be delivered into the stomach, but a small intestinal tube may be required in the setting of food intolerance. Current evidence favours enteral over parenteral nutrition.

16.8.2 Trauma

The principles of nutrition in trauma patients are the same as in any critical illness with early commencement of enteral nutrition (within 24–48 h) provided that the patient is hemodynamically stable.

16.8.3 Open Abdomen

An open abdomen is deemed equivalent to a wound involving 40% of the body surface area. While general principles of nutrition once again apply, careful monitoring of fluid losses is needed as these patients require an extra 15–30 g protein for every litre of exudate lost from the abdominal cavity.

16.8.4 Burns

Predictive equations for nutritional needs are particularly unreliable in burns patients due to an associated hypermetabolic state. Modern management with debridement of non-viable tissue and skin grafting tends to ameliorate this effect, but indirect calorimetry remains the most accurate method to assess energy needs. Burns guidelines recommend provision of high protein loads, about 1.5–2.0 g/kg/day.

16.9 Accessing the Gut for Enteral Feeding

Feeding through a nasogastric tube is the simplest means of enteral access. After insertion, the correct position of the tip should be verified radiologically as aspiration of gastric contents and measurement of the pH is not sufficiently accurate. The X-ray only needs to be repeated if the tube becomes displaced.

Positioning a tube with the tip beyond the pylorus is indicated in the setting of poor tolerance of intragastric feeds or when there is otherwise a high risk of aspiration. This can be achieved endoscopically, radiologically or with electromagnetic guidance (Cortrak® system). Feeding into the small intestine is associated with a lower frequency of pneumonia than the intragastric route, but no differences in mortality or length of stay have been reported.

If enteral nutrition is required for over 4 weeks, percutaneous access should be considered. This recommendation is not absolute, but prolonged transnasal tube feeding is associated with nasal and oesophageal ulceration, aspiration pneumonia and sinusitis (the latter less so with oro-gastric tubes). If long-term feeding into the small intestine is needed (e.g. due to gastroparesis), the best option is a jejunostomy. This may be placed surgically or endoscopically depending on local expertise and patient characteristics. A jejunal extension tube positioned through a gastrostomy is less satisfactory as these frequently become displaced although this complication may be less frequent with newer modifications.

When placing a gastrostomy, care should be taken to avoid an excessively tight external bolster which risks the development of "buried bumper syndrome". In addition, the tube should be kept perpendicular to the plane of the skin in order to avoid side torsion and excessive enlargement of the tract. Blocked tubes should be flushed back and forth with warm water and, if necessary, pancreatic enzymes dissolved in bicarbonate. Mechanical unblocking with wires or brushes should only be attempted with extreme care to avoid perforating either the tube or the gut. Excessive granulation tissue at the stoma can be treated with the topical application of silver nitrate on a stick or a topical steroid. Infection is best treated empirically with antibiotics as cultures are rarely helpful. Leakage from the stoma should be managed with high-dose acid suppression, with wound care including barrier ointments and sometimes by placement of a jejunal extension/gastric aspiration tube. Leaking is never resolved by attempting to replace the tube with one of larger diameter. Occasionally, the tube needs to be removed, the stoma is allowed to heal, and a new gastrostomy is placed at a different site. In the event of inadvertent tube removal within 7–10 days of initial placement, immediate endoscopic or radiological replacement should be performed through the same tract. Beyond this period, when the tract has matured, the tube can be replaced blindly, but its correct position should be confirmed radiologically.

Indications for placement of a percutaneous gastrostomy tube need careful consideration in certain circumstances including discussions with patients and their families. In advanced dementia, gastrostomy feeding is not likely to improve the quality of life, reduce the risk of aspiration pneumonia, heal pressure sores or reduce mortality. In other terminally ill patients, thirst or hunger does not usually cause suffering if nutrition is not provided. Sometimes the placement of a gastrostomy for symptom relief (e.g. decompression of intestinal obstruction) is indicated in terminal malignancy. In motor neurone disease, gastrostomy insertion has been shown to reduce coughing and choking, avoid prolonged mealtimes and facilitate administration of medications. Survival is prolonged if the procedure is carried out before the forced vital capacity falls below a predicted level of 50%.

16.10 Indications for Parenteral Nutrition

Although the enteral route is preferred for the delivery of nutrients, intravenous (parenteral) feeding is a safe and suitable alternative in special situations. Absolute indications for intravenous feeding include mechanical obstruction of the gastrointestinal tract, uncontrolled peritonitis, ischaemic gut, short gut syndrome and some cases of high output fistulas. Intravenous feeding may also be needed in esophageal perforation or rupture, prolonged ileus and persistent intolerance to enteral feeding. However, if the patient is well nourished at baseline, there is no clinical benefit in commencing intravenous feeding during the first 7–10 days while waiting for enteral nutrition to become established.

16.11 Prescription and Management of Parenteral Nutrition

Parenteral nutrition within and outside the hospital should be prescribed and managed by a nutrition support team which typically comprises a medical specialist with a special interest in nutrition, a dietitian, a nurse and a pharmacist. This team can manage line access requirements and complications as well as the appropriate prescription of fluid volume and nutrients.

Parenteral nutrition provides all nutritional requirements including energy (glucose, lipid, and protein), vitamins (both fat and water soluble), electrolytes and trace elements. It must be delivered via a dedicated line into a central vein as additions to the line or bag increase the risk of sepsis. The provision of lipid as an energy source provides essential free fatty acids, reduces the requirement for glucose and helps to avoid hyperglycemia. There has also been a recent trend to prescribe greater protein delivery than previously, but, as for enteral feeding, robust data to support this practice are lacking. In order to improve shelf-life, parenteral nutrition is now usually provided in a 2- or 3-chamber bag, with mixing of the substrates occurring just before administration.

16.12 Complications of Parenteral Nutrition

Complications of parenteral nutrition include infections, particularly blood-stream infections related to the line. All intravenous lines can become infected, but those delivering parenteral nutrition are particularly at risk, presumably because of high glucose concentrations. Line management needs to be meticulous and the line site assessed frequently for signs of infection.

Metabolic complications are also frequent. Hyperglycemia often occurs, particularly in patients who are prone to glucose intolerance. This can be managed by reducing the amount of glucose or providing insulin. The latter can be added to the bag in the pharmacy rather than at the bedside. Refeeding syndrome (associated with hypokalemia, hypophosphatemia and hypomagnesemia) may occur, and, because of this, parenteral nutrition is always initiated slowly, particularly in at-risk patients such as those who have undergone prolonged fasting or those with recent weight loss, a low body mass index or a history of alcohol abuse.

Hypertriglyceridemia occasionally occurs during delivery of parenteral nutrition and can be treated with reduction or cessation of parenteral lipids. Infusion of lipid may also result in changes in liver function tests because of hepatic steatosis or intrahepatic cholestasis. There is also gallbladder inactivity that often results in gallbladder sludge and may result in cholelithiasis. How closely this relates to acalculous cholecystitis, which sometimes complicates critical illness, is not known.

16.13 Recent Improvements in Parenteral Nutrition

Older studies comparing enteral nutrition to parenteral nutrition often demonstrated worse outcomes with the use of parenteral nutrition. However, recent reports suggest that parenteral nutrition is a safe alternative when enteral nutrition cannot be given. This may be due to changes in the composition of parenteral nutrition solutions or to changes in how their delivery is managed. One change is in the type of lipid. Older parenteral nutrition solutions used soy-based lipids, and, while the evidence is not yet compelling, expert opinion now recommends the use of non-soy-based lipid when available. This appears to reduce the risk of liver dysfunction. Another change has been in the management of hyperglycemia with high-level evidence indicating that blood glucose should be kept below 10 mmol/L in critically ill patients in order to reduce complications. Intravenous catheters for delivering parenteral nutrition solutions have also undergone improvements over recent years, reducing the risk of line-related blood stream infections. Catheters are now frequently impregnated with antibiotics or antiseptics, and peripherally inserted central catheters (PICCs), placed under ultrasound and/or image intensifier guidance by radiologists, are now recommended for intravenous access in patients requiring parenteral nutrition for longer than a few days.

16.14 Cessation of Parenteral Nutrition

Patients who are not malnourished should cease parenteral nutrition as soon as they are able to take nutrients enterally. It needs to be remembered that parenteral nutrition diminishes appetite and reduces the intake of fluids. However, it should not be discontinued suddenly because of the risk of rebound hypoglycemia. Rather, it should be weaned over 24 h, and blood glucose should be monitored for a further 24 h thereafter.

Recommended Reading

Ali Abdelhamid Y, Chapman MJ, Deane AM. Peri-operative nutrition. Anaesthesia. 2016;71(Suppl 1):9–18.

American Society of Anesthesiologists Committee. Practice guidelines for preoperative fasting and the use of pharmacologic agents to reduce the risk of pulmonary aspiration: application to healthy patients undergoing elective procedures: an updated report by the American Society of Anesthesiologists Committee on Standards and Practice Parameters. Anesthesiology. 2011;114:495–511.

Besselink MG, van Santvoort HC, Buskens E, et al. Probiotic prophylaxis in predicted severe acute pancreatitis: a randomised, double-blind, placebo-controlled trial. Lancet. 2008;371:651–9.

Casaer MP, Mesotten D, Hermans G, et al. Early versus late parenteral nutrition in critically ill adults. N Engl J Med. 2011;365:506–17.

Doig GS, Simpson F, Sweetman EA, et al. Early parenteral nutrition in critically ill patients with short-term relative contraindications to early enteral nutrition: a randomized controlled trial. JAMA. 2013;309:2130–8.

Finfer S, Chittock DR, Su SY, et al. Intensive versus conventional glucose control in critically ill patients. N Engl J Med. 2009;360:1283–97.

Harvey SE, Parrott F, Harrison DA, et al. Trial of the route of early nutritional support in critically ill adults. N Engl J Med. 2014;371:1673–84.

Heyland DK, Dhaliwal R, Jiang X, Day AG. Identifying critically ill patients who benefit the most from nutrition therapy: the development and initial validation of a novel risk assessment tool. Crit Care. 2011;15:R268.

Itkin M, DeLegge MH, Fang JC, et al. Multidisciplinary practical guidelines for gastrointestinal access for enteral nutrition and decompression from the Society of Interventional Radiology and American Gastroenterological Association (AGA) Institute, with endorsement by Canadian Interventional Radiological Association (CIRA) and Cardiovascular and Interventional Radiological Society of Europe (CIRSE). Gastroenterology. 2011;141:742–65.

McClave SA, DiBaise JK, Mullin GE, Martindale RG. ACG clinical Guideline: nutrition therapy in the adult hospitalized patient. Am J Gastroenterol. 2016a;111:315–34.

McClave SA, Taylor BE, Martindale RG, et al. Guidelines for the Provision and Assessment of Nutrition Support Therapy in the Adult Critically Ill Patient: Society of Critical Care Medicine

(SCCM) and American Society for Parenteral and Enteral Nutrition (A.S.P.E.N.). JPEN J Parenter Enteral Nutr. 2016b;40:159–211.

Osland E, Yunus RM, Khan S, Memon MA. Early versus traditional postoperative feeding in patients undergoing resectional gastrointestinal surgery: a meta-analysis. JPEN J Parenter Enteral Nutr. 2011;35:473–87.

Peake SL, Davies AR, Deane AM, et al. Use of a concentrated enteral nutrition solution to increase calorie delivery to critically ill patients: a randomized, double-blind, clinical trial. Am J Clin Nutr. 2014;100:616–25.

Reintam Blaser A, Starkopf J, Alhazzani W, et al. Early enteral nutrition in critically ill patients: ESICM clinical practice guidelines. Intensive Care Med. 2017;43:380–98.

Taylor BE, McClave SA, Martindale RG, et al. Guidelines for the Provision and Assessment of Nutrition Support Therapy in the Adult Critically Ill Patient: Society of Critical Care Medicine (SCCM) and American Society for Parenteral and Enteral Nutrition (A.S.P.E.N.). Crit Care Med. 2016;44:390–438.

Weimann A, Braga M, Carli F, et al. ESPEN guideline: clinical nutrition in surgery. Clin Nutr. 2017;36:623–50.

White JV, Guenter P, Jensen G, Malone A, Schofield M. Consensus statement of the Academy of Nutrition and Dietetics/American Society for Parenteral and Enteral Nutrition: characteristics recommended for the identification and documentation of adult malnutrition (undernutrition). J Acad Nutr Diet. 2012;112:730–8.

The Non-surgical Acute Abdomen

17

Ian C. Roberts-Thomson

17.1 Introduction

Acute abdominal pain is a common cause for visits to emergency departments throughout the world. The percentage of patients with abdominal pain as the major symptom varies in different surveys but is usually between 5% and 10%. Some of these patients have major surgical emergencies, but others have various abdominal symptoms with negative investigations that improve or resolve spontaneously over hours to days. The latter patients are usually categorized as "non-specific abdominal pain" in surgical reports and as "functional abdominal pain syndromes" in medical reports. Despite some variation in categorization, these non-surgical patients are a relatively large group of up to one-third of the total with abdominal pain.

Although these non-surgical patients are often categorized as a single group, there is substantial variation in the site and severity of pain and the presence of additional gastrointestinal symptoms. The most common functional syndromes are the irritable bowel syndrome and non-ulcer dyspepsia. These have been discussed in detail in Chapter 1. For most of these patients, pain is of mild to moderate severity and is mostly investigated outside the emergency service. However, biliary-type pain syndromes can be severe and are discussed in more detail in this chapter along with other functional syndromes such as the levator ani syndrome.

The assessment of acute abdominal pain also needs to include the possibilities that pain is arising from disorders outside the abdominal cavity or from more generalized disorders with abdominal pain as one of several manifestations. Most of these disorders do not require surgery. There are also a number of well-defined causes of abdominal pain that may well require hospital admission but do not require surgery. Some of these are briefly discussed at the end of this chapter under

I. C. Roberts-Thomson (✉)
Adelaide Medical School, University of Adelaide, Adelaide, SA, Australia
e-mail: ian.robertsthomson@adelaide.edu.au

M. W. Wichmann et al. (eds.), *Gastroenterology For General Surgeons*,
https://doi.org/10.1007/978-3-319-92768-8_17

Table 17.1 Extra-intestinal and more generalized disorders that may result in acute abdominal pain

Cardiac, vascular and respiratory disease
• Myocardial infarction
• Pneumonia with pleurisy
• Pulmonary embolism with infarction
• Aortic dissection
• Esophageal rupture [Boerhaave's syndrome]
Metabolic and endocrine disorders
• Diabetic ketoacidosis
• Familial Mediterranean fever
• Porphyria
• Addison's disease
• Hyperlipidemia
• Hypercalcemia
Hematologic and immunologic disorders
• Sickle cell crisis
• Systemic lupus erythematosus
• Henoch-Schönlein purpura
• Hemolytic uremic syndrome
• Food allergy
• Hereditary angioneurotic edema
Infections
• Herpes zoster
• *Yersinia enterocolitica* gastroenteritis
• Malaria
• Typhoid fever
• Tabes dorsalis
Neurologic, psychiatric and miscellaneous disorders
• Functional abdominal pain
• Spinal degeneration or injury
• Lead poisoning
• Cocaine abuse
• Psychiatric disorders

the heading, non-functional, non-surgical causes of acute pain. Extra-intestinal and more generalized disorders that may result in acute abdominal pain are listed in Table 17.1.

17.2 Pathogenesis of Functional, Non-surgical Pain

The pathogenesis of both acute and chronic functional abdominal pain has been debated for decades and has been discussed in Chapter 1. Nevertheless, there is general agreement on the presence of a "brain-gut axis" that involves continuous communication between the enteric nervous system in the gut and pain perception in the central nervous system. The axis also includes stress and emotional responses through the hypothalamic-pituitary-adrenal pathway and the autonomic nervous system. Superimposed on this complex framework are issues such as personality profiles, previous physical and sexual abuse, dysfunctional family relationships, cultural factors and health beliefs.

Reasons for the development of acute pain or acute on chronic pain remain unclear for many patients with functional syndromes. For some patients, however, predisposing factors include recent stress, poor social supports, unhappiness with current medical care, fear of serious disease and drug-seeking behaviour. A small minority may also have abdominal pain because of the use of opioids for other pain problems such as back pain [see Chapter 24].

Various attempts have also been made to correlate pain events with changes in gastrointestinal motility and changes in visceral sensitivity. In relation to motility, patients with pain do have changes in colonic, small bowel and gastric motility, but similar changes are sometimes observed in control subjects. Similarly, many patients with pain have evidence of increased visceral sensitivity [but not somatic pain thresholds], but the pain response may be more closely associated with psychological factors than with variation in visceral sensitivity.

17.3 Clinical Features of Functional, Non-surgical Pain

The typical patient who attends the emergency service with acute functional pain is a woman between the ages of 20 and 50 years. Reasons for the female predominance may include greater concerns in relation to health issues, a greater willingness to discuss symptoms and the higher likelihood of previous abuse. Whether levels of female sex hormones are also relevant is debated although both acute and chronic symptoms usually improve after the menopause. A non-hormonal explanation is that the menopause is often a marker for reduced personal and family stress.

A detailed history of current and previous abdominal symptoms is central to a provisional diagnosis of functional pain. The site of acute functional pain is highly variable between patients but is usually consistent within an individual patient. For most patients, pain is located in the lower mid-abdomen, left iliac fossa, epigastrium or right upper quadrant. Additional abdominal symptoms may include nausea, vomiting, abdominal distension and changes in bowel habit. There may also be non-abdominal symptoms such as malaise, headaches, dizziness and urinary symptoms. Other information may also be helpful including previous medical disorders, psychiatric diagnoses and social issues.

On physical examination, most patients appear to be in reasonable health despite reporting severe pain. Pulse, blood pressure and temperature are usually normal. On abdominal examination, pain is poorly localized, perhaps apart from tenderness over the lower colon in some patients with pain in the left iliac fossa. One interesting sign is that patients with functional pain usually close their eyes during abdominal palpation in contrast to those with abdominal inflammation. Abdominal rigidity and rebound tenderness are normally absent.

Screening blood tests are usually normal including hemoglobin, white cell count, urea and electrolytes and liver function tests. A normal C-reactive protein level can also exclude inflammation if pain has been present for more than 6 h. Additional investigations may be performed depending on the site and severity of symptoms and results from any previous studies. In the emergency service setting, an abdominal ultrasound or computed tomography [CT] scan may be appropriate although, in general, care should be taken to avoid repeat investigations.

17.4 Acute Biliary-Type Pain Syndromes

An interesting group of patients are those with episodes of biliary-type pain and a normal upper abdominal ultrasound study. These are usually women [80%] with a mean age of approximately 30 years. The presenting symptom is one or more episodes of severe pain in the epigastrium or right upper quadrant of the abdomen, usually lasting for several hours. Most of these patients do not have background features of an irritable bowel syndrome. Some have evidence of impaired gallbladder emptying as assessed by cholescintigraphy after the administration of cholecystokinin.

This appears to be a heterogeneous group of patients. In those proceeding to cholecystectomy, approximately one-third have microscopic cholelithiasis, while the remainder have either a normal gallbladder, cholesterolosis or a narrow cystic duct. After cholecystectomy, approximately 70% of patients are free of pain in the longer term.

Sphincter of Oddi dysfunction is a term applied to patients with continuing episodes of pain after cholecystectomy in the absence of other causes for pain such as retained bile duct stones. The group includes those who have had a cholecystectomy with a normal ultrasound study as well as patients who had a cholecystectomy for known gallstones. Some have evidence of sphincter dysfunction including dilatation of the bile duct [presumably related to impaired bile flow] and elevation of liver enzymes, either persistently or after episodes of pain. Another distinctive feature is induction of pain by intramuscular morphine, sometimes accompanied by elevation of liver enzymes and amylase [see Chapter 23]. Motility in the sphincter of Oddi has also been assessed by passage of a thin manometry catheter through the channel of a side-viewing endoscope and into the sphincter. Again, a minority have a persistent elevation of basal pressure in the sphincter while others have motility changes of uncertain significance. Division of the biliary component of the sphincter can be performed by endoscopic sphincterotomy and results in improvement in symptoms in approximately 60–70% of patients, particularly those with a high basal pressure at manometry. After division of the sphincter, repeat morphine tests induce either no or only mild pain, and there are no changes in liver enzymes. As endoscopic sphincterotomy for sphincter of Oddi dysfunction is associated with a significant risk of pancreatitis, the procedure should be restricted to experienced endoscopists, usually working in tertiary centres.

For almost all patients, pain induced by morphine is identical to that experienced with spontaneous episodes. The major effect of morphine on sphincter motility is an increase in the frequency of phasic contractions. This reduces the flow of bile through the sphincter and results in an increase in intrabiliary pressure, particularly after cholecystectomy. Similar increases in intrabiliary pressure are also likely in those patients with spontaneous episodes of pain associated with elevation of liver enzymes. Elevation of the basal pressure in the sphincter would also be expected to raise intrabiliary pressure although the pathogenesis of a high basal pressure remains unclear. Possible explanations include idiopathic hypertrophy of sphincter muscle and sphincter fibrosis caused by inflammation or operative trauma. It is also unclear whether patients with biliary-type pain syndromes have a lower threshold for induction of pain caused by spontaneous or morphine-induced rises in intrabiliary pressure.

17.5 Unexplained Anal and Rectal Pain

Anal symptoms are a common reason for surgical evaluation. Disorders such as hemorrhoids, fissures and anal stenosis have been discussed elsewhere. Anal pruritis can sometimes be difficult once local anal and rectal problems have been excluded including pinworm infections [*Enterobius vermicularis*].

Another issue is unexplained episodes of rectal pain. One syndrome involves episodes of discomfort or pain in the upper rectum. These episodes can last for 20 min or more and are sometimes precipitated or aggravated by defecation. Symptoms may also be aggravated by sitting and improved by walking. On examination the levator ani muscle is tender in some patients, a feature that has given rise to the term, levator ani syndrome. The syndrome is probably common but only a minority of patients seek medical advice.

Similar issues exist in relation to proctalgia fugax. In this syndrome, patients have recurrent pains in the rectum that normally last from seconds to minutes. Men and women are equally affected, mostly in middle age. Pains can be severe, are usually described as sharp or stabbing and sometimes wake the patient from sleep. Some authors consider this to be a variant of the levator ani syndrome, but other pelvic muscles may be involved. Management is usually restricted to reassurance as symptoms improve spontaneously in most patients.

17.6 Non-functional, Non-surgical, Acute Abdominal Pain

Although functional syndromes constitute the majority of patients attending emergency services with non-surgical acute pain, there are a number of other diagnoses to be considered. Some of these relate to abdominal pain as a feature of disease outside the abdomen, while others are abdominal disorders that do not require surgery. The following list attempts to place these in an order that includes both frequency and importance.

17.6.1 Myocardial Infarction

The pain of myocardial infarction is largely located in the epigastrium in up to 10% of patients, particularly those with inferior infarction. Furthermore, up to 50% of patients have additional symptoms such as nausea, vomiting and sweating. These symptoms can be similar to those of acute pancreatitis and biliary colic. The diagnosis of myocardial infarction is usually confirmed by an electrocardiogram and serum levels of cardiac troponin 1.

17.6.2 Pneumonia and Pulmonary Embolism

Inflammation or infarction that extends to the pleural surface typically causes pain that is aggravated by deep breathing or coughing. However, basal pleurisy may cause pain in the left or right upper quadrants with only a minimal pleural component. This may raise the possibility of disorders such as acute cholecystitis. Pneumonia can usually be excluded with a chest radiograph, but more detailed investigations will be necessary to confirm pulmonary embolism.

17.6.3 Diabetic Ketoacidosis

The symptoms of diabetic ketoacidosis normally include polyuria, polydipsia, vomiting, weight loss and dehydration. Acute abdominal pain can also be a feature, particularly in children. In almost all patients, pain improves with rehydration and correction of metabolic abnormalities. Early laparotomy has been performed in some patients but has been associated with significant morbidity and mortality.

17.6.4 Pyelonephritis and Nephrolithiasis

Renal pain is typically located in the costovertebral angle but can be localized to the right or left flank or, rarely, the right or left upper quadrants. Pyelonephritis often has an acute onset with pain, fever, malaise and urinary symptoms such as frequency, dysuria and urgency. Susceptible groups include infants and children [especially girls], pregnant women and older men with prostatic hypertrophy. Pain with renal colic may remain localized to the costovertebral angle or may spread downwards into the abdomen and groin as stones pass through the ureter.

17.6.5 Inflammatory Bowel Disease

Crohn's disease is an important cause of strictures in the small bowel. Some of these patients present with acute abdominal pain due to a partial or complete small bowel obstruction. Symptoms usually improve with conservative measures or medication, but some will eventually need correction of the stricture with an operative procedure. Severe inflammatory bowel disease is usually accompanied by significant abdominal pain, but most patients have at least moderate diarrhea.

17.6.6 Vasculitis

Mesenteric vasculitis is an unusual cause of acute abdominal pain. In adults, systemic lupus erythematosus [SLE] is the most frequent underlying disorder, but this can also occur with systemic vasculitis and scleroderma. In children, the most likely cause is Henoch-Schönlein purpura. Abdominal pain is almost always associated with active disease. Characteristic findings on CT scans include focal or diffuse thickening of the bowel wall, dilated bowel loops, mesenteric edema and abnormal bowel wall enhancement [target sign].

17.6.7 Acute Salpingitis

In women, the differential diagnosis of acute abdominal pain needs to include gynecological disorders. One non-surgical cause is acute salpingitis, often caused by gonorrhea or chlamydial infections. Although early abdominal pain may be located in the mid-abdomen, subsequent pain is largely in the lower abdomen, often favouring the left or right side. Additional features include an abnormal vaginal discharge, urinary symptoms and fever. These features can be similar to those of acute appendicitis although differentiation is usually possible with ultrasonography or a CT scan.

17.6.8 Mesenteric Adenitis

This is an important cause of acute abdominal pain in children, largely between the ages of 2 and 12 years. Abdominal pain may be diffuse or localized to the right iliac fossa and is usually accompanied by fever, nausea, vomiting and diarrhea. The disease is self-limiting in most patients although suppuration and abscess formation have been reported. Several infectious agents appear to be responsible including viruses, bacteria and mycobacteria. Ultrasonography and CT scans usually assist with the diagnosis and help to exclude acute appendicitis.

17.6.9 Familial Mediterranean Fever

This inherited disorder mostly affects people of Jewish, Turkish, Arabic and Armenian ancestry. The disease is characterized by recurrent episodes of abdominal pain, fever and joint pain that typically last for 3–5 days. Most patients have their first attack prior to the age of 20 years. Abdominal pain is mild in some patients, but others have severe pain with muscle rigidity and rebound tenderness. Upright abdominal radiographs may show dilatation of the small bowel and air-fluid levels that raise the possibility of a small bowel obstruction. Treatment with colchicine is helpful during acute episodes and is usually recommended as long-term therapy to prevent recurrent episodes.

17.6.10 Acute Intermittent Porphyria

Acute intermittent porphyria is another genetic disorder that results in acute episodes that are more common in women than in men. Almost all the acute episodes are accompanied by abdominal pain [usually severe], but other features may include urinary symptoms, dark urine, anxiety, delusions, hallucinations, seizures, tremor, nausea and excessive sweating. Some episodes are precipitated by hormonal changes or by drugs. Treatment includes cessation of possible offending drugs and intravenous infusions of 10% glucose.

17.7 Non-surgical Acute Abdominal Pain at the Extremes of Age

The causes of non-surgical, acute abdominal pain vary with age. In infants less than 2 years, the differential diagnosis needs to include infantile colic, gastroenteritis, urinary tract infection and constipation. In older children [<12 years], additional diagnoses need to be considered such as mesenteric adenitis, Henoch-Schönlein purpura, sickle cell crisis, pharyngitis and functional pain. For teenagers, gynecological disorders become more important including dysmenorrhea, ovulation pain [Mittelschmerz] and pelvic inflammatory disease.

In patients over 65 years, episodes of functional pain still occur but are less frequent. There are also fewer patients with urinary infections and gastroenteritis as a cause of significant abdominal pain. The majority of admissions in this group have a surgical orientation and include intestinal obstruction, gallstone disease, diverticular disease and malignancy.

Recommended Reading

Arowojolu AO, Bakare RA, Oni AA, Ilesanmi AO. Laparoscopic and microbiological features of acute salpingitis in developing countries. J Obstet Gynaecol. 1998;18:164–8.

Barut K, Sahin S, Adrovic A, et al. Familial Mediterranean fever in childhood: a single-center experience. Rheumatol Int. 2018;38:67–74.

de Buriet K, Lam A, Larsen P, Dennett E. Acute abdominal pain-changes in the way we assess it over a decade. N Z Med J. 2017;130:39–44.

Irvin TT. Abdominal pain: a surgical audit of 1190 emergency admissions. Br J Surg. 1989;76:1121–6.

Royal Children's Hospital Melbourne. Abdominal pain. www.rch.org.au.

Toouli J, Baker RA. Innervation of the sphincter of Oddi: physiology and considerations of pharmacological intervention in biliary dyskinesia. Pharmacol Ther. 1991;49:269–81.

Vijayaraghavan MD, Kurup D, Singh A. Imaging of acute abdomen and pelvis: common acute pathologies. Semin Roentgenol. 2009;44:221–7.

Liver and Gastrointestinal Disorders During Pregnancy

18

William M. Hague and Ian C. Roberts-Thomson

18.1 Introduction

The emergence of medical and surgical problems during pregnancy can present challenges for the general surgeon. These include a desire to minimise investigations in the interests of woman and baby, a desire to defer surgery until after delivery of the baby and constraints on the use of medication with potential effects on fetal development. Decision-making is also constrained by the absence of prospective, controlled trials during pregnancy for disorders, such as biliary colic or pancreatitis, where options include early or later surgical intervention. Nevertheless, management algorithms have now been developed for many pregnancy-related disorders based on careful clinical studies that have included morbidity and mortality data for both pregnant women and their babies.

Liver and gastrointestinal disorders during pregnancy have been appropriately categorised as those that are unique to pregnancy and those that complicate pregnancy. The latter category includes disorders, such as esophageal reflux and acute hepatitis, that can develop during pregnancy, together with the effect of pregnancy on known chronic disorders, such as cirrhosis and inflammatory bowel disease. Disorders that are unique to pregnancy include hyperemesis gravidarum, pre-eclampsia, intrahepatic cholestasis of pregnancy and acute fatty liver of pregnancy. In this chapter, disorders that complicate pregnancy will be restricted to those that involve the gastrointestinal tract and liver.

W. M. Hague (✉)
Women's and Children's Hospital, Adelaide, SA, Australia
e-mail: bill.hague@adelaide.edu.au

I. C. Roberts-Thomson
Adelaide Medical School, University of Adelaide, Adelaide, SA, Australia
e-mail: ian.robertsthomson@adelaide.edu.au

M. W. Wichmann et al. (eds.), *Gastroenterology For General Surgeons*,
https://doi.org/10.1007/978-3-319-92768-8_18

18.2 Gastrointestinal and Liver Disorders Unique to Pregnancy

18.2.1 Hyperemesis Gravidarum

Approximately 60% of women have at least some nausea and vomiting during the first trimester of pregnancy. Hyperemesis gravidarum is a term used for severe nausea and vomiting that usually results in one or more hospital admissions for dehydration, electrolyte disturbances and nutritional therapy. The frequency is approximately 1 in 200 pregnancies and is more common with the first pregnancy and in women who are overweight or obese. There is also an association with the gestational trophoblastic disease, hydatidiform mole, and ovarian hyperstimulation for induction of ovulation.

Laboratory abnormalities include hypokalemia, hyponatremia and ketonuria that may be accompanied by mild increases in serum aminotransferases and bilirubin. There are also increased free thyroxine and reduced thyroid-stimulating hormone concentrations in 60% of patients, but these spontaneously revert to normal with resolution of hyperemesis. Changes in thyroid function tests probably reflect the mild thyrotrophic effect of placental β human chorionic gonadotropin. The pathogenesis of hyperemesis gravidarum is still poorly understood but may be associated with increases in serum concentrations of oestrogens. Other potential factors include autonomic dysfunction, delayed gastric emptying and psychological issues.

Treatment is symptomatic and supportive with the cautious infusion of intravenous fluids and the use of antiemetic agents including metoclopramide, prochlorperazine, ondansetron and [very occasionally] oral steroids. In addition, small amounts of concentrated albumin (20%) may be required to maintain the intravascular volume. Prophylactic measures to reduce the risk of thrombosis are recommended in women largely confined to bed, including wearing compression stockings and the use of low molecular weight heparin. For those patients unable to tolerate oral antiemetics, options include intramuscular or intravenous metoclopramide, rectal prochlorperazine, intramuscular promethazine and intravenous ondansetron. All these drugs appear to be relatively safe.

18.2.2 Pre-eclampsia

Pre-eclampsia is a common complication of the second half of pregnancy, and is characterised by maternal hypertension, involvement of other organ systems [often proteinuria] and effects on the fetus. Although up to 10% of pregnancies can be affected by mild disease, severe complications, such as eclampsia and the HELLP syndrome [hemolysis, elevated liver enzymes and low platelets], are rare [0.1%] in higher-income countries. Several risk factors have been identified, including prior hypertension, diabetes mellitus, older age and obesity. There are also associations with primipaternity and multiple pregnancy. The pathogenesis appears to lie in the placenta with inadequate remodelling of the maternal uterine spiral arteries in the face of the invading trophoblast. Maternal and fetal manifestations can be present in varying proportions ranging from profound maternal hypertension without fetal compromise to severe fetal growth restriction with maternal normotension. Early-onset disease is associated with increased rates of both maternal and perinatal morbidity and mortality.

In addition to proteinuria, laboratory investigations associated with more severe pre-eclampsia include increases in serum creatinine and aminotransferases and a platelet count of less than 100×10^9/L. Increases in serum aminotransferases are sometimes accompanied by abdominal pain and may reflect hepatic hypoperfusion caused by vasoconstriction. Rare complications relevant to the surgeon include hepatic infarction and subcapsular or intrahepatic hemorrhage. Some of these patients have disseminated intravascular coagulopathy and can be managed with recombinant factor VIIa, while others require surgical procedures. The definitive treatment for pre-eclampsia is delivery of the baby, including the placenta, from the maternal environment. The timing of delivery is crucial and attempts to balance risks to the mother that increase with time with risks to the baby that are largely determined by prematurity. Mothers with pre-eclampsia have a higher than expected frequency of delivery by cesarean section. Recurrence of pre-eclampsia is common, especially in early-onset disease, where the risk may be as high as 30–40%. This risk can be reduced to some extent by the prophylactic use of low-dose aspirin and calcium supplements that need to begin early in pregnancy.

18.2.3 Intrahepatic Cholestasis of Pregnancy

Intrahepatic cholestasis of pregnancy usually develops in the third trimester [although it can occur earlier] and affects approximately 0.7% of pregnancies. The major symptom is pruritus, but this can be severe in a minority of women resulting in skin excoriation, profound sleep disturbance and significant psychopathology. The disorder is associated with interruption of the enterohepatic circulation of bile acids with increased concentrations of bile acids in blood. This appears to be linked to increased concentrations of oestradiol, progesterone and progesterone metabolites that affect bile acid pathways via effects on farnesoid X receptors. Changed activities of other enzymes and transporter proteins may explain why cholestasis only develops in a small minority of individuals.

Laboratory tests reveal elevated serum concentrations of alkaline phosphatase, aminotransferases and bile acids and, in a minority of patients, increased concentrations of bilirubin. In contrast to patients with biliary obstruction, levels of gamma-glutamyltranspeptidase [GGT] are usually normal. There is an association with cholelithiasis. In patients with at least moderate pruritus, drug-therapy with ursodeoxycholic acid may be helpful. Additional or alternative drugs include cholestyramine and rifampicin. In patients with severe disease [serum bile acids >40 μmol/L], there are small but significant risks to the fetus including preterm labour, passage of meconium into the liquor and stillbirth. Because of this, patients with severe disease often have an induced delivery at 37 weeks, although, thus far, there are no randomised trials showing benefit from this approach.

18.2.4 Acute Fatty Liver of Pregnancy

This is a serious but rare disease with a frequency of 1 in 5000–10,000 pregnancies. The typical presentation is in the third trimester with malaise, anorexia, nausea, vomiting and neurological features of hepatic encephalopathy. Some episodes appear to follow an intercurrent infection such as a respiratory or urinary tract infection. Most patients develop jaundice and some [50%] develop transient diabetes insipidus. The disorder is more common with male fetuses and there is an association with multiple gestation.

Laboratory investigations reveal a marked neutrophil leucocytosis, mild thrombocytopenia, prolongation of prothrombin and activated partial thromboplastin times, reduced antithrombin, hypoglycemia and elevated concentrations of hepatic aminotransferases, bilirubin, creatinine, uric acid, lactate and, in severe disease, ammonia. There are some links with pre-eclampsia and the HELLP syndrome, but distinctive features include hypoglycemia and more striking increases in serum aminotransferases, bilirubin and creatinine. A minority of patients develop pancreatitis. Treatment consists of stabilisation of the patient, correction of any hypoglycemia and coagulopathy and urgent delivery of the fetus. This is followed by supportive treatment for hepatic failure and renal impairment, as well as oral or parenteral desmopressin, if necessary, for diabetes insipidus. Occasionally, milder forms of acute fatty liver of pregnancy are managed by delayed delivery to facilitate maturation of the fetus. In most patients, delivery is followed by a slow but steady improvement in laboratory parameters over several weeks. Maternal mortality is low, but fetal mortality ranges from 5% to 10%.

18.3 Gastrointestinal and Liver Disorders That Complicate Pregnancy but Are Not Unique to Pregnancy

18.3.1 Gastro-esophageal Reflux Disease

Approximately 40% of pregnant women report problems with reflux and heartburn, particularly during the third trimester. This is related to an increase in intra-abdominal pressure and a decrease in resting lower oesophageal sphincter pressure. Life-style measures are sometimes helpful, including elevation of the head of the bed, cessation of smoking and avoidance of fatty foods, coffee and chocolate. Those with persistent and more severe symptoms can be safely treated with H_2 receptor antagonists [apart from cimetidine] or proton pump inhibitors.

18.3.2 Constipation

This is an issue for 10–40% of pregnant women and may be related to the effects of progestagen on colonic motor activity. Management includes an increase in dietary fibre or the use of bulk-forming agents such as psyllium. Resistant constipation can be treated with an osmotic laxative such as lactulose.

18.3.3 Hemorrhoidal Disease

Hemorrhoids may enlarge in the third trimester of pregnancy and cause pain, bleeding or anal pruritus. Several local preparations are available, but the most helpful measure may be correction of constipation. Rarely, patients are referred for injection sclerotherapy or rubber band ligation.

18.3.4 Gallstone Disease

Pregnancy, particularly multiple gestation, increases risks for the development of stones in the gallbladder. The mechanism includes cholesterol supersaturation due to changes in biliary bile acids as well as impaired emptying of the gallbladder. Approximately 1 in 500 pregnancies is complicated by symptomatic gallstone disease with biliary colic, biliary pancreatitis, acute cholecystitis and choledocholithiasis in decreasing order of frequency. Patients with isolated episodes of biliary colic are likely to be managed conservatively with a low-fat diet and avoidance of surgery during pregnancy. This also applies to biliary pancreatitis unless investigations support persisting stones in the bile duct. However, in the setting of acute cholecystitis, the evidence appears to favour early laparoscopic cholecystectomy rather than the alternative option of intravenous fluids and antibiotics with delayed cholecystectomy. Patients with stones in the bile duct, with or without pancreatitis, can usually be managed by ERCP and endoscopic sphincterotomy with appropriate shielding of the fetus during radiological screening. Symptomatic gallstone disease during pregnancy is associated with a minor increase in maternal morbidity and with preterm birth and neonatal morbidity.

18.3.5 Peptic Ulcer Disease

Persuasive evidence supports the view that peptic ulcers are less frequent in pregnancy than in non-pregnant controls. The causes remain unclear but may include hormonal effects on gastric acid secretion, hormonal effects on mucosal growth and mucus production and avoidance of ulcerogenic factors such as smoking and non-steroidal, anti-inflammatory drugs.

18.3.6 Acute Appendicitis

Pregnancy does not appear to affect the frequency of acute appendicitis but has been associated with a higher rate of negative [non-appendicitis] appendectomies, perhaps because of difficulty with the interpretation of ultrasound studies. In addition, there is debate on the relative merits of laparoscopic versus open appendectomy as the laparoscopic procedure has been associated with a greater risk of fetal loss.

18.3.7 Inflammatory Bowel Disease

Pregnancy does not appear to have a major effect on the course of inflammatory bowel disease, perhaps apart from effects related to changes in medication. Occasionally, the first symptoms of ulcerative colitis develop in early pregnancy, but this appears to be extremely rare in Crohn's disease. In general, patients who are in remission at the start of pregnancy are likely to remain in remission throughout pregnancy. For those with active disease, aminosalicylates [sulphasalazine and mesalazine] are useful and safe during pregnancy, as are oral and rectal steroids. Methotrexate should not be used. Several studies show that good control of active disease throughout pregnancy results in the best outcomes for mother and baby. This includes continuation of thiopurines, such as azathioprine and 6-mercaptopurine, and, in special circumstances, the use of biologics. There is a small risk of an exacerbation of bowel inflammation in the post-partum period. Treatment may be continued during breast feeding, including the use of thiopurines.

18.3.8 Viral Hepatitis

Pregnancy does not appear to affect the outcomes of acute hepatitis A, B or C. However, the development of acute hepatitis E, particularly in the third trimester, is associated with a high risk of fulminant hepatitis with a maternal mortality rate of up to 20%. This infection is rare in Western countries but is more common in India, Pakistan and the Middle East. Hepatitis due to herpes simplex virus is also a rare cause of fulminant hepatitis, again largely in the third trimester.

18.3.9 Chronic Liver Disease

A much more common problem is pregnancy in the setting of chronic hepatitis B or C. There is no clear evidence that pregnancy adversely affects the activity of hepatitis, but a critical issue is the prevention of maternal to fetal transmission of hepatitis B during and after delivery. This is usually achieved by vaccination beginning on day 1 as well as administration of hepatitis B immunoglobulin at birth to infants born to mothers with higher serum concentrations of virus, as determined by the presence of hepatitis B e-antigen or higher titres of hepatitis B DNA. Maternal to fetal transmission of hepatitis C is extremely rare, perhaps largely due to low concentrations of virus in blood. Women with cirrhosis [from whatever cause] often have impaired fertility, but, if pregnancy develops, risks of variceal bleeding may increase because of pressure on the inferior vena cava and increased flow through the azygous venous system. This is sometimes aggravated by coagulation abnormalities associated with cirrhosis. The initial therapy for bleeding varices will usually be endoscopic band ligation, but whether there is a role for prophylactic band ligation remains unclear.

18.3.10 Budd-Chiari Syndrome

Pregnancy is associated with a relatively hypercoagulable state, particularly at delivery, which may be amplified by additional hypercoagulable disorders, such as the antiphospholipid syndrome and inherited thrombophilias. The Budd-Chiari syndrome is a rare disorder, usually caused by thromboses in hepatic veins, that may result in hepatomegaly, abdominal pain, ascites and liver failure. Anticoagulants are effective as prophylaxis against this and other thrombotic syndromes in some of these higher-risk women.

Recommended Reading

Akbari M, Shah S, Velayos FS, Mahadevan U, Cheifetz AS. Systematic review and meta-analysis on the effects of thiopurines on birth outcomes from female and male patients with inflammatory bowel disease. Inflamm Bowel Dis. 2013;19:15–22.

Athwal R, Bhogal RH, Hodson J, Ramcharan S. Surgery for gallstone disease during pregnancy does not increase fetal or maternal mortality: a meta-analysis. Hepatobiliary Surg Nutr. 2016;5:53–7.

Date RS, Kaushal M, Ramesh A. A review of the management of gallstone disease and its complications in pregnancy. Am J Surg. 2008;196:599–608.

Geenes V, Chappell LC, Seed PT, Knight M, Williamson C. Association of severe intrahepatic cholestasis of pregnancy with adverse pregnancy outcomes: a prospective population-based case-control study. Hepatology. 2014;59:1482–91.

Joshi D, James A, Quaglia A, Westbrook RH, Heneghan MA. Liver disease in pregnancy. Lancet. 2010;375:594–605.

Knight M, Nelson-Piercy C, Kurinczuk JJ, Spark P, Brockelhurst P, Obstetric Surveillance System UK. A prospective national study of acute fatty liver of pregnancy. Gut. 2008;57:951–6.

Ovadia C, Williamson C. Intrahepatic cholestasis of pregnancy: recent advances. Clin Dermatol. 2016;34:327–34.

Shihab Z, Yeomans ND, De Cruz P. Anti-tumour necrosis factor therapies and inflammatory bowel disease pregnancy outcomes: a meta-analysis. J Crohns Colitis. 2016;10:979–88.

Westbrook RH, Dusheiko G, Williamson C. Pregnancy and liver disease. J Hepatol. 2016;64:933–45.

Wilasrusmee C, Sukrat B, McEvoy M, Attia J, Thakkinstian A. Systematic review and meta-analysis of safety of laparoscopic versus open appendectomy for suspected appendicitis in pregnancy. Br J Surg. 2012;99:1470–8.

Won RP, Friedlander S, Lee SL. Management and outcomes of appendectomy during pregnancy. Am Surg. 2017;83:1103–7.

Intestinal Failure

19

Timothy K. McCullough and Matthias W. Wichmann

19.1 Definition and Classification

Intestinal failure (IF) is the inability to achieve adequate nutritional, water or electrolyte balance, as a result of insufficient length or function of the gastrointestinal tract. It is life-threatening in some forms and may impact very severely upon quality of life if occurring as a chronic condition. The frequency with which it occurs has been difficult to quantify. Implicit in the name of the condition is the potential need to either supplement or replace the function of the gut acutely or long-term but also to address the potential cause, assess the patient from a wide perspective and approach treatment in the most appropriate fashion. In complex cases, this is best done as a team-based discipline with IF rightly regarded as a subspecialty in its own right. For the purpose of this chapter, and of most salience to the general surgeon, intestinal failure may be categorized broadly as follows:

- Type 1. Transient, frequent, usually self-limiting, lasting less than 28 days but may need treatment, supplementation or nutritional support. Ileus, by far the most frequently encountered version of IF, may be minimized, but there is no widely accepted single treatment for this commonly seen phenomenon amongst general surgeons.
- Type 2. This type is severe, often complex and longer-term and requires nutritional support during expectant or conservative management. This type may arise from acute episodes of medical illness but increasingly from surgery or surgical complications. The outcome from this situation may include complete recovery, but the course of disease, treatment and restoration of function takes more than 28 days and should involve a multimodal, phasic approach and wherever possible, a multi-disciplinary team. This type of IF is of most interest to

T. K. McCullough (✉) · M. W. Wichmann
Department of Surgery, Mount Gambier General Hospital, Mount Gambier, SA, Australia
e-mail: timothy.mccullough@sa.gov.au; matthias.wichmann@sa.gov.au

M. W. Wichmann et al. (eds.), *Gastroenterology For General Surgeons*,
https://doi.org/10.1007/978-3-319-92768-8_19

general surgeons since surgery is often pivotal in the etiology, stabilization and the ultimate rectification of the problem. Surgical issues giving rise to type 2 IF are anastomotic leak and ensuing sepsis, extensive resections for ischemia or trauma or entero-cutaneous fistulas arising from intraoperative bowel injury.

- Type 3. This type describes a more chronic situation where the causative pathology or event has been stabilized or is slow-moving. Supplementation or chronic parenteral nutrition is required. It may be irreversible. Type 2 may progress to Type 3.

19.2 Etiology

Increasingly, surgery or its complications lead to short gut conditions, but the cause may be congenital, such as gastroschisis. The end result may be reached cumulatively or suddenly, for example, by the need for multiple resections in Crohn's or massive resection for infarction. Surgical injuries resulting in short gut and high output stomas or fistulas are common causes for Type 2 IF. Obstruction, either mechanical or from dysmotility disorders, may be the causative agents. Mucosal or absorption defects may result in IF.

19.3 Early Management

It may be counterintuitive that IF is not always obvious, but in early stages especially, this is true. For example, the clinician might have difficulty discerning the difference between a patient who is recovering postoperatively within normal timeframes and parameters and someone who is not regaining expected function in appropriate time or fashion. The time to initiate investigation is a subject of preference or habit. It should be contemplated in the context of the individual case, but early consideration of the question is rarely regretted. The initial targets for further investigation would appropriately be focused clinical examination for sepsis or obstruction, electrolyte and water balance assessment and imaging to check for surgical complication. Essentially, the initial goal should be to stop deterioration, correct the correctable and allow stabilization of the situation whilst preserving vulnerable other organs such as the skin, liver and vasculature pending a planned reversal of the causation if possible. Immediate measures to address any physiological deficit, sepsis or shock should be instituted. It is of benefit to anticipate early whether recovery is imminent or whether parenteral nutrition should be initiated. If the interval to recovery is likely to be more than 1 week, parenteral nutrition is likely to be of benefit.

The treatment of sepsis is a conspicuous target in IF management not only because of obvious local effects, such as abscess drainage to facilitate fistula treatment, but also because of the systemic barriers to recovery, which are caused, perpetuated or exacerbated by systemic sepsis. With regard to eliminating intra-abdominal sepsis and, bearing in mind, the recent surgery which has often preceded the episode, there has been an important and widely adopted move towards radiological drainage wherever possible. This is eminently preferable to reoperation. The benefits are avoidance of the massive physiological insult to a potentially compromised patient of repeat laparotomy or laparoscopy, the likely lower risk of further traumatization of a friable gastrointestinal tract, preservation of the abdominal wall and avoidance of further anesthetics. Sepsis control frequently resurges as a priority in the course of the treatment of type 2 IF. This may involve an overt target or be suspected from a more subtle and vague pattern of lack of progress, or poor correction of inflammatory markers and electrolytes, despite best efforts to do so. Laparotomy might be unavoidable for further resection of infarcted bowel, to form a controlled proximal stoma or to treat obstruction, for example, but the risk of further injury in the hostile post-complication abdomen is to be stressed. If reoperation cannot be avoided, a minor procedure to eliminate sepsis should be the goal as complex or intricate reconstruction is prone to failure. Stoma formation or defunctioning should be liberal.

Suspected fistula ought to be allowed to establish in the absence of sepsis needing drainage, and the temptation to reoperate early resisted. Remaining early considerations include establishment of reliable robust long-term venous access.

With resuscitation, fluid and electrolyte repletion and maintenance, nutrition and sepsis management established, there may then follow stages of physiological recovery, anatomical investigation, planning of surgical reconstruction or restoration and subsequent rehabilitation.

During the initial phase of management, histamine 2-receptor antagonist or proton-pump inhibitor should be administered to reduce gastric hypersecretion and reduce fluid losses.

19.4 Nutrition and Issues of Venous Access

In establishing conditions to allow resolution of the IF episode, nutritional support is pivotal. Successful total nutrition or supplementation will either permit spontaneous healing or restore the patient to anabolism and allow investigation, planning and ultimately surgical restoration of intestinal continuity or sufficiency where feasible. Enteral feeding should be the goal, as immunological and local (mucosal) benefits are widely accepted, and bacterial translocation will be reduced. Patency and function of the gut will be preserved, and once established, fistulas will not be worsened by enteral feeding, nor is there evidence that healing is impaired. The benefit of being allowed to eat upon the psychological well-being of the patient is a very important consideration in what is often an extremely distressing, debilitating and protracted condition. The composition of fluids taken by mouth to those with a high-output fistula needs careful attention. Water and hypotonic solutions may dramatically increase fistula output, and very strict water restriction is usually needed. Strong electrolyte solutions (double strength Dioralyte) replace high salt losses and will reduce massive water loss by diminishing stoma output. These patients are at risk of dehydration and should be advised to drink 1–3 L of oral rehydration solution daily. Small volumes of water may be offered mainly for comfort. Enteral feeding distal to a fistula is used in specialist units, to encourage distal bowel patency, to preserve mucosal health and to augment nutrition. Feeding catheter placement may be achieved through the stoma bag, but this is normally outside the normal scope of nurse-administered enteral feeding in a general surgical unit and therefore may be problematic to achieve.

Whatever the extent to which enteral feeding may be used, parenteral nutrition is effectively used to cover the shortfall in requirements and allows targeted correction of micronutrients. Parenteral nutrition improves the chance of fistula closure without surgery and better prepares the patients who will need corrective surgery, improving outcome and survival very significantly in entero-cutaneous fistula. In Type 3 IF, parenteral nutrition is life-prolonging.

Parenteral nutrition requires long-term venous access, the evolution of which has decreased the infective complications, but central venous catheter-related bloodstream infections remain a major source of morbidity in Type 2 and 3 IF patients. Making the diagnosis of line infection should be done carefully using clinical and examination findings and microbiological testing with appropriate interpretation of the results. Complex recommended pathways to diagnose line infection have been proposed, for example, those by the European Society for Parenteral and Enteral Nutrition, but these employ methods not widely available, and the standard for diagnosis or confirmation varies. The consequences are significant variation in antibiotic use which is often inappropriate in respect of type or purpose or needless removal of lines. Antibiotic use is often a therapeutic trial and test of the diagnosis of line infection. There are recent reports of high rates of line salvage using antibiotics, but fungal line infections remain usually unsalvageable. Line removal for infection is at least a major hindrance and may lead to the complete exhaustion of venous access options, an infrequent indication for intestinal transplant. Line care and sterility standards must be prioritized. Other venous catheter complications include tunnel-section infections, kinking and occlusion and venous thrombosis.

Intestinal failure-associated liver disease (IFALD) is the main cause of death in those on long-term parenteral nutrition. It is a distinct entity from non-alcoholic fatty liver disease (NAFLD) with distinguishing histological features, but the two may coexist. The etiology of IFALD is not well understood, but parenteral nutrition, lipid use for calorific intake, micronutrient lack, poly vinyl chloride infusion lines, gallstones, steatohepatitis, sepsis and medication are known contributors. It occurs in 5% of adults on parenteral nutrition but in a much higher proportion of children on parenteral nutrition. The longer a patient remains on parenteral nutrition, the higher the risk of IFALD, and it is a bigger problem for Type 3 than other forms of IF.

Patients with stabilized nutritional regimes may be able to continue their treatment at home, for example, if home parenteral nutrition is available or if supplementation is all that is required. This is associated with benefits to the patients' psychological and emotional welfare.

19.5 Fistulas and Stomas

Stoma and fistula care may present serious challenges to management and might be the reason for transfer to a specialist unit. Pain caused by skin damage from leaking stoma or wound manager appliances may be severe, with a high requirement for analgesics, especially, in those with extensive entero-cutaneous fistulas. Involvement of experienced stoma nurses is imperative, and appliance manufacturers may help on an individual basis in complex cases, such as laparostomy with fistula.

19.6 Planning Reconstruction

The assessment of the GI tract in IF may be a simple matter of visualizing an upstream segment and a downstream segment in a single fistula situation, or it may be far more complicated. Axial imaging is a mainstay, and a radiologist with a keen interest and experience is key to the process. In cases of multiple fistulae, contrast and endoscopic visualization add much detail. The anatomical statuses in terms of length of remaining bowel, height of entero-cutaneous fistula, presence of entero-enteric or other fistula, anatomy of involved other organs, urinary or gynaecological tracts, complications of treatment, ongoing sepsis, distal obstruction, active Crohn's and the state of the abdominal wall are concerns to the planning of any corrective surgery in Type 2 IF. Planned, sequential investigation, with close communication between radiologist and potentially other specialists, may require an IF unit with a dedicated MDT and access, for example, to theatre time with vascular, urological, plastic or other surgical attendance.

19.7 Intestinal Restoration

The important question of whether to attempt to restore intestinal continuity should be answered considering the benefit of possibly eliminating fistula and reducing or ceasing parenteral nutrition against the risks of surgery. If deemed best to proceed, it is important to do so at the best time, which is not too early for a peritoneal cavity to have reformed or the patient to have regained nutritional repletion, but not so late as to have repeated complications from parenteral nutrition or other treatments or to have lost the patients cooperation and trust. The physical examination should reveal a pliable, soft abdomen reflective of the mobile viscera and pouting mucosa or prolapsing bowel at the site of fistulation. This may take several months to achieve. Operation before this time is to be avoided.

The approach to surgery is to anticipate a long adhesiolysis and mobilization. Extra caution to avoid enterotomy and in the fashioning of anastomoses is advisable, and there is some evidence that two-layered sewn anastomoses may be superior to staples in this setting. Defunctioning of anastomoses should be considered. Closure of the abdomen should be performed with any future planned procedures in mind.

19.8 Abdominal Wall

The abdominal wall closure is a major facet of restorative surgery in IF. Effective treatment can decrease the chance of reforming fistulas, decrease postoperative cardiorespiratory complications, reduce the incidence of debilitating massive abdominal wall herniation and improve the cosmetic result. Returning massive hernia contents to the abdomen and effecting closure may not be immediately possible or may embarrass ventilation and subsequent breathing, and whilst primary suture of the abdominal closure is the most desirable method, severe attenuation of the recti and anterior abdominal wall may preclude this. Component separation and mesh use may be necessary. The use of non-absorbable mesh is associated with a higher infection and refistulation rate, and non-absorbable meshes should not be placed intraperitoneally. Biological meshes (non-crosslinked) are useful in the setting of complex fistula surgery with its potential for wound sepsis and may be used, ideally extraperitoneal.

19.9 Other Options in Intestinal Failure

There has been work on hormonal manipulation in the past to reduce parenteral nutrition requirements or eliminate the need for parenteral nutrition in Type 3 IF, but none has had any enduring effect. There has been more recent experimental use of glucagon-like peptide agonists and growth hormone, which in higher doses seem to be able to reduce calorie and parenteral nutrition requirements by up to 40%.

Surgical procedures to lengthen a short bowel are the only surgical alternative to transplantation. These, briefly, aim to fashion two narrower lengths of small bowel from one normal calibre length and to join them end-to-end (Bianchi procedure), make a spiral incision around a length of small bowel and re-sutured to increase length (Spiral Incision Lengthening and Tailoring) or to perform incomplete transverse incisions, re-sutured to increase length and create brakes in the small intestine (Serial Transverse EnteroPlasty, STEP). None increases absorptive area, and there are only small numbers available in the literature. Some patients have been able to decrease parenteral nutrition or rarely discontinue it, but some have required transplant or have not survived.

At present, intestinal transplantation has a lower 5-year survival than parenteral nutrition. The indications for transplant include catastrophic complications of parenteral nutrition, loss of venous access by thrombosis or infection and liver disease or severe dehydration episodes despite parenteral nutrition. Rejection, sepsis, antirejection complications, graft-versus-host disease and surgical complication lead to 1-, 5-, and 10-year survival rates as low as 76%, 56% and 43% in small bowel-only transplants. Intestinal transplant may be part of a multivisceral transplant including the liver, and this is the more likely option in those with established or impending liver failure. Another consideration, especially in rural areas, is the high level of medical and surgical supervision required post-transplantation because of rejection, antirejection therapy or surgical complications.

19.10 Conclusion

Intestinal failure is uncommon, but is potentially a very serious, long-term condition to be managed variously by surgical and non-surgical means. In its mildest form, it is a transient and self-limiting disorder. In its most severe form, it is profoundly life-altering or fatal. Surgical rescue from abdominal catastrophe or surgical catastrophe is increasingly the cause of Type 2 IF, and its management is often slow, demanding, complicated and reliant on many specialties. The multi-disciplinary team of a specialist unit is best placed to provide optimal outcomes in severe cases and ought to be consulted as early as possible. New treatment options are emerging, but the established sequence of stabilization, sepsis management, nutritional optimization and planning of repair remains the standard.

Recommended Reading

Carlson G, Gardiner K, McKee R, MacFie J, Vaizey C. The Surgical Intestinal Failure Working Party on behalf of the Association of Surgeons of Great Britain and Ireland. Surg Manage Patients with Acute Intestinal Failure. London: Association of Surgeons of Great Britain and Ireland; 2010.

Datta V, Engledow A, Chan S, Forbes A, Cohen CR, Windsor A. The management of enterocutaneous fistula in a regional unit in the United Kingdom: a prospective study. Dis Colon Rectum. 2010;53(2):192–9.

Grainger JT, Maeda Y, Donnelly SC, Vaizey CJ. Assessment and management of patients with intestinal failure: a multidisciplinary approach. Clin Exp Gastroenterol. 2018;(11):233–41.

Hodgkinson JD, Maeda Y, Leo CA, Warsavitarne J, Vaizey CJ. Complex abdominal wall reconstruction in the setting of active infection and contamination: a systematic review of hernia and fistula recurrence rates. Colorectal Dis. 2017;19(4):319–30.

NHS England. https://www.england.nhs.uk/wp-content/uploads/2013/06/a08-intestinal-failure-adult.pdf. Accessed 25 May 2018.

Oke S, Lloyd D, Nightingale J, Gabe S. OC-022 Factors that affect survival in type 3 intestinal failure; the largest single centre experience of 978 patients over 36 years. Gut. 2017;66(Suppl 2):A11–2.

Vaizey CJ, Maeda Y, Barbosa E, et al. European Society of Coloproctology consensus on the surgical management of intestinal failure in adults. Colorectal Dis. 2016;18(6):535–48.

Ischemic Enteritis/Colitis

20

Matthias W. Wichmann and Timothy K. McCullough

20.1 Epidemiology/Risk Factors/Pathogenesis

Ischemic injury of the large and small intestine results from insufficient delivery of oxygen and nutrients. Collateral blood supplies as well increased oxygen extraction can allow for compensation in slowly progressing disease (atherosclerosis).

The two major causes of acute mesenteric arterial occlusion are mesenteric arterial embolism and mesenteric arterial thrombosis.

The large diameter and small takeoff angle of the superior mesenteric artery (SMA) make it susceptible to embolism. The embolus usually lodges 3 to 10 cm distal to the origin of the SMA. The middle segment of the jejunum is most distant from the collateral blood supply out of the celiac trunk and the inferior mesenteric artery and therefore is most often involved in ischemia.

Thrombosis of the mesenteric artery is usually superimposed on a preexisting stenosis (atherosclerotic plaque) and usually occurs at the origin of the vessel.

Ischemic colitis is caused by an initial nonocclusive acute change in colonic microvasculature with acute damage to the cellular structure and subsequent reperfusion injury.

20.1.1 Risk Factors

The risk of embolism is increased due to cardiac arrhythmia, cardiac valvular disease, endocarditis, atherosclerosis of the aorta and aortic aneurysm.

The risk of thrombotic occlusion is increased with peripheral artery disease, age, low cardiac output, and trauma. Atherosclerosis is more commonly observed in patients who smoke and suffer from hypertension, hyperlipidemia, and diabetes.

M. W. Wichmann (✉) · T. K. McCullough
Department of Surgery, Mount Gambier General Hospital, Mount Gambier, SA, Australia
e-mail: matthias.wichmann@sa.gov.au; timothy.mccullough@sa.gov.au

M. W. Wichmann et al. (eds.), *Gastroenterology For General Surgeons*,
https://doi.org/10.1007/978-3-319-92768-8_20

The major risk factors for ischemic colitis are age, hypertension, hyperlipidemia, coronary artery disease and diabetes. Some drugs (digoxin, diuretics, NSAIDs, cocaine, laxatives, antihypertensives) may contribute to the risk of ischemic colitis through mesenteric vasoconstriction or volume depletion.

20.1.2 Symptoms

Any patient with acute-onset abdominal pain, minimal findings on examination, and metabolic acidosis should be considered as having acute intestinal ischemia until proven otherwise. The triad of older patient with atrial fibrillation and severe abdominal pain out of proportion of the clinical examination can be observed in up to 50% of the patients with acute embolic occlusion.

Patients with ischemic colitis usually present with abdominal pain, diarrhea, rectal blood loss (self-limiting), and abdominal distension. Only rare patients with ischemic colitis present with bowel perforation.

Most patients with atherosclerotic mesenteric vascular disease are asymptomatic due to an extensive collateral blood supply. Symptomatic patients with chronic mesenteric ischemia are usually older than 60 and female and have a history of smoking. The symptoms are described as intestinal angina with recurrent episodes of acute abdominal pain after eating. The pain can be variable in intensity and location and may radiate to the back.

20.2 Diagnosis/Differential Diagnosis

The timely diagnosis of acute mesenteric ischemia depends on a high level of clinical suspicion, and a definitive diagnosis can only be made by demonstrating the occlusion within the mesenteric arteries on imaging (CT angiography).

In ischemic colitis, CT may demonstrate colitis but is not diagnostic. Colonoscopy can show evidence of colitis, and ischemia can be confirmed on biopsies.

For the diagnosis of chronic mesenteric ischemia, vascular imaging (CT angiogram, conventional arteriography) must demonstrate stenosis of at least two of the major mesenteric vessels (celiac axis, superior mesenteric artery, inferior mesenteric artery).

20.3 Nonsurgical Management

Emergency management of patients with acute mesenteric ischemia requires gastric decompression (nasogastric tube), intravenous fluids, antithrombotic therapy (unfractionated heparin), broad-spectrum antibiotics, proton pump inhibitors, and oxygen. Vasopressors should be avoided to prevent additional mesenteric vasoconstriction.

Some patients can be observed with the above measures in place. Watch-and-wait is indicated if the patient is hemodynamically stable and has no clinical signs of advanced bowel ischemia.

Poor-risk surgical patients with extensive ischemia and transmural infarction should be considered for palliative management.

Ischemic colitis can usually be treated conservatively. This includes intravenous antibiotics, intravenous fluids, gastrointestinal decompression, bowel rest, and oxygen. There is no evidence for the use of anticoagulation or antiplatelet therapy in patients presenting with ischemic colitis.

Patients with an incidental diagnosis of chronic mesenteric occlusive disease are managed with smoking cessation and secondary prevention measures (antiplatelet therapy). Nutritional support may be needed to treat malnutrition resulting from "food fear" associated with intestinal angina.

20.4 Surgical Management

Good-risk surgical candidates who present with indications for immediate laparotomy (free air, extensive pneumatosis intestinalis) should be taken directly to theater for exploration. Bowel resection is ideally delayed until after revascularization. In a situation where appropriate vascular expertise is not available, resection of necrotic or perforated bowel is appropriate (damage control surgery). A subsequent transfer for revascularization (bypass for mesenteric thrombosis, embolectomy for mesenteric embolism) and bowel anastomosis is also an acceptable option.

Up to one quarter of patients presenting with ischemic colitis require resection of the ischemic bowel. Indications for surgery are gangrenous disease, fulminant colitis, peritonitis, perforation, persisting hemorrhage, mucosal necrosis on colonoscopy, and non-resolution over 2 weeks despite adequate conservative treatment. Ischemic strictures can develop in up to one quarter of all patients; most of these are asymptomatic and require no treatment.

The indication for revascularization in chronic mesenteric ischemia is the presence of symptoms (pain, weight loss). The aim of treatment is to prevent future bowel infarction. Recurrent vascular stenosis after successful revascularization occurs in up to 15% of all patients, and regular follow-up after treatment is necessary.

20.4.1 Surgery Versus Endovascular Intervention

During recent years, endovascular intervention has developed as an alternative treatment option with acute mesenteric arterial occlusion. Treatment consists of pharmacologic or mechanical thrombectomy as well as balloon angioplasty plus stent insertion. So far no randomized trials are available to help with the treatment decision. Endovascular intervention is only an option in patients who are hemodynamically stable and do not show signs of advanced intestinal ischemia (peritonitis, free air).

A second-look operation after 24–48 h is needed in most patients after successful revascularization to reevaluate the bowel. Up to one quarter of patients require additional bowel resection at the time of second-look operation.

Mortality from acute mesenteric ischemia in patients undergoing procedures for revascularization can be as high as 60%. Perioperative mortality is similar for surgical and endovascular interventions.

Ischemic colitis carries an overall mortality of approximately 10%. Right-sided ischemic colitis is more likely to require emergency surgery and has a mortality of up to 50%.

Long-term medical management after successful surgical/nonsurgical treatment aims at prevention of recurrent events. This includes reduction of risk factors as well as anticoagulation (vitamin K antagonists, novel oral anticoagulants).

20.5 When to Transfer

Non-operative management of acute mesenteric ischemia may require endovascular intervention. If this is not available, transfer to a center offering endovascular intervention must be considered. In patients having emergency surgery, post-operative care will require admission to an HDU or ICU. These patients may also benefit from transfer to a centre that offers the full complement of radiological and vascular surgical options.

Ischemic colitis can be treated in most surgical centers even if no access to vascular surgery or endovascular intervention is available.

Treatment of chronic mesenteric ischemia is elective and should always be performed in a dedicated vascular surgical unit which offers conventional surgical as well as endovascular treatment options.

Recommended Reading

Nikolic AL, Keck JO. Ischaemic colitis: uncertainty in diagnosis, pathophysiology and management. ANZ J Surg. 2018;88:278–83.

UpToDate®: Acute mesenteric arterial occlusion

UpToDate®: Chronic mesenteric ischemia

21 Genetics of Inherited Gastrointestinal Tumors

Nicola K. Poplawski

21.1 Background

Approximately 1–3% of gastric cancer is due to an inherited cancer predisposition. Around 5–10% of colorectal carcinoma (CRC) is due to a germline mutation in a high-penetrance cancer predisposition gene. Depending on the number and histological type of colorectal polyps, an inherited colorectal polyposis syndrome may explain the colonic findings. A family history of CRC increases a person's probability of developing CRC, with part of this increased susceptibility being attributable to genetic factors.

Although inheriting a disease-causing variant (mutation) in a GI cancer predisposition gene increases the lifetime risk of GI cancer, most inherited GI cancer syndromes do not confer a 100% risk of cancer. Other non-genetic factors contribute to cancer development, including aging, diet, lifestyle factors and chance. This means that counselling about cancer risk for a mutation carrier is probabilistic (not binary). For most mutation carriers, cancer risk management is multifaceted and includes strategies for prevention, risk reduction and early detection.

21.2 Diagnosis

There are four key components in the diagnosis of an inherited GI cancer syndrome;

1. A patient's personal cancer and polyp experience
2. The family history of cancer and colorectal polyps
3. DNA mismatch repair studies in tumor tissue
4. Diagnostic genetic testing in constitutional DNA

N. K. Poplawski (✉)
Adult Genetics Unit, Royal Adelaide Hospital, Adelaide, SA, Australia

Discipline of Paediatrics, Adelaide Medical School, University of Adelaide, Adelaide, SA, Australia
e-mail: Nicola.Poplawski@sa.gov.au

M. W. Wichmann et al. (eds.), *Gastroenterology For General Surgeons*,
https://doi.org/10.1007/978-3-319-92768-8_21

21.2.1 Personal and Family History

A family cancer history is a record of the cancer and tumor diagnoses for an individual and his/her genetic relatives. Ideally the history includes at least three generations (parents, children, sibs, nieces, nephews, aunts and uncles, grandparents). The family history should be updated regularly as new diagnoses may be made (or remembered) over time. Reported histories may be inaccurate, so where possible the cancer/tumor diagnoses should be confirmed via histopathology reports, medical records, cancer registry records, or death certificates (see Lu et al.).

A general surgeon should be able to recognize the red flags that raise the possibility that there is an inherited genetic component to a patient's personal and family history of GI cancers and/or tumors (Box 21.1).

Box 21.1: Red Flags

Personal factors

- Has a genetic relative with a mutation in a cancer predisposition gene
- CRC at age <50 years
- CRC and a second LS-cancer[a] at any age (including two CRC)
- Intra-abdominal or abdominal wall desmoid tumor at age <60 years
- Gastric fundic gland polyposis in the absence of proton pump inhibitor therapy
- Gastric cancer and colorectal polyposis

Tumour factors

- CRC with abnormal MMR immunohistochemistry[b]
- Diffuse-type gastric cancer
- Two or more hamartomatous colorectal polyps at any age
- Two or more juvenile colorectal polyps at any age
- Any number of Peutz-Jeghers polyps (any site) at any age
- Twenty or more (cumulative) adenomatous colorectal polyps at any age
- Ten or more (cumulative) adenomatous colorectal polyps by age 30 years
- Twenty or more (cumulative) serrated colorectal polyps at any age

Family history factors

- Personal history of CRC
  and FmHx meets Amsterdam I or II criteria (see Box 21.2)
- Personal history of CRC
  and FmHx of one or more first/second-degree relatives with CRC or endometrial cancer *and* at least one of the cancers is diagnosed at age <50 years
- Personal history of CRC
  and FmHx of two or more first- or second-degree relatives with LS-cancer, regardless of age

CRC colorectal carcinoma, *FmHx* family history, *LS* Lynch syndrome, *LS-cancer* Lynch syndrome-associated cancer, *MMR* mismatch repair

[a]Lynch syndrome-associated cancers include adenocarcinoma of the colorectum, endometrium, small intestine, stomach, ovary, or pancreas; urothelial cancer; cholangiocarcinoma; brain tumor (usually glioblastoma); keratoacanthoma or sebaceous gland tumor of the skin

[b]Except where a tumor has loss of expression of MLH1 and either hypermethylation of the MLH1 promoter or the BRAF V600E mutation is detected in the tumor, and there are no high-risk factors for a constitutional epimutation (see Fig. 21.1)

Box 21.2: Amsterdam Criteria[a]

Amsterdam I criteria (1991)

A family who meets **ALL** the following:

- At least three members of the family with colorectal cancer AND
- At least one affected relative is a first-degree relative of both of the other two AND
- At least two generations of the family have colorectal cancer AND
- At least one of the cases of colorectal cancer was diagnosed under the age of 50

Amsterdam II criteria (1998)

A family with three or more relatives with a LS-associated cancer[b] plus **ALL** of the following:

- At least one affected relative is a first-degree relative of both of the other two AND
- At least two generations of the family have a LS-associated cancer AND
- At least one of the cases of cancer was diagnosed under the age of 50 AND
- Familial adenomatous polyposis has been excluded in relatives with colorectal cancer AND
- Tumors have been verified by pathological examination

Vasen et al. The International Collaborative Group on Hereditary Non-Polyposis Colorectal Cancer (ICG-HNPCC). Dis *Colon Rectum* 1991;34(5):424–425; Vasen et al. New clinical criteria for hereditary nonpolyposis colorectal cancer (HNPCC, Lynch syndrome) proposed by the International Collaborative group on HNPCC. Gastroenterology 1999;116(6):1453–1456

[a]The Amsterdam criteria were developed to identify families that should be clinically classified as having Lynch syndrome (LS). The criteria were developed before LS was shown to be due to abnormal mismatch repair and before the identification of the causatives genes. Many LS families do not meet Amsterdam criteria. Many families that meet Amsterdam criteria have MMR-proficient colorectal cancer (i.e., not LS) or MMR-deficient colorectal cancer without a MMR-gene mutation (Lynch-like syndrome). LS should be diagnosed on the basis of molecular studies of the MMR genes not the Amsterdam criteria

[b]Lynch syndrome-associated cancers include adenocarcinoma of the colorectum, endometrium, small intestine, stomach, ovary, or pancreas; urothelial cancer; cholangiocarcinoma; brain tumor (usually glioblastoma); keratoacanthoma or sebaceous gland tumor of the skin

21.2.2 Mismatch Repair Studies

DNA mismatch repair (MMR) is an intracellular process that corrects replication errors in newly synthesized DNA, as well as repairing some types of acquired DNA damage. Inactivation of both alleles of one of the four MMR genes leads to defective MMR. This bi-allelic inactivation of a MMR gene in a cell causes an increased mutation rate (genomic instability) and increases the probability that that cell will accumulate sufficient mutations to transform into a cancer cell.

Tumor tissue can be screened for MMR deficiency using either microsatellite instability (MSI) or immunohistochemistry (IHC) testing. The discussion in this chapter focuses on MMR-IHC. MMR-IHC uses antibodies to detect loss of expression (LOE) of the MMR proteins MLH1, MSH2, MSH6 and PMS2 in tumor tissue. Absent or reduced nuclear staining of one or more MMR protein suggests that there may be a constitutional mutation in a gene encoding one of these proteins, i.e. Lynch syndrome (LS).

Until recently most centres targeted MMR-IHC screening of CRC to people with a personal or family cancer history meeting revised Bethesda guidelines (RBG). Multiple publications have shown that RBG has low sensitivity for LS and that over-reliance on RBG leads to significant underdiagnosis of LS. Universal MMR-IHC of all CRC, irrespective of age at diagnosis or family history, has been proposed. An alternative is to test all CRC diagnosed under age 70 years regardless of family history, plus all CRC diagnosed at age 70 or older where RBG is met.

Although abnormal MMR-IHC raises the possibility of LS it is not diagnostic of the condition. Acquired MMR deficiency is relatively common in CRC, and MMR-IHC cannot differentiate inherited MMR deficiency (due to LS) from sporadic somatic MMR deficiency that is acquired by and confined to the tumor.

In CRC the most common MMR-IHC abnormality is combined LOE of *MLH1* and *PMS2*. This pattern of LOE increases in frequency with age and is usually due to acquired somatic hyper-methylation of the *MLH1* promoter leading to silencing of the *MLH1* gene.

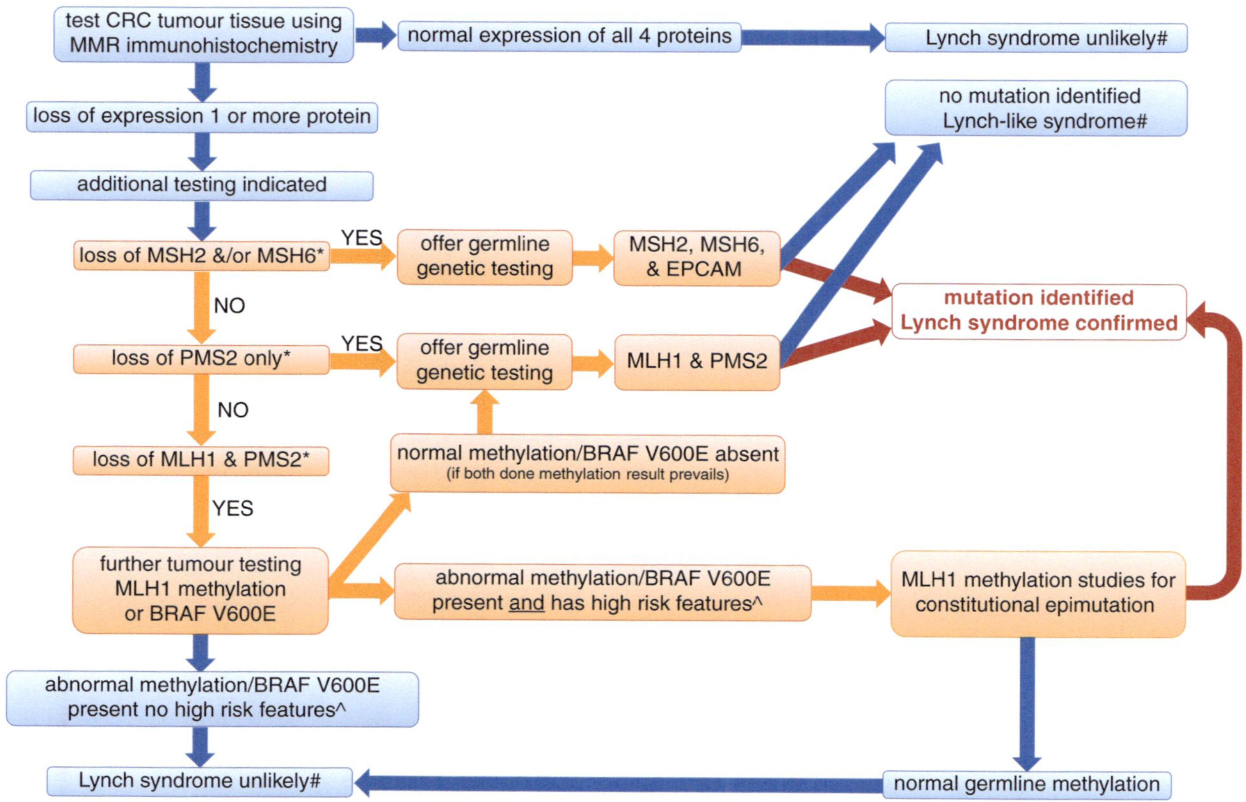

Fig. 21.1 Immunohistochemistry to guide genetic testing for Lynch syndrome. ∗For patterns of loss not covered by this algorithm consider referral to clinical genetics. ^High-risk factors for *MLH1* constitutional epimutation are *MLH1* promoter methylation in tumor **and** one or more of (a) <50 at diagnosis of CRC; (b) multiple Lynch syndrome-associated cancers in that individual; (c) family history of Lynch syndrome-associated cancers meeting Amsterdam criteria. #See Fig. 21.2

There are several methods available to screen tumor DNA for promoter hyper-methylation including CpG pyrosequencing, methylation-specific PCR and methylation-specific MLPA. These methods can also be used to screen for constitutional *MLH1* promoter hyper-methylation (i.e. a constitutional *MLH1* epimutation).

An alternative is to test tumor tissue for the *BRAF* V600E mutation, as presence of the mutation is a proxy marker for *MLH1* promoter hyper-methylation in a CRC displaying LOE of *MLH1*. PCR- and IHC-based approaches to detect *BRAF* V600E are available. These methods are not suitable for screening for constitutional *MLH1* promoter hyper-methylation.

Local availability and processes will influence which method is more commonly used to screen CRC for *MLH1* promoter hyper-methylation (methylation studies or PCR-based detection of *BRAF* V600E or IHC-based detection of *BRAF* V600E).

Figures 21.1 and 21.2 outline the general approach to the interpretation of MMR-IHC results, taking into account the association between age and somatic *MLH1* promoter methylation, the most common patterns of MMR-IHC loss and the small chance of a constitutional epimutation. Scenarios that do not fit the algorithms should be discussed with expert colleagues and, depending on the personal and family history of cancer and polyps, and the tumor IHC, BRAF and methylation results, referral to a clinical genetics service may be indicated.

21.2.3 Diagnostic Genetic Testing

In a healthcare setting genetic testing refers to the laboratory analysis of DNA or RNA looking for variations that disrupt the normal function of a gene, causing or increasing the risk of disease. *Diagnostic* genetic testing refers to the first test done in a family, in a person who is affected by the clinical disorder under investigation (a "new" mutation search). In contrast, *predictive* genetic testing is testing for the presence or absence of the specific mutation identified in a genetic relative, where the person being tested has no features of the disorder at the time of testing.

The medical implications and the ethical, emotional and social consequences of diagnostic and predictive genetic testing differ. In acknowledgement of these differences the Australian National Pathology Accreditation Advisory Council (NPAAC) guidelines classify a predictive test as a level 2 DNA test "… for which professional genetic counselling should precede and accompany the test". Most Australian genetic laboratories will only accept predictive test requests from appropriately trained healthcare providers working in clinical genetic or familial cancer clinics.

Diagnostic genetic testing is an integral part of precision medicine and mainstream diagnostic genetic testing of cancer-predisposition genes is now the standard of care for many cancer types. Genetic testing may have a number of benefits for the person being tested, as well as their genetic relatives, but it can also create dilemmas which need sensitive management. With appropriate training, a general surgeon can provide pretest counselling, order the appropriate mainstream diagnostic genetic test, interpret and disclose the result, arrange appropriate patient follow-up and initiate family management (Figs. 21.1, 21.2, 21.3, 21.4, 21.5, Box 21.3, 21.4 and 21.5).

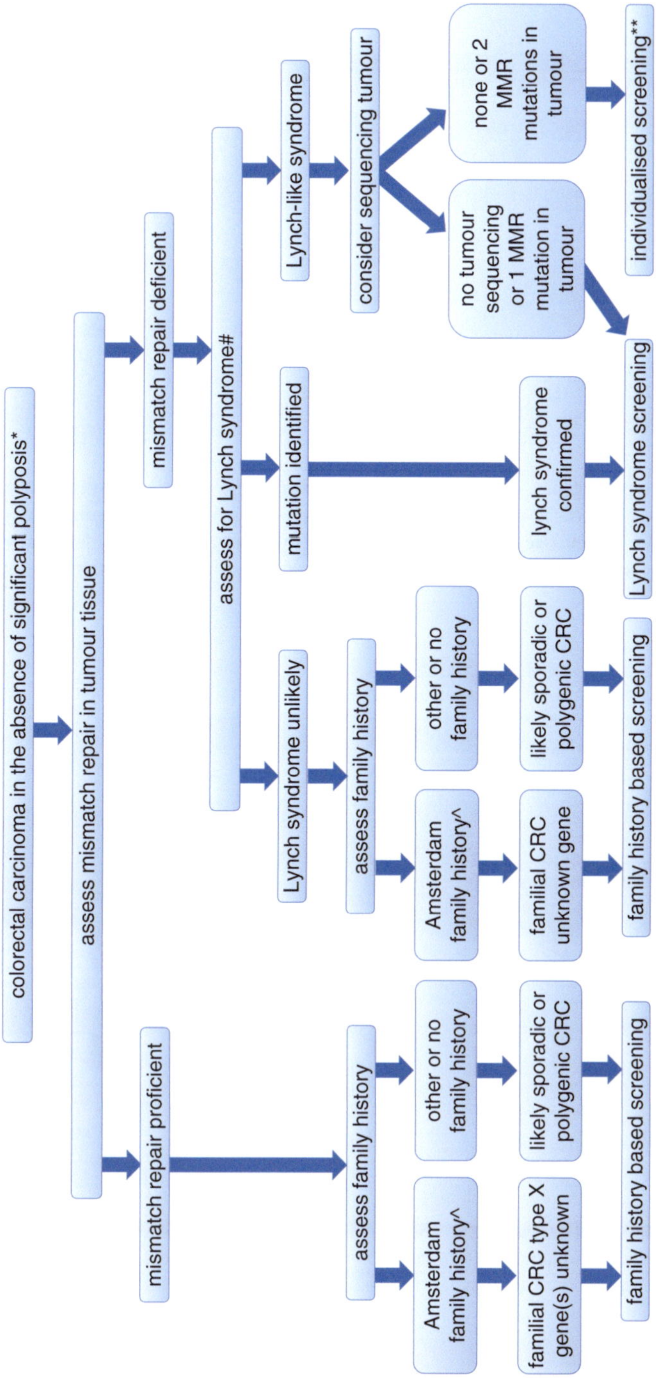

Fig. 21.2 Colorectal cancer. *If ≥10 adenomas or serrated polyps, more than two hamartomatous polyps or any number of Peutz-Jeghers polyps refer to Fig. 21.3. ^See Box 21.2. #See Fig. 21.1. **Guided by personal and family history of CRC and other cancers, genetic test results and tumor test results

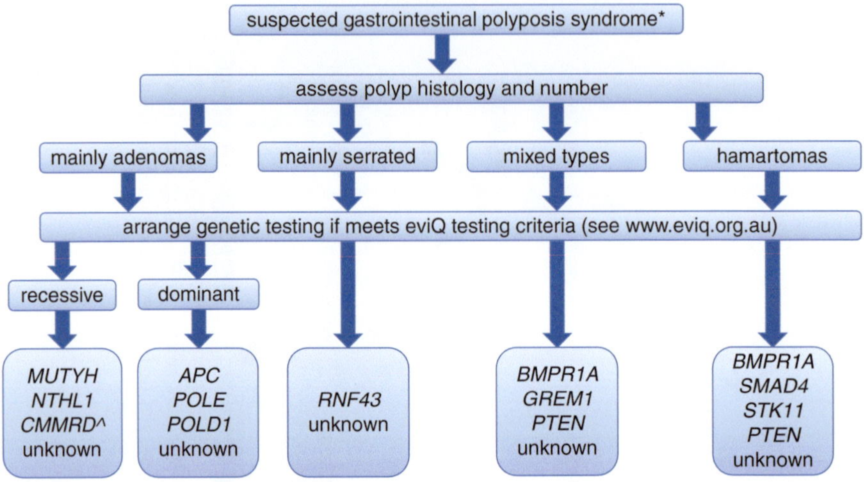

Fig. 21.3 Colorectal polyposis genes. ∗ ≥10 adenomas or serrated polyps (cumulative) before age 30 years ***or*** ≥20 adenomas or serrated polyps (cumulative) at any age ***or*** two or more hamartomatous polyps ***or*** any number of Peutz-Jeghers polyps. ^CMMRD = constitutional MMR deficiency due to bi-allelic MMR gene mutations (causative genes MLH1, MSH2, MSH2 and MSH6)

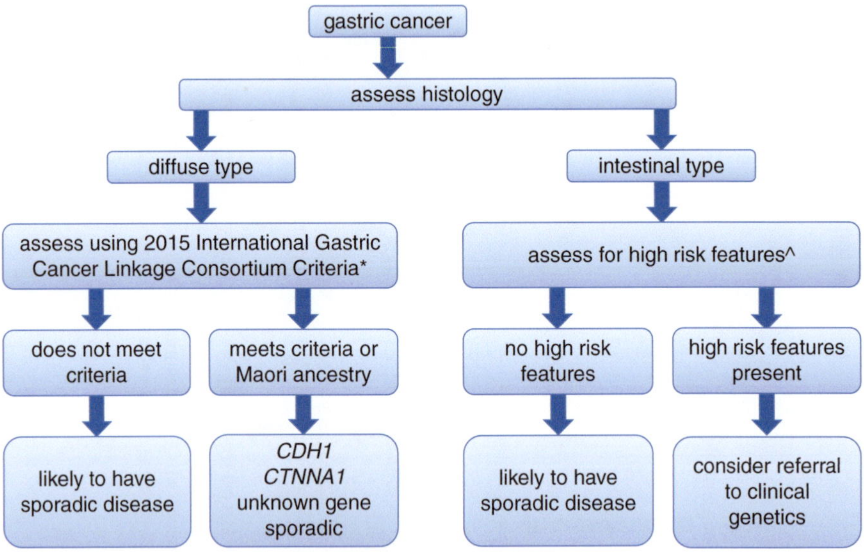

Fig. 21.4 Genetic assessment of gastric cancer. ∗See van der Post et al., J Med Genet 2015;52:361–374. ^High-risk features include diagnosis <40 years, colorectal adenomas, fundic gland polyps in the absence of proton pump inhibitor therapy, family history of gastric cancer and family history of colorectal carcinoma

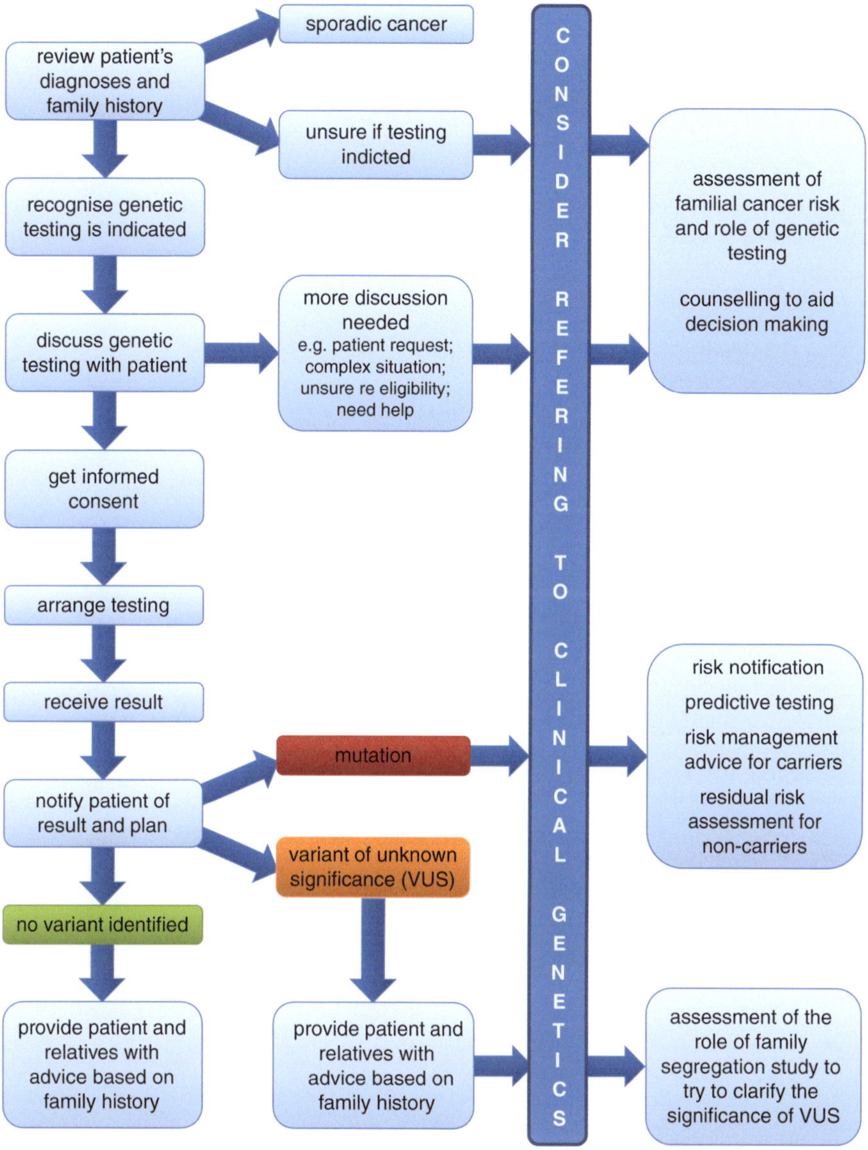

Fig. 21.5 Overview of mainstream genetic testing for a familial cancer predisposition

New genetic testing technology has dramatically reduced the cost of diagnostic genetic testing. Rather than examining one gene at a time (the historical approach using Sanger sequencing) it is now common to interrogate a number of relevant genes at the same time using a massive parallel sequencing platform. Sequencing multiple genes in parallel (a gene panel) increases the chance of identifying a disease-causing mutation, with lower cost than sequential sequencing. However, gene panels have the disadvantage of a higher probability of detecting a variant of unknown

Box 21.3: Checklist when Obtaining Consent for a Diagnostic Genetic Test

- After counselling patients should have the option to decline testing.
- If testing is declined it may be appropriate to offer DNA storage so a sample is available for future testing (provided that appropriate (future) consent is given).
- If the situation is complex consider referral to a clinical geneticist or genetic counsellor.

Condition being tested for

- The condition, its prognosis and management
- Likely inheritance pattern

Test process

- Type of sample(s) required (e.g. blood, buccal swab, skin biopsy)
- Consent needed
- What will be tested
- Turnaround time for result
- How the result will be disclosed (e.g. letter, phone, face to face)
- When results can be disclosed to others (e.g. other health services, health insurance providers)
- Cost (if any) to the person being tested

Possible test results

- The possible outcomes (for details see Box 21.5)
- What each result means for the individual and their family

Potential benefits

- May confirm a specific condition or diagnosis
- May rule out some conditions
- May influence clinical management of a cancer
- May provide information about cancer risk
- May reduce uncertainty
- May influence relatives' healthcare

Risks of the test

- Physical risks (e.g. pain, bleeding)
- Implications for insurance premiums and/or eligibility
- Emotional, social and financial consequences of the result
- Potential for genetic discrimination
- Result may increase uncertainty

Limitations of genetic testing

- False-negative result
- Variants of unknown significance
- Result may confirm a risk of a condition but not if or when that condition will develop
- In some situations an uninformative result cannot confirm or rule out a specific condition

Family implications

- Result may impact on reproductive decisions.
- Need for family risk notification if a mutation is identified.
- Relatives may still need enhanced cancer screening if no mutation is identified.

Box 21.4: Some Genetic Terminology

Mainstream genetic testing	Genetic testing in a patient with a condition (e.g. colorectal cancer) which is arranged by their non-genetic healthcare professional
Diagnostic genetic testing	Genetic testing in a patient suspected to have a particular condition because they have physical signs and symptoms of the condition
Predictive genetic testing	Testing a healthy (unaffected) person for the presence/absence of a specific mutation that has been identified in a genetic relative
Allele	Version of a gene or DNA sequence at a single locus
Locus	The unique chromosomal location defining the position of a gene or DNA sequence
Phenotype	The observable characteristics of a cell or an individual
Genotype	The genetic composition of an individual either overall or at a particular locus
Genetic variant	A DNA sequence that is different from the most common DNA sequence in the population
Polymorphism	A genetic variant that is common in the population
Benign variant	A genetic variant that has no impact on health
Variant of unknown significance (VUS)	A genetic variant whose significance to the health of an individual is not known; the VUS could be benign or could be disease causing
Mutation	A genetic variant that is disease causing
Epimutation	A change in chromatin organisation that causes a change in the expression (activity) of one or more genes, without any change in the DNA sequence of that gene(s)
Germline variant	A genetic variant that is present in sperm or oocytes; can be transmitted to offspring
Somatic variant	A genetic variant that arises in a somatic cell after conception; cannot be transmitted to offspring
Constitutional variant	A genetic variant that is present in every cell; is present in somatic and germ cells so could be transmitted to offspring
Mosaic variant	A variant that is present in some cell lines but not others; may or may not involve germline cells

Box 21.5: Understanding Genetic Test Results for Familial Cancer Syndromes

Classification of genetic variants

Variant class	Class 1	Class 2	Class 3	Class 4	Class 5
Plain language terms	Not a genetic error Normal variation Benign variant		VUS[a]	Genetic error Gene fault Disease-causing variant Mutation	
ACMG classification	Benign	Likely benign	Equivocal	Likely pathogenic	Pathogenic
ACMG probability of being pathogenic[b]	<0.1%	0.1–9.9%	10–90%	90.1–99%	>99%
IARC probability of being pathogenic[c]	<0.1%	0.1–4.9%	5–94.9%	95–99%	>99%

[a]Variant of unknown significance

[b]ACMG = American College of Medical Genetics. See Richards et al., Genet Med. 2015 Jan;17(1):68–9

[c]IARC = IARC Unclassified Genetic Variants Working Group; See Plon et al., Hum Mutat 2008;29:1282–1291

A mutation is found

- The gene/mutation causing the disorder has been identified.
- The result may influence clinical management.
- Reproductive options may be available to prevent future affected children.
- Predictive genetic testing is available to close relatives.
- Confirmatory genetic testing is available for clinically affected relatives.
- There may be insurance implications for family members.
- Referral to a clinical genetics service is recommended.

A mutation is not found

- A genetic cause for the disorder has not been identified.
- The clinical diagnosis may be unchanged.
- Predictive genetic testing of relatives is not possible.
- The genetic implications for other family members may be unchanged.
- At-risk relatives may need cancer surveillance depending on the family cancer history.

A variant of unknown significance (VUS) is found

- A variant has been identified but its significance is not known.
- The clinical diagnosis may be unchanged.
- Predictive genetic testing of relatives is not possible.
- The genetic implications for other family members may be unchanged.

- At-risk relatives may need cancer surveillance depending on the family cancer history.
- Testing of other family members may sometimes be recommended as part of a segregation analysis to help determine the significance of the variant.
- Referral to a clinical genetics service is recommended.

significance. Also, if gene selection is broad rather than focused, there is a risk of identifying variants in genes with unproven casual association with GI tumor risk.

In a mainstream setting, this author recommends selecting a panel of genes that have both clinical validity and clinical utility for the cancer phenotype of concern. In other words, limit the genes tested to those which have proven association with the cancer and/or tumor(s) your patients have, and where mutations in that gene are a well-established cause of an inherited GI cancer syndrome for which there are evidence-based risk management guidelines. Refer to clinical genetic or familial cancer clinic if you think testing of less well-established genes or "off-phenotype" genes may be indicated.

Just as genes are "shared" by a family—so are mutations. A cancer-affected patient is effectively being tested as "a representative of the family". Clinicians who order mainstream diagnostic genetics tests must remember that the result will have implications for relatives, not just the patient being tested. Therefore, mainstream diagnostic genetic tests should only be ordered by medical professionals who are part of or linked to a service which has the resources to manage the familial implications of the result.

21.2.4 Consent for Diagnostic Genetic Testing

As with all medical testing, before a person has a genetic test they must give their informed consent. "Informed" means the person has enough information to make an educated decision about genetic testing; "consent" means the person gives their voluntary agreement to have the test done. It is important that he or she understands the testing procedure; the potential benefits, risks and limitations of genetic testing; and the possible consequences of the genetic test result (Box 21.3 and 21.5). Most laboratories will require evidence that a patient has given their consent for testing.

Genetic discrimination occurs when people are treated differently by their employer or insurance company because they have a gene mutation that causes or increases the risk of an inherited disorder. Fear of insurance discrimination is a common concern among people considering genetic testing for cancer predisposition, and should be discussed as part of the consent process. Written information relevant to the Australian context is available online from the Centre for Genetics Education (NSW).

If there is local mainstreaming of genetic testing, consent can be obtained by the managing clinician; otherwise referral to a clinical genetics or familial cancer clinic is needed (Fig. 21.5). These services provide assistance and support for mainstream testing—and can also arrange the genetic test if the managing clinician feels that they do not have the required knowledge, expertise or time for mainstream testing.

For some patients their personal and family situation introduces complexities to their decision about testing. Referral to a clinical geneticist or genetic counsellor is recommended if a patient is struggling with their decision, if the genetic test result has the potential to lead to complex clinical issues or if a patient requests additional information or counselling.

21.2.5 Managing the Family

A diagnostic genetic test may identify a mutation in a relevant gene and confirm a suspected inherited GI cancer syndrome (Box 21.5). Most inherited GI cancer syndromes are dominantly inherited. If a mutation is identified the person's first-degree relatives have up to a 50% chance of inheriting the mutation and having an increased cancer risk. A critical component of family care is predictive genetic testing of relatives who may have inherited the mutation. Genetic counsellors have specific expertise in this area, and all families that have a mutation identified should be referred to a clinical genetics or familial cancer clinic for family risk notification and predictive testing of at-risk relatives.

Men and women of reproductive age should be aware of the availability of preimplantation and prenatal genetic diagnosis.

21.2.6 Limitations of Genetic Testing

Genetic testing technology is imperfect and current knowledge of the genes underlying inherited GI cancer predisposition is incomplete. Failure to identify a disease-causing mutation may not rule out an inherited GI cancer syndrome and this type of result is better regarded as uninformative rather than normal. If a mutation is not identified the family history can be used to assess the gastrointestinal cancer risk for close relatives, and guide their cancer screening recommendations.

21.2.7 Family History-Based Management of Colorectal Cancer Risk

Provided that a cancer-unaffected person is not known to have or to be at risk of an inherited GI cancer syndrome (see below), their family history of CRC can be used to estimate their individual CRC risk. Personal screening recommendations can then be based on this estimate (Table 21.1).

21.3 Specific Inherited GI Cancer Predisposition Syndromes (Table 21.2)

The clinical care of a cancer-affected person with an inherited GI cancer predisposition syndrome should be individualised taking their cancer diagnoses and current health status into account. In most instances these patients should be referred to a tertiary-level service for management.

Table 21.1 Population colorectal cancer screening based on family history[a]

	category 1	category 2	category 3*
	at or slightly above average risk	moderately increased risk	high risk
family history	no first or second-degree relatives with CRC one first or one second-degree relative with CRC diagnosed at or over 55y one second-degree relative with CRC diagnosed under 55y two second-degree relatives with CRC both diagnosed at or over 55y (same or different sides of the family) one first and one second-degree relative with CRC both diagnosed at or over 55y (same or different sides of the family)	consult Cancer Australia for details example family histories include one first-degree relative with CRC diagnosed under 55y two second-degree relatives with CRC both diagnosed under 55y (same or different sides of the family) two first-degree relatives with CRC both diagnosed at or over 55y (same or different sides of the family) one first and 2 or more second-degree with CRC all diagnosed at or over 55y (same or different sides of the family)	consult Cancer Council Australia for details example family histories include two first-degree relative with CRC both diagnosed under 55y 3 or more first or second degree with CRC with at least one diagnosed under 55y (same or different sides of the family) 3 or more first degree relatives with CRC all daignosed at or over 55y (same or different sides of the family)
relative risk	no family history - 10% lower than average history as above - up to 2 X average risk	3-6 X average risk	7-10 X average risk
lifetime risk to age 75y	5-10%	15-30%	30-40%
	recommendations	**recommendations**	**recommendations**
aspirin	consider low dose aspirin from age 50y (100-300mg/day)	consider low dose aspirin from age 50y (100-300mg/day)	consider low dose aspirin from age 50y (100-300mg/day)
FOBT	FOBT every 2 years from 50y if one first-degree >55y consider starting at 45y	FOBT every 2 years from 40y	FOBT every 2 years from 35y
colonoscopy	not recommended	5 yearly colonoscopy from 50y	5 yearly colonoscopy from 45y

Based on Cancer Council Australia Clinical practice guidelines for the prevention, early detection and management of colorectal cancer

See https://wiki.cancer.org.au/australia/Guidelines:Colorectal_cancer

[a]Excludes confirmed high-risk colorectal cancer syndromes which have their own screening guidelines (e.g. Lynch syndrome, juvenile polyposis syndrome, FAP)

Table 21.2 Inherited gastrointestinal tumor syndromes

Syndrome	Gene(s)	inheritance	Gastrointestinal features	Extra-intestinal features	Surveillance
Lynch syndrome	*MLH1*	Dominant	Colorectal carcinoma	Endometrial carcinoma	PMS2/MSH6: Annual colonoscopy; start from age 30y[a]
	PMS2		Gastric carcinoma	Epithelial ovarian cancer	MLH1/MSH2/EPCAM: Annual colonoscopy; start from age 25y[b]
	MSH2		Small intestinal carcinoma	Urothelial cancer	All genes: If family history of gastric cancer or high ethnic risk second-yearly UGIE; start from age 30y
	MSH6			Cholangiocarcinoma	All genes: Hysterectomy after childbearing complete or from age 40y
	EPCAM			Brain tumors	All genes: Consider bilateral oophorectomy at the time of hysterectomy
				Sebaceous gland tumors	
				Keratoacanthomas	
Classical FAP	*APC*	Dominant	Colorectal adenomas	Desmoid tumor	Annual screening of colon; start from age 10 to 12y
			Colorectal carcinoma	Papillary thyroid cancer	Flexible sigmoidoscopy adequate initially; colonoscopy once first adenoma identified
			Gastric fundic gland polyps	Brain tumor	UGIE 1–5 yearly depending on Spigelman criteria; start from age 25y
			Duodenal adenoma	Hepatoblastoma	
			Duodenal cancer	CHRPE	
Attenuated FAP	*APC*	Dominant	Colorectal adenomas	Desmoid tumor	Annual colonoscopy; start from age 18 to 20y
			Colorectal carcinoma	Papillary thyroid cancer	UGIE 1–5 yearly depending on Spigelman criteria; start from age 25y
			Gastric fundic gland polyps	Brain tumor	
			Duodenal adenoma	Hepatoblastoma	

			Duodenal cancer	CHRPE	
Clinical FAP	Unknown	Dominant	Colorectal adenomas	Desmoid tumor	Annual colonoscopy; start from age 10 to 15y
(No APC mutation identified)			Colorectal carcinoma	Papillary thyroid cancer	If no polyps by age 25y change to every 2y
			Gastric fundic gland polyps	Brain tumor	If no polyps by age 35y change to every 3y
			Duodenal adenoma	Hepatoblastoma	If no polyps by age 45y every 3–5y thereafter
			Duodenal cancer	CHRPE	If adenomas detected, change to classical FAP surveillance
MUTYH-associated polyposis	*MUTYH*	Recessive	Colorectal adenomas	Unclear	Second-yearly colonoscopy; start from age 30y; increase to annually if polyps detected
			Duodenal adenoma		UGIE 1–5 yearly depending on Spigelman criteria; start from age 25y
			Duodenal cancer		
Serrated polyposis syndrome	Unknown	Unknown	Serrated polyps	Nil known	Frequent colonoscopy with polypectomy until all polyps >5 mm removed
			Colorectal carcinoma		Then colonoscopy 1–3 yearly with frequency determined by number, size and dysplasia of polyps
Juvenile polyposis syndrome	*BMPR1A*	Dominant	Hamartomatous polyps	SMAD4 mutation: Features of HHT	Second yearly colonoscopy; start from age 15y; increase to annually if polyps detected
	SMAD4		Colorectal carcinoma		Second yearly UGIE start from age 25y; increase to annually if polyps detected
			Small intestinal carcinoma		SMAD4 mutation carriers also need HHT surveillance
			Gastric cancer		
Peutz-Jeghers syndrome	*STK11*	Dominant	Hamartomatous polyps	Breast cancer	Baseline colonoscopy, UGIE and small bowel imaging at age 8y
			Colorectal carcinoma	Rare gonadal tumors	If no polyps repeat at 18y, then repeat at least every 3y depending on polyp burden

(continued)

Table 21.2 (continued)

Syndrome	Gene(s)	inheritance	Gastrointestinal features	Extra-intestinal features	Surveillance
			Small intestinal carcinoma	Pancreatic adenocarcinoma	Annual breast MRI ± mammography; start from age 30y
			Gastric cancer	Adenoma malignum of the cervix	Annual endocervical smear; start from age 18y
				Mucocutaneous pigmentation	
PTEN hamartoma syndrome	*PTEN*	Dominant	Colorectal polyps (hamartoma, adenoma, serrated)	Macrocephaly	Colonoscopy: Follow screening guidelines based on the family history of CRC
				Mucocutaneous papillomatosis	Annual breast MRI ± mammography; start from age 30y
				Intellectual disability	
				Autism	
				Trichilemmoma	
				Breast cancer	
				Endometrial cancer	
				Soft-tissue hamartoma	
				Renal cancer	
Polymerase proofreading	*POLE*	Dominant	Colorectal adenomas	Unknown	Colorectal screening inferred from attenuated FAP
Associated polyposis	*POLD1*		Colorectal carcinoma		
NTHL1-associated polyposis	*NTHL1*	Recessive	Colorectal adenomas	Unknown	Colorectal screening inferred from attenuated FAP
			Colorectal carcinoma		
GREM1-associated polyposis	*GREM1*	Dominant	Colorectal polyps (mixed) Colorectal carcinoma	Unknown	Colorectal screening inferred from attenuated FAP

RNF43-associated polyposis	*RNF43*	Dominant	Serrated polyps	Unknown	Inferred from serrated polyposis syndrome
			Colorectal carcinoma		
CDH1-associated HDGC	*CDH1*	Dominant	Diffuse gastric cancer	Lobular breast cancer	No effective screening for gastric cancer; refer for total gastrectomy in early adulthood
				Cleft lip and/or palate	Annual breast MRI; start from age 30y
				Blepharocheilodontic syndrome	
CTNNA1-associated HDGC	*CTNNA1*	Dominant	Diffuse gastric cancer	Unknown	Inferred from CDH1-associated HDGC

CHRPE congenital hypertrophy of the retinal pigment epithelium, *CRC* colorectal carcinoma, *FAP* familial adenomatous polyposis, *HDGC* hereditary diffuse gastric cancer, *HHT* hereditary haemorrhagic telangiectasia, *UGIE* upper gastrointestinal endoscopy, *y* years

[a]In a family with a CRC diagnosed <35 years begin screening 5 years before the youngest affected

[b]In a family with a CRC diagnosed <30 years begin screening 5 years before the youngest affected

Genetic relatives of mutation carriers should be referred to a clinical genetics service for predictive genetic testing, with the age for testing depending on the particular GI cancer predisposition syndrome. In general, predictive testing of children is only done if there is a risk of cancer or tumors in childhood, or where prevention or surveillance strategies are recommended to begin in childhood.

Healthy (cancer unaffected) mutation carriers should be offered a cancer prevention and surveillance programme. Evidence-based "risk management guidelines" have been suggested by a number of organisations including the Australian national eviQ program (www.eviq.org.au) and Cancer Australia. (wiki.cancer.org.au/australia/Clinical_question:Family_history_and_CRC_risk). Risk management may be complex and in most instances mutation carriers should be referred to tertiary-level services for management.

21.3.1 Lynch Syndrome

LS is a dominantly inherited cancer predisposition syndrome that accounts for 3–5% of colorectal cancers. The historical name hereditary non-polyposis colorectal cancer or HNPCC is misleading as LS is associated with a risk of a broad range of cancers (Table 21.2). For men the key cancer risk is CRC and for women CRC and endometrial cancer. For both men and women there is also an increased risk of a number of other cancers and tumors although the absolute risk of these is much smaller than for CRC and endometrial cancer.

LS-associated tumors are MMR deficient and both MMR-IHC screening of tumors and good cancer family history taking are keys to recognising LS (Fig. 21.1).

LS is usually due to a mutation in one of four MMR genes (*MLH1*, *MSH2*, *MSH6* or *PMS2*) or a deletion in the distal part of the *EPCAM* gene that leads to epigenetic inactivation and silencing of *MSH2*. Typically there is a strong family history of LS-associated cancers, including diagnoses at younger than average ages. However, small family size and incomplete penetrance may result in an "unimpressive" family cancer history.

Rarely LS is caused by a primary constitutional epimutation, with most reported cases occurring in individuals with young-onset CRC (under 50 years) or a personal history of multiple LS-associated cancers. As methylation is "erased" during meiosis most primary constitutional epimutations segregate in a non-Mendelian fashion and are seldom associated with a strong family history of cancer.

21.3.1.1 Managing the Family

Predictive genetic testing should be offered to adults. The average cancer risk varies by the gene involved, family cancer history and gender; these factors should be taken into account when discussing cancer surveillance and risk-reducing strategies.

21.3.2 Lynch-Like Syndrome

Lynch-like syndrome (LLS) is an emerging term for the situation where a person has a MMR-deficient CRC but no MMR gene mutation is identified in constitutional DNA, and if there is LOE of MLH1 there is no evidence of *BRAF* V600E or *MLH1* promoter methylation in their tumor. The genetic mechanism underlying LS is not known. Possible explanations include mosaic MMR gene mutations that do not involve the lymphocyte cell line, constitutional MMR gene mutations not detected by current assays (a false-negative result), mutation(s) in currently unknown genes that impair formation and/or function of the MMR gene complex and sporadic tumor MMR gene mutations.

Up to 70% of LLS CRC have bi-allelic MMR gene mutations, but it is currently unclear if these somatic events are secondary to unknown heritable genetic defects or are "true" sporadic tumor events. It is likely that the LLS group represents a heterogeneous group ranging from sporadic MMR-deficient patients to true LS patients with cryptic MMR gene mutations.

LLS patients have a mean age of diagnosis that is similar to LS patients, suggesting that there is a genetic component to their experience. However, while their relatives have a higher CRC and extra-colonic cancer risk than in a sporadic setting, they have a lower risk of cancer compared to LS families. This suggests that relatives at risk of LLS may not require as extensive screening as those with LS.

Current National Comprehensive Cancer Network (NCCN) guidelines include tumor sequencing when no constitutional MMR gene is identified. If bi-allelic tumor mutations are identified, family history-based screening is recommended for relatives. If only one or no somatic mutations are identified, LS surveillance is recommended. If tumor and diagnostic genetic test results are complex and/or LLS is suspected, referral to clinical genetics should be considered.

21.3.3 Constitutional Mismatch Repair Deficiency

Constitutional mismatch repair deficiency (CMMRD) is due to bi-allelic germline mutations in any one of the MMR genes. People with CMMRD have no DNA MMR activity in normal tissue which results in a high risk of a broad range of tumors particularly colorectal and small-bowel adenoma and carcinoma, brain tumors and haematological cancers (leukaemia and lymphoma). Atypical café au lait macules are common and may be misdiagnosed as features of neurofibromatosis type 1. Patients often present with malignancy in the first two decades of life. MMR-IHC demonstrates MMR deficiency in tumor and normal tissue (in contrast to LS where MMR-IHC is retained in normal tissue).

There is no consensus on the optimal surveillance, although expert opinion-based recommendations have been published.

21.3.3.1 Managing the Family

The parents of a child with CMMRD are obligate carriers of a MMR gene mutation and should be offered LS surveillance. It should be noted that most people with CMMRD do not have an immediate family history of LS-associated cancers as their parents are usually young and so have not yet developed a LS-associated cancer despite having a mono-allelic mutation in a MMR gene.

Siblings are at 25% risk of CMMRD and 50% risk of LS. On average, one in four siblings will inherit two normal MMR genes and not have either condition. Siblings should be offered predictive genetic testing in early childhood.

21.3.4 Familial Adenomatous Polyposis

Familial adenomatous polyposis (FAP) is a dominantly inherited disorder due to mutations in the *APC* gene. It accounts for less than 1% of all CRC. Patients with a classical phenotype develop 100s to 1000s of colorectal adenomas with the polyposis beginning at a young age. The lifetime CRC risk approaches 100%. In attenuated or atypical FAP, fewer adenomas develop, onset of polyposis is later and CRC risk is lower. There is also an increased risk of other cancers including upper GI, brain, thyroid and liver (Table 21.2).

A diagnosis of FAP should be suspected in patients with a cumulative adenoma count of 10 or more before age 30 years, or more than 20 at any age. If an APC gene mutation is identified this confirms a diagnosis of FAP.

21.3.4.1 Managing the Family

Predictive genetic testing should be offered from early childhood.

Failure to identify an *APC* mutation does not rule out FAP. Surveillance guidelines have been developed for first-degree relatives of a patient with a clinical diagnosis of FAP where a mutation has not been identified (see www.eviq.org.au).

21.3.5 MUTYH-Associated Polyposis

MUTYH-associated polyposis (MAP) is due to bi-allelic mutations in the *MUTYH* gene (Table 21.2). In MAP there is predisposition to adenomatous colorectal polyps and early-onset CRC. Affected patients commonly have between 20 and 100 adenomas but may have a phenotype mimicking classical FAP. Less commonly oligopolyposis is seen. Some patients develop both adenomatous and serrated polyps, but current data indicates that the adenomatous polyps almost always dominate. Approximately 20% of patients with MAP develop duodenal polyposis and these polyps may undergo malignant transformation.

Extra-intestinal cancers have been reported in patients with MAP but whether they are part of the phenotype or coincidental sporadic cancers is debated.

MAP should be suspected in patients with a cumulative adenoma count of 10 or more before age 30 years, or more than 20 at any age.

21.3.5.1 Managing the Family

Predictive genetic testing should be offered to adult siblings of bi-allelic mutation carriers as they may have inherited two mutations and have MAP.

There is no consensus on the management of mono-allelic *MUTYH* mutation carriers. On average mono-allelic *MUTYH* mutations confer 1.5- to 2-fold increase in the risk of CRC. One option is to offer colonoscopy 5 yearly from 10 years younger than the earliest CRC diagnosis in the family.

21.3.6 Juvenile Polyposis Syndrome

Juvenile polyposis syndrome (JPS) is an autosomal dominant disorder due to mutations in either the *BMPR1A* or the *SMAD4* gene (Table 21.2). JPS is characterised by multiple hamartomatous gastrointestinal polyps with "juvenile" histology. This is a misleading name as juvenile polyps often develop in adulthood. There is an increased risk of CRC and other gastrointestinal cancers. Patients with *SMAD4* mutations may also manifest features of hereditary hemorrhagic telangiectasia.

The generally accepted clinical criteria for a diagnosis of JPS is at least five confirmed juvenile polyps in the colorectum, or two or more juvenile polyps involving at least two different sites.

21.3.6.1 Managing the Family

Predictive genetic testing should be offered in childhood.

21.3.7 Peutz-Jeghers Syndrome

Peutz-Jeghers syndrome (PJS) is an autosomal dominant disorder due to mutations in the *STK11* gene (Table 21.2). PJS is characterised by multiple hamartomatous gastrointestinal polyps, mucocutaneous melanocytic pigmentation and an increased risk of gastrointestinal and other cancers. Peutz-Jeghers polyps have distinct histological features including extensive smooth muscle arborisation throughout the polyp. Although the gastrointestinal cancer risk is for adult-onset cancers, GI surveillance should begin in childhood as polyps can act as a fulcrum for intussusception.

There is also an increased risk of a number of rare tumors including ovarian sex cord tumors with annular tubules (SCTAT), testicular large calcifying Sertoli cell tumors (LCST) and adenoma malignum of the cervix. Adenoma malignum, also known as minimal deviation adenocarcinoma, is difficult to diagnose because tumor cells are usually well differentiated. Cervical cancer screening programmes based on detection of HPV DNA do not detect this subtype of cervical cancer and specific surveillance is required (Table 21.2).

A clinical diagnosis of PJS is made in patients with one or more of the following criteria: (1) two or more histologically confirmed PJS polyps; (2) any number of PJS polyps in a person who also has characteristic mucocutaneous pigmentation; (3) any number of PJS polyps in a person who has a close relative with PJS; and (4) characteristic mucocutaneous pigmentation in a person who has a close relative with PJS.

21.3.7.1 Managing the Family

Predictive genetic testing should be offered in childhood.

21.3.8 PTEN

Mutations in the *PTEN* gene cause a group of related clinical phenotypes that are collectively called PTEN hamartoma tumor syndrome (PHTS). The PHTS phenotypes include Cowden syndrome, Bannayan-Riley-Ruvalcaba syndrome and PTEN-related Proteus syndrome, all of which have different key clinical features. There is considerable variation in the clinical features that develop from person to person, even within the same family (Table 21.2). Published estimates of the lifetime risk of developing specific features of PHTS are biased by descriptions of families with florid manifestations of the condition.

There may be an increased risk of colorectal cancer in some families. However, there is insufficient evidence to recommend routine colonoscopy to all individuals with PHTS.

21.3.8.1 Managing the Family

Predictive genetic testing should be offered in childhood.

21.3.9 Serrated Polyposis Syndrome

Serrated polyposis syndrome (SPS) is currently diagnosed in patients meeting one of the three 2010 World Health Organisation (WHO)-defined criteria: (1) five or more serrated polyps proximal to the sigmoid colon, at least two 10 mm or more in size; (2) any number of serrated polyps proximal to the sigmoid colon in an individual who has a first-degree relative with SPS; or (3) more than 20 serrated polyps throughout the colon (regardless of size). Some patients also have conventional colorectal adenomas and their presence increases the CRC risk further. It is currently debated whether patients with smaller numbers of serrated polyps (e.g. 10–20 cumulative) should be managed in the same way as those meeting WHO criteria for SPS.

Most cases of SPS occur in the absence of a family history of serrated polyps and are of unknown genetic basis (Table 21.2). Rare familial cases due to dominant germline mutations in the *RNF43* gene have been reported.

21.3.9.1 Managing the Family

Regular colonoscopy should be offered to first-degree relatives of a patient with SPS. The optimal surveillance for relatives has not been clearly defined. Some experts suggest colonoscopy 5 yearly from age 40 years, or from 10 years before the age of the youngest diagnosis of SPS or CRC in the family, whichever is earliest. Screening should be individualised if polyps are identified.

21.3.10 Emerging Colorectal Cancer Syndromes

In more recent years a number of novel genes have been found to be associated with cases of familial colorectal polyposis and/or familial CRC. For most of these genes there is a lack of compelling evidence for a causal relationship to polyposis or CRC. Testing of these genes should remain in a research setting.

For a small number of genes the evidence of a causal relationship is robust, and testing of these genes is now moving from a research to a clinical/routine setting (Table 21.2). As few families with mutations in these "new" genes have been identified, evidence-based surveillance recommendations for mutation carriers are not available. Suggested surveillance is largely inferred from the better known syndromes and will need to be refined as additional mutation carriers are identified and reported.

21.3.11 Hereditary Diffuse Gastric Cancer

Mutations in the *CDH1* gene cause the dominant cancer predisposition syndrome hereditary diffuse gastric cancer (HDGC). The penetrance of diffuse gastric cancer is high with the cumulative risk to age 80 years estimated to be 70% for men and 56% for women. Female mutation carriers also have an increased risk of lobular breast cancer (cumulative risk 42% by age 80 years). There are uncommon families who co-segregate cleft lip and/or palate (Table 21.2).

Recently mutations in a second diffuse cancer gene, *CTNNA1*, were identified. Cancer penetrance in *CTNNA1* mutation carriers is unknown.

Decisions about the management of the diffuse gastric cancer risk are difficult. Endoscopic surveillance strategies are of unproven benefit. It is clear that mutation carriers develop multiple foci of in situ or stage T1a diffuse gastric carcinoma that is not visible endoscopically and may be missed histologically despite multiple gastric biopsies. An advanced asymptomatic invasive cancer can also be missed despite multiple gastric biopsies at the time of surveillance endoscopy. Risk-reducing total gastrectomy is the only intervention proven to prevent the development of diffuse gastric cancer in *CDH1* mutation carriers. However, the gastric cancer risk while high is not 100% and gastrectomy has significant morbidity and mortality.

The sensitivity of mammography for lobular breast cancer is low, so breast MRI should be used for breast cancer surveillance in female CDH1 mutation carriers.

21.3.11.1 Managing the Family

Predictive genetic testing should be offered in late adolescent/early adulthood.

21.3.12 Gastric Adenocarcinoma and Proximal Polyposis of the Stomach

In the absence of proton pump inhibitor treatment, extensive polyposis of the gastric body and fundus raises the possibility of the rare syndrome gastric adenocarcinoma and proximal polyposis of the stomach (GAPPS), due to mutations in promoter 1B of the *APC* gene. Cancer and polyp penetrance is unknown. As less than ten families have been reported, evidence-based surveillance recommendations for mutation carriers are not available.

21.3.12.1 Managing the Family

The optimal age for predictive genetic testing is not known. The age for testing should be individualised taking family preference into account.

21.4 Online Evidence-Based Resources

21.4.1 National eviQ Program (Australia)

https://www.eviq.org.au/

The eviQ online resource provides evidence-based, consensus-driven cancer treatment protocols and information, for use at the point of care. The protocols are regularly reviewed and updated. There are three types of protocols directly relevant to cancer genetics:

1. Referral protocols
2. Genetic testing protocols
3. Risk management protocols

21.4.2 Cancer Council Australia Colorectal Cancer Wiki

https://wiki.cancer.org.au/australia/Guidelines:Colorectal_cancer

This wiki-guideline includes two sections with particular relevance to familial and inherited gastrointestinal cancer.

1. A section on inherited colorectal cancer syndromes: https://wiki.cancer.org.au/australia/Guidelines:Colorectal_cancer/High-risk_familial_syndromes
2. A section on family history-based colorectal cancer screening: https://wiki.cancer.org.au/australia/ Guidelines: Colorectal_cancer/Risk_and_ screening_ based_ on_ family_ history

Reference: Cancer Council Australia Colorectal Cancer Guidelines Working Party. Clinical practice guidelines for the prevention, early detection and management of colorectal cancer. Sydney: Cancer Council Australia. [Version URL: https://wiki.cancer.org.au/australiawiki/index.php?oldid=180618, cited 2018 Mar 17].

Available from https://wiki.cancer.org.au/australia/Guidelines:Colorectal_cancer. Approved by NHMRC 27 October 2017.

21.4.3 Centre for Genetics Education (NSW, Australia)

An on-ine resource of information about genetics including

1. Fact sheets: http://www.genetics.edu.au/publications-and-resources/facts-sheets
2. Information about cancer and family history: http://www.genetics.edu.au/individuals-and-families/cancer-in-the-family
3. Information about genetic testing and insurance: http://www.genetics.edu.au/publications-and-resources/facts-sheets/fact-sheet-20-life-insurance-products-and-genetic-testing-in-australia

21.4.4 GeneReviews (USA)

https://www.ncbi.nlm.nih.gov/books/NBK1116/

GeneReviews is an international point-of-care resource that provides clinically relevant information about inherited conditions in a standardised journal-style format. Individual chapters are regularly reviewed and updated.

21.4.5 The National Comprehensive Cancer Network (USA)

https://www.nccn.org/professionals/physician_gls/pdf/genetics_colon.pdf

The NCCN guideline for the diagnosis and management of genetic colorectal cancer syndromes. It is regularly reviewed and updated.

Guideline name: NCCN guidelines for detection, prevention, and risk reduction. Genetic/familial high-risk assessment: colorectal.

21.4.6 National Institute for Health and Care Excellence (United Kingdom)

https://www.nice.org.uk/guidance/dg27

The NICE guideline for testing colorectal cancer tissue to screen for Lynch syndrome.

Guideline name: Molecular testing strategies for Lynch syndrome in people with colorectal cancer Diagnostics guidance [DG27]. Published February 2017.

21.4.7 Canadian Agency for Drugs and Technologies in Health

https://www.cadth.ca/mismatch-repair-deficiency-testing-colorectal-cancer-patients

The CADTH guideline for testing colorectal cancer tissue to screen for Lynch syndrome.

Guideline name: Mismatch Repair Deficiency Testing for Colorectal Cancer Patients. Published September 2015.

21.4.8 Genetics Home Reference: Your guide to understanding genetic conditions

https://ghr.nlm.nih.gov

Genetics Home Reference is hosted by the US National Library of Medicine, and is regularly updated and consumer-friendly information about the effects of genetic variation on human health.

Recommended Reading

Family History

Lu KH, et al. American Society of Clinical Oncology Expert Statement: collection and use of a cancer family history for oncology providers. J Clin Oncol. 2014;32:833–41.

Reviews of GI Tumour Syndromes

Lorans M, et al. Update on hereditary colorectal cancer: improving the clinical utility of multigene panel testing. Clin Colorectal Cancer. 2018;17(2):e293–305. https://doi.org/10.1016/j.clcc.2018.01.001.

Stoffel EM, Mangu PB, Gruber SB, et al. Hereditary colorectal cancer syndromes: American Society of Clinical Oncology Clinical Practice Guideline endorsement of the familial risk-colorectal cancer: European Society for Medical Oncology Clinical Practice Guidelines. J Clin Oncol. 2015;33:209–17.

Syngal S, Brand RE, Church JM, Giardiello FM, Hampel HL, Burt RW. ACG clinical guideline: genetic testing and management of hereditary gastrointestinal cancer syndromes. Am J Gastroenterol. 2015;110:223–62.

Lynch Syndrome and CMMRD

Peltomaki P. Update on lynch syndrome genomics. Familial Cancer. 2016;15:385–93.

Rubenstein JH, Enns R, Heidelbaugh J, Barkun A. American Gastroenterological Association Institute Guideline on the Diagnosis and Management of Lynch Syndrome. Gastroenterology. 2015;149:777–82.

Vasen HF, et al. Guidelines for surveillance of individuals with constitutional mismatch repair-deficiency proposed by the European Consortium "Care for CMMR-D" (C4CMMR-D). J Med Genet. 2014;51:283–93.

Serrated Polyposis

East JE, et al. British Society of Gastroenterology position statement on serrated polyps in the colon and rectum. Gut. 2017;66:1181–96.

Gastric Cancer

Li J, et al. Point mutations in exon 1B of APC reveal gastric adenocarcinoma and proximal polyposis of the stomach as a familial adenomatous polyposis variant. Am J Hum Genet. 2016;98(5):830–42.

van der Post RS, et al. Hereditary diffuse gastric cancer: updated clinical guidelines with an emphasis on germline CDH1 mutation carriers. J Med Genet. 2015;52:361–74.

22 Gastrointestinal Stromal Tumors: An Update for the General Surgeon

Markus I. Trochsler and Harsh A. Kanhere

22.1 Introduction

Gastrointestinal stromal tumors (GIST) affect only 1% of patients diagnosed with neoplasms of the gastrointestinal (GI) tract. Despite their relative rarity compared to epithelial tumours, these are the most frequent neoplasms of mesenchymal origin in the GI tract. GISTs in fact are the most commonly diagnosed subtype of sarcomas overall. Other soft tissue tumours of the GI tract include lipomas, liposarcomas, leiomyomas, desmoid tumours, schwannomas and peripheral nerve sheet tumours.

GIST was recognized as a specific entity in the late 1980s based on clinical, histopathological and immunohistochemical features and was thought to be derived from smooth muscle cells given the spindle cell appearance at light microscopy. Today, a more likely derivation is the interstitial cells of Cajal (ICC).

22.2 Epidemiology and Clinical Features of GIST

The incidence of GIST is estimated at 7–15 new cases per million population per year. Autopsy studies do suggest though the incidence of subcentimetre gastric GIST (micro-GIST) might be as high as 30%. These lesions typically do not show any mitotic activity. The mean age at diagnosis lies at approximately 60 years with a slight predominance for the male gender.

GIST may arise anywhere in the gastrointestinal tract from the esophagus to the rectum. The stomach (40–60%) followed by the jejunum and ileum (25–30%) are the most common sites of origin. GIST of the duodenum (5%), esophagus (<1%), colon and

M. I. Trochsler (✉) · H. A. Kanhere
Discipline of Surgery, University of Adelaide, Adelaide, SA, Australia
e-mail: markus.trochsler@sa.gov.au; Harsh.Kanhere@sa.gov.au

M. W. Wichmann et al. (eds.), *Gastroenterology For General Surgeons*,
https://doi.org/10.1007/978-3-319-92768-8_22

rectum (5–15%) are rare. Due to accidental dispersion during embryogenesis, GIST can originate outside the gastrointestinal (<5%) tract, in the abdominal cavity, greater omentum and retroperitoneum. Tumors reach a median size of 5–7 cm at the time of diagnosis. Asymptomatic patients with much larger lesions are not uncommon.

An increasing number of GIST are asymptomatic and diagnosed accidentally by endoscopy or cross-sectional imaging (Fig. 22.1). Patients often present with nonspecific symptoms such as bloating, early satiety, unspecific abdominal pain or pain related to other pathologies. Fifty percent of patients with gastric GIST present with overt or occult bleeding due to erosion of the gastric mucosa over the subepithelial tumour (Fig. 22.2). Tumor rupture into the peritoneal cavity causing significant hemorrhage is rare.

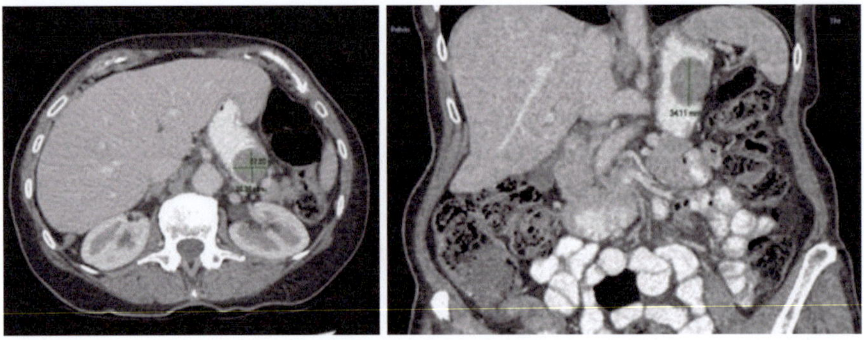

Fig. 22.1 Typical appearance of gastric GIST with endophytic growth pattern

Fig. 22.2 Endoscopic view on a gastric GIST. Typical submucosal tumor with smooth surface without ulceration

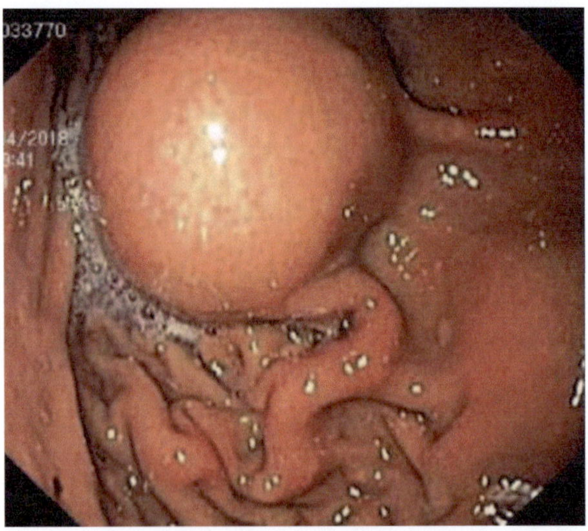

Common sites of metastasis are the liver and the peritoneal cavity. Metastatic disease to the lung is uncommon in contrast to most soft tissue sarcomas. Lymph node metastasis is rare. Hypothyroidism and non-islet cell tumor hypoglycemia in a paraneoplastic setting have been described in isolated cases.

22.3 Molecular Features and Targets

The KIT proto-oncogene and its protein product, the KIT tyrosine kinase receptor (c-KIT, CD 117), are central for diagnosis and management of GIST. c-KIT is a transmembrane receptor with an extracellular binding site for stem cell factor (SCF). Binding of SCF to c-KIT leads to activation of multiple intracellular signalling cascades controlling cell proliferation, adhesion, apoptosis, survival and differentiation. "Gain of function" mutations in KIT lead to overexpression of the receptor tyrosine kinase KIT and subsequent tumorgenesis. The detection of overexpressed c-KIT receptors on the cell surface by immunohistochemistry and KIT mutations by DNA sequencing has contributed to discriminating GIST from other soft tissue neoplasms. Anoctamin 1 (DOG1) is a transmembrane chloride ion channel protein constitutively expressed in ICC and in the majority of GIST, including many KIT-negative GIST. CD34, a hematopoietic progenitor cell antigen, can be present on GIST but is less specific than KIT and DOG1. Commercial antibodies are available for epitopes on both proteins and present a helpful adjunct for diagnosing GIST.

Nearly 80% of GIST carry mutations in the KIT gene. Mutations in the KIT gene are usually limited to 1 of 4 of the 21 exons. Mutations in exon 11 are described in two thirds of GIST followed by exon 9 (7%), exon 13 (1%) and exon 17 (1%). About 10% of newly diagnosed GIST do not carry any mutations in the KIT gene but have mutations in the platelet-derived growth factor receptor alpha (PDGFRA) gene. PDGFRA is a receptor tyrosine kinase similar to c-KIT. Activating mutations in exon 12, 14 and 18 leads to histologically indistinguishable tumours compared to KIT mutation carriers. The remaining group of "wild-type" GIST has no detectable KIT or PDGFRA mutations. This group continues to shrink as gene mutations in BRAF, SDHF and neuro-fibromatosis 1 (NF1) have been discovered. Figure 22.3 shows structures, mutation sites and frequency of c-KIT and PDGFRA.

The type of mutation and the mutated gene has clinical relevance for diagnostic and more importantly treatment purposes. Anatomical tumor location, affected patient group and drug sensitivity are influenced by these factors as outlined in Table 22.1. The discovery of mutations in the KIT oncogene led to the ability to target the overexpressed c-KIT receptors. In 2001, Joensuu reported the first successful treatment of GIST using tyrosine kinase inhibitor (TKI) STI571 (imatinib mesylate, Gleevec™). This favourable result was confirmed in a larger cohort of patients, and GIST became the first solid tumour to be treated using a small molecule tyrosine kinase inhibitor.

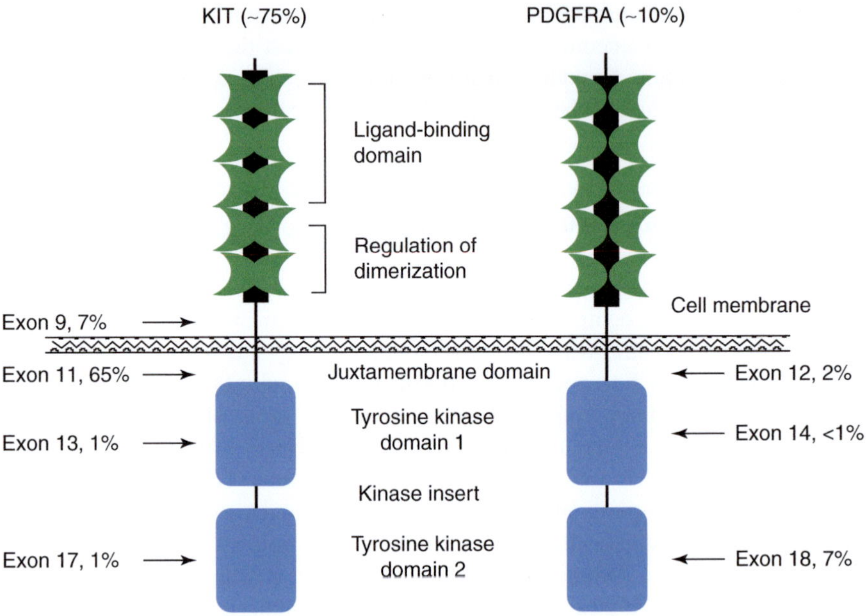

Fig. 22.3 Schematic structure of KIT and PDGFRA. The percentage indicate the frequency of mutations detected in each exon of the gene

Table 22.1 Classification of GISTs. Only the most common gene mutations are shown

Type of GIST	Incidence	Mutated gene	Clinical features	Imatinib sensitivity
Sporadic GIST				
KIT mutation				
Exon 9	~7%	*KIT*	Most non-gastric	Yes
Exon 11	~65%	*KIT*	Gastric or non-gastric	Yes
Exon 13	~1%	*KIT*		Variable
Exon 17	~0.5%	*KIT*		Variable
PDGFRA mutation				
Exon 12	~1.5%	*PDGFRA*	Most gastric	Yes
Exon 14	~0.1%	*PDGFRA*		Yes
Exon 18	~7%	*PDGFRA*	Most gastric	D842V insensitive. Most other sensitive
Wild-type (wt)	~10%	*KIT* wt, *PDGFRA* wt, sometimes *BRAF*, *SDHA*, *SDHB* or *SDHC* mutation	Gastric or non-gastric	Variable

22.4 Prognostic Determinants and Risk Stratification

GISTs often do not show classical histopathological features such as invasion and anaplasia/pleomorphism of cells and nuclei characteristic of many other cancers. Nearly all GISTs have the potential for malignant behaviour, and therefore a division into benign and malignant tumours is not useful in determining clinical management. As surgical resection remains the main pillar of GIST treatment, most risk stratification models are based on factors determined after resection of the tumors. These models predict progression-free survival based on factors described below. Güller et al. additionally found that nodal involvement, distant metastasis, older age, male gender and single marital status were associated with significant worse overall survival in a large population-based study including more than 5000 patients (see recommended reading).

Primary tumor site, tumor size and mitotic index independently predict risk of tumor recurrence after resection. In essence, tumors greater than 5 cm in diameter, with more than 5 mitotic figures per 50 high-powered fields and located outside the stomach (non-gastric GISTs), are associated with worse outcomes (Table 22.2).

Imaging is not routinely used to stratify recurrence risk. Several authors have reported computed tomography (CT) or endoscopic ultrasound (EUS) findings such as heterogenous enhancement, lobulated and/or exophytic growth pattern, mesenteric fat infiltration, ulceration and regional lymphadenopathy to be associated with higher risk of metastatic spread. Tumor rupture either spontaneous or intraoperative is an independent risk factor with a negative impact on disease-free survival.

The exact impact of the tumor genotype and kinase mutation status is confounded by the variable sensitivity of each gene mutation to imatinib. GIST with mutations in exons 9 and 11 seem to show a more aggressive phenotype compared to other mutation locations on the KIT gene. KIT exon 9 mutations are often found in non-gastric GIST. PDGFR gene mutations are nearly always found in gastric GIST and have a better outcome.

Table 22.2 Rates of progression-free survival for GISTs of the stomach and small intestine depending on tumour size and mitotic index

		Patients (%) with long-term progression-free survival	
Tumour size (cm)	Mitotic index (HPFs)	Gastric $n = 1055$	Small intestine $n = 629$
≤2	≤5/50	100	100
	>5/50	100	50
2–5	≤5/50	98.1	95.7
	>5/50	84	27
5–10	≤5/50	96.4	76
	>5/50	45	15
>10	≤5/50	88	48
	>5/50	14	10

22.5 Diagnostic Work-Up

Most GIST are now diagnosed by CT scan. Contrast (intravenous and oral)-enhanced CT of the abdomen and pelvis is the main imaging modality for staging. A typical GIST appears as a homogenous enhancing mass within the stomach wall or lumen (Fig. 22.1). Larger tumors might show intrinsic necrosis which appears as heterogenous enhancing mass. Large fungating and hyper-vascular lesions of the stomach might mimic primary liver lesions. MR imaging is reserved for specific anatomic locations such as rectum or duodenum. Assessment of extent of GIST metastasis in the liver is an indication for MRI.

Some gastric GIST might initially be found at endoscopy. The presence of a smooth submucosal mass in the stomach with or without overlying ulcer is pathognomonic (Fig. 22.2). The submucosal location direct biopsies are often not sufficient. Endoscopic ultrasound (EUS) allows for guided deeper fine needle aspiration (FNA) or core biopsies. GIST appear typically as hypoechoic, homogenous lesions with well-defined margins with EUS. Most GISTs originate from the muscularis propria (layer 4), but smaller lesions may arise from the muscularis mucosae (layer 2). EUS-guided core biopsies allow definite diagnosis of GIST by immunohistochemistry for KIT receptor presence and further allow assessment of KIT and other gene mutations. This is relevant for lesions where neoadjuvant treatment is considered due to anatomical location (esophagus, gastroesophageal junction, peripancreatic, rectum) in order to prevent potentially morbid or multivisceral resections. If the radiological appearance is typical and the perioperative risk is reasonable, histological confirmation by biopsy is not necessary prior to surgery.

Positron emission tomography using fluorodeoxyglucose (FDG-PET) is highly sensitive (86–100%) due to high glucose metabolism in GIST. However, specificity and anatomical definition are too low to consider FDG-PET as a primary diagnostic tool. Its main role is in accessing treatment response. Marked decreased glycolytic tumor metabolism can be detected as early as 24 h after treatment initiation with imatinib.

22.6 Principles of Surgery and Organ-Specific Aspects

Surgical resection of GIST remains the only established curative approach and is the treatment of choice. According to the long-term ACOSOG Z9001 trial, up to 70% patients with primary GIST of 3 cm and larger were cured by surgery alone. In general primary surgical resection is recommended for GIST larger than 2 cm in patients with life expectancy greater than 5 years and a reasonable perioperative risk profile. The natural history of GIST between 1 and 2 cm diameters is being researched regarding growth rate and metastatic potential. Kim et al. followed 948 patients with gastric subepithelial tumours smaller than 3 cm in a large retrospective study. Only 8.5% of these lesions ≤3 cm showed growth or changes in morphology over a median observation period of 24 months. Of the 25 patients who underwent surgical resection of the gastric subepithelial lesions, GIST was confirmed in 19. It is acceptable to observe subepithelial lesions of 2 cm or less in diameter with no concerning morphological features using endoscopy or imaging. The optimal frequency of follow-up and specific risks of this approach, however, remains uncertain.

The goal of surgical treatment is resection of the tumour including its pseudocapsule. The aim is to achieve negative microscopic resection margins, but its positive impact on recurrence-free survival is not proven. It seems that other factors such as mitotic index and tumour size play a more significant role in determining the risk of recurrence irrespective of imatinib treatment. As previously mentioned, lymph node metastasis is rare (1%), and therefore regional lymph node resection is not warranted. GIST mostly show a displacing rather than invasive growth pattern independent from their size. At larger sizes, GIST induce significant growth of vasculature with large supplying arteries and veins. Even large GISTs may still have only a small attachment to the organ of origin and therefore can relatively be easily resected without affecting the adjacent organs. At larger sizes and following neoadjuvant treatment, GIST become increasingly friable and prone to rupture. Dissection should be performed with great care to prevent rupture associated with almost inevitable peritoneal tumor recurrence.

GIST of the esophagus are rare. Most submucosal lesions in the distal oesophagus are leiomyomas and not GIST. Well-circumscribed mesenchymal lesions that are >2 cm should undergo EUS and biopsy to confirm diagnosis due to the scope of operation needed to resect these tumors. Further consideration needs to be given to neoadjuvant imatinib to downstage these lesions. Due to the need of multimodal treatment, a referral and discussion within a multidisciplinary team are recommended. Local enucleation of GIST in the esophagus has been reported but has not been widely adopted due to lack of prospective outcome data using this approach.

Gastric GIST may arise from anywhere in the stomach but are most commonly found in the fundus. Laparoscopic resections have been widely adopted into surgical practice for resection of gastric GIST. Tumors up to a diameter of 6–8 cm are usually well suited for laparoscopic resection. Any surgical approach to the stomach starts with a careful assessment of the peritoneal surfaces and liver to assess for metastatic disease. A no-touch surgical technique and a plastic specimen retrieval bag are used to avoid peritoneal tumor seeding. An intraoperative resection margin of 1 cm is sufficient to achieve microscopic negative resection margins. Tumors arising from the anterior surface of the body/fundus and greater curvature are often amendable to resection with a wedge of stomach using an appropriate stapling device. Lesions originating from the posterior gastric surface or with an endoluminal growth pattern might need a trans-gastric approach via an open or laparoscopic gastrotomy. In both situations we find the simultaneous use of an endoscope to verify appropriate resection margins and as a guide for the stapling device to verify a patent stomach lumen very helpful. Resection of lesions in the antrum, at the incisura, lesser curvature, and gastroesophageal junction are more challenging due to the risk of luminal narrowing. In this setting additional strategies are may need to be considered including use of a bougie (50Fr), neoadjuvant imatinib for downstaging or a formal (partial) gastrectomy. These patients are often better managed by an experienced upper gastrointestinal surgical team with access to multimodal treatment options.

The small intestine is the second most common site of GIST. Jejunal and ileal GIST are removed with the tumor-containing segment of small bowel. Formal segmental lymph node resection is not indicated. Laparoscopic approaches with intracorporal stapled or extracorporeal small bowel anastomosis are the preferred approach. Management of duodenal GIST is more challenging from a surgical point of view. A multidisciplinary team approach and consideration of multimodal treatment in an experienced centre are warranted. Careful assessment of the tumor location in relation to the pancreas and the papilla of Vater is crucial. Preoperative downstaging with imatinib is often used to minimize the extent of resections. Small lesions away from the pancreas might be amendable to resection with a disc of duodenal wall. Depending on the extent of duodenal resection, direct tension-free closure might be achieved without compromising the lumen. Alternatively, a duodeno-jejunostomy in a Roux-en-Y configuration will need to be performed. Lesions in the third and fourth part of the duodenum are often amendable to segmental duodenal resection after a generous Kocher manoeuvre and division of the ligament of Treitz. Reconstruction can either be performed by direct end-to-end anastomosis to the proximal jejunum or as above, by a duodeno-jejunostomy with closure of the distal duodenum.

Rectal GIST benefit from additional imaging with a pelvic MRI to define local involvement due to the missing serosal layer of the rectum and proximity to the anal sphincter. Neoadjuvant imatinib can downstage the tumor and improve outcomes when compared to rectal surgery alone. Standard open and laparoscopic resection strategies as well as trans-anal resection approaches have been described.

22.7 Neoadjuvant and Adjuvant Imatinib Mesylate

GIST respond poorly to almost all standard chemotherapy agents and radiotherapy. Imatinib mesylate (STI571, Gleevec) is the first agent to exhibit a significant activity in GIST. Imatinib inhibits tyrosine kinases such as KIT and PDGFR and is now considered the standard first-line treatment for advanced GIST. At a usual dose of 400 mg orally once daily, the treatment is well tolerated with common adverse effects that include periorbital edema, muscle cramps, diarrhea and anemia. Approximately 15% of GIST are resistant to imatinib such as carriers of KIT exon 9 mutations. Response to imatinib can be estimated by mutation analysis or observed by imaging. GIST typically respond by transformation from dense lesion into cyst-like structures under imatinib treatment. This morphologic transformation is often the only sign of response exhibited by the tumour and is especially important in accessing the response of imatinib in the neoadjuvant setting.

There have been no trials comparing surgery first with neoadjuvant imatinib followed by surgery. It is a common practice nowadays to consider neoadjuvant treatment in the setting of locally advanced lesions to prevent extensive organ or multivisceral resections as aforementioned. The goal is to downstage tumors to allow for safer and less morbid surgical interventions. Standard chemotherapy response criteria (RECIST) do not work well in GIST. Despite often immediate metabolic changes within the tumour seen in FDG-PET scans, decreased tumor size will only be seen after several weeks of treatment. In practice, a CT and FDG-PET 4 weeks after treatment initiation with imatinib might not show significant tumor shrinkage but often shows a decrease in tumor density, a morphologic cystic transformation and a decreased metabolic activity. Failing this, tyrosine kinase inhibitor resistance needs to be considered. Unlike other chemotherapy agents, imatinib can be continued up to the time of surgery and restarted straight after as there are no immunosuppressive effects and no negative impact on wound healing.

Adjuvant imatinib was established in the landmark ACOSOG Z9001 trial. In this study, over 700 patients with operable GIST (diameter > 3 cm) were randomized to either receive placebo or imatinib 400 mg daily for 1 year following surgical resection. The trial was stopped at interim analysis due to significantly improved progression-free survival in the imatinib group. One-year recurrence-free survival was 98% in the imatinib group and 83% in the placebo group. Adjuvant imatinib was well tolerated with a low rate of serious adverse events in the treatment group. As demonstrated in Fig. 22.4, the progression-free survival curves seem to converge after 3 years. This might indicate that imatinib is effective in controlling

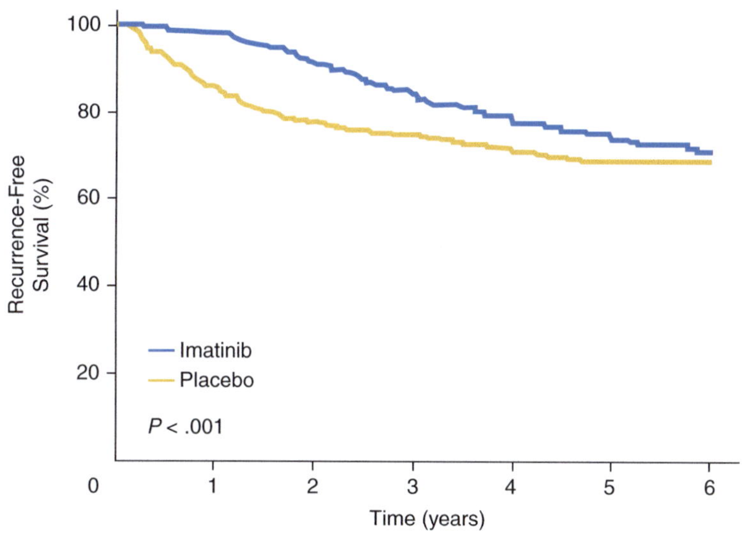

No. at risk							
Imatinib 400 mg	359	296	261	230	199	143	74
Placebo	354	278	243	218	186	132	64

Fig. 22.4 Recurrence-free survival of patients with primary GIST of 3 cm or greater after complete resection, randomized to 1 year of adjuvant imatinib vs. placebo

residual disease but is not able to clear it. Further studies are underway to clarify the optimal duration of adjuvant treatment with imatinib. Current recommendations are for adjuvant therapy with imatinib for 3 years following primary resection of high-risk lesions.

22.8 Role of Surgery in Metastatic and Recurrent GIST

Although imatinib has become the first-line treatment for recurrent and metastatic disease, there remains a role for surgery. In the setting of recurrent diseases, median progression-free survival with imatinib is 24 months. Development of secondary mutations in tumour subclones is thought to be responsible for imatinib resistance. Second- (sunitinib) and third-line (regorafenib) tyrosine kinase inhibitors (TKI) are indicated but show less durable response rates. The goal of secondary metastasectomy or debulking surgery is to remove tumour mass before resistance to second- and third-line TKI develops and to stop disease progression by eliminating resistant clones. This approach has not been tested in prospective randomized trials due difficult accrual of patients. Several retrospective single-institution studies report long-term disease control and longer overall survival in selected patient groups (i.e. stable disease, focal progression only, partial responders and isolated sites of progression) with this approach.

The liver and the peritoneum are the most common sites of metastatic disease. It is estimated that around 25–30% of patients presenting with recurrent/metastatic disease are technically resectable. The ideal timing for surgery is unknown. The median time to best response is 3.5 months, and little further tumour downsizing is reported after 9 months. TKI treatment should continue after metastasectomy or debulking procedures. Liver metastasis is approached similar to colorectal liver metastasis. Treatment is focused on clearing the liver from any disease using resectional and/or ablative techniques. Limited data is available on long-term outcomes of hepatic artery embolization, chemoembolization or radioembolization using yttrium-90-tagged microspheres in patients with unresectable liver disease. Removal of peritoneal metastasis might necessitate en bloc resection with other intra-abdominal organs.

22.9 Summary

GIST is a rare neoplastic disease affecting the entire gastrointestinal tract only known as specific entity for the last 40 years. Discovery of molecular mechanisms involved in the pathogenesis of this tumour has led to the development of targeted therapies. Disease pathology ranges from clinically irrelevant micro-GIST to highly aggressive neoplasms presenting with widespread metastasis and therapy-resistant genetic mutations. Given the complex clinical behaviour and highly variable genetic background, a multidisciplinary team approach is warranted for these patients. Figure 22.5 summarizes the therapeutical approach to primary and recurrent/metastatic GIST.

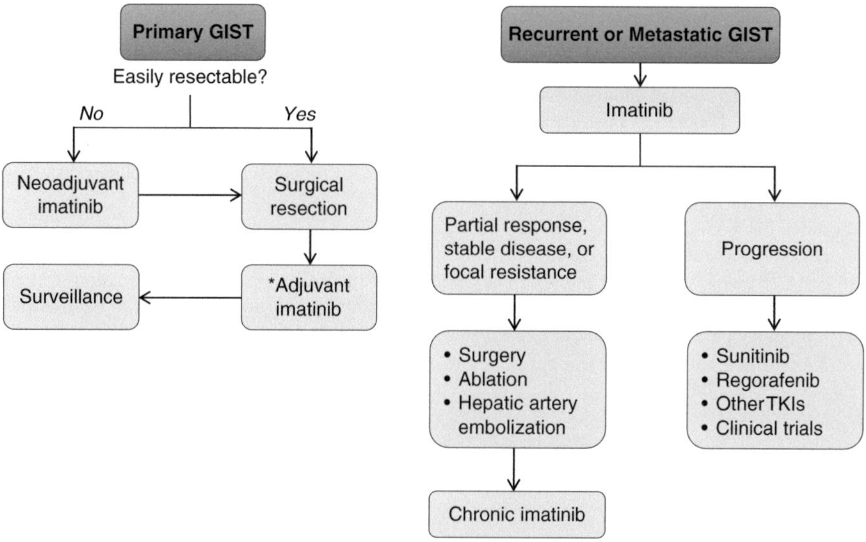

Fig. 22.5 Summarized approach to primary and metastatic/recurrent GIST

Recommended Reading

Cameron S. Long-term adjuvant treatment of gastrointestinal stromal tumors (GIST) with imatinib-a comment and reflection on the PERSIST-5 study. Transl Gastroenterol Hepatol. 2018;3:16.

Cavnar MJDRP. The management of gastrointestinal stromal tumors. In: Cameron JLCAM, editor. Current surgical therapy. 12th ed. Philadelphia, PA: Elsevier; 2017. p. 104.

Corless CL, Ballman KV, Antonescu CR, Kolesnikova V, Maki RG, Pisters PW, et al. Pathologic and molecular features correlate with long-term outcome after adjuvant therapy of resected primary GI stromal tumor: the ACOSOG Z9001 trial. J Clin Oncol. 2014;32(15):1563–70.

Cost of imatinib Australia 2018 [Cost of imatinib]. https://www.yourdiscountchemist.com.au/glivec-400mg-tablets-30-imatinib.html.

DeMatteo RP, Ballman KV, Antonescu CR, Corless C, Kolesnikova V, von Mehren M, et al. Long-term results of adjuvant imatinib mesylate in localized, high-risk, primary gastrointestinal stromal tumor: ACOSOG Z9000 (Alliance) intergroup phase 2 trial. Ann Surg. 2013;258(3):422–9.

Fairweather M, Balachandran VP, Li GZ, Bertagnolli MM, Antonescu C, Tap W, et al. Cytoreductive surgery for metastatic gastrointestinal stromal tumors treated with tyrosine kinase inhibitors: a 2-institutional analysis. Ann Surg. 2018;268(2):296–302.

Gold JS, Dematteo RP. Combined surgical and molecular therapy: the gastrointestinal stromal tumor model. Ann Surg. 2006;244(2):176–84.

Guller U, Tarantino I, Cerny T, Schmied BM, Warschkow R. Population-based SEER trend analysis of overall and cancer-specific survival in 5138 patients with gastrointestinal stromal tumor. BMC Cancer. 2015;15:557.

Hirota S, Isozaki K, Moriyama Y, Hashimoto K, Nishida T, Ishiguro S, et al. Gain-of-function mutations of c-kit in human gastrointestinal stromal tumors. Science. 1998;279(5350):577–80.

Joensuu H, DeMatteo RP. The management of gastrointestinal stromal tumors: a model for targeted and multidisciplinary therapy of malignancy. Annu Rev Med. 2012;63:247–58.

Joensuu H, Roberts PJ, Sarlomo-Rikala M, Andersson LC, Tervahartiala P, Tuveson D, et al. Effect of the tyrosine kinase inhibitor STI571 in a patient with a metastatic gastrointestinal stromal tumor. N Engl J Med. 2001;344(14):1052–6.

Kim MY, Jung HY, Choi KD, Song HJ, Lee JH, Kim DH, et al. Natural history of asymptomatic small gastric subepithelial tumors. J Clin Gastroenterol. 2011;45(4):330–6.

Maynard MA, Marino-Enriquez A, Fletcher JA, Dorfman DM, Raut CP, Yassa L, et al. Thyroid hormone inactivation in gastrointestinal stromal tumors. N Engl J Med. 2014;370(14):1327–34.

Miettinen M, Lasota J. Histopathology of gastrointestinal stromal tumor. J Surg Oncol. 2011;104(8):865–73.

Miettinen M. Gastrointestinal stromal tumors. An immunohistochemical study of cellular differentiation. Am J Clin Pathol. 1988;89(5):601–10.

Miettinen MLJ. Gastrointestinal stromal tumors: pathology and prognosis at different sites. Semin Diagn Pathol. 2006;23(2):70–83.

Nilsson B, Bumming P, Meis-Kindblom JM, Oden A, Dortok A, Gustavsson B, et al. Gastrointestinal stromal tumors: the incidence, prevalence, clinical course, and prognostication in the preimatinib mesylate era—a population-based study in western Sweden. Cancer. 2005;103(4):821–9.

Gastrointestinal Disorders Induced by Medication

23

Ian C. Roberts-Thomson

23.1 Introduction

Adverse drug reactions (ADRs) can be defined as harmful or unpleasant reactions caused by taking a medication. Many are known side effects related either to individual sensitivity or to augmented pharmacologic effects caused by variation in drug metabolism. The term "intolerance" can be used for patients with very low thresholds for side effects or for nonspecific symptoms (e.g., generally unwell) that accompany use of specified drugs. A minority of ADRs are related to drug allergy, while others are unexplained and labelled as idiopathic or idiosyncratic. Severe reactions that follow a single dose of medication are often related to allergy, but more common ADRs usually appear after days or weeks of medication or the use of combinations of two or more drugs.

ADRs are often classified as mild, significant, or serious. A serious ADR is usually defined as one that requires hospitalization, prolongs hospitalization, is permanently disabling, or results in death. The category, possible ADR, reflects the difficulty of attributing an outcome to a drug in the presence of other major medical issues. One area of difficulty is complications from anticancer drugs in the presence of advanced cancer. Yet another issue is use of the term ADR for intentional or unintentional noncompliance with medication. Unintentional noncompliance is usually included as an ADR if higher than recommended doses are taken that result in side effects. Excluded are patients with drug abuse, suicide attempts, and alcohol intoxication.

In all developed countries, ADRs are a significant cause of morbidity and mortality. For example, ADRs have been estimated to cause approximately 100,000 deaths per year in the USA and may rank as the sixth leading cause of death after heart disease, cancer, stroke, pulmonary disease, and accidents. Surveys have shown that

I. C. Roberts-Thomson (✉)
Adelaide Medical School, University of Adelaide, Adelaide, SA, Australia
e-mail: ian.robertsthomson@adelaide.edu.au

M. W. Wichmann et al. (eds.), *Gastroenterology For General Surgeons*,
https://doi.org/10.1007/978-3-319-92768-8_23

Table 23.1 Groups of drugs causing adverse effects of special relevance to general surgeons

• Antibiotics
• Non-steroidal anti-inflammatory drugs
• Antithrombotic agents
• Opioids
• Chemotherapeutic drugs
• Glucocorticoids
• Biologicals
• Laxatives
• Biophosphonates
• Cannabinoids

up to 5% of admissions to adult hospitals and 2% of admissions to pediatric hospitals are related to ADRs. For adults, these events commonly involve anticancer drugs, antibiotics, anticoagulants, sedatives, and opiates. For children, the drugs most frequently involved are anticancer drugs and antibiotics. The mortality for an admission with an ADR is approximately 4%, while a similar or higher mortality applies to patients who develop an ADR during hospitalization.

This chapter will outline ADRs of particular relevance to general surgeons. The focus is on complications from ten groups of drugs that may result in admission to hospital under surgical units or may develop in patients already in hospital (Table 23.1).

23.2 Antibiotics

Antibiotics are widely prescribed in the community and are a common cause of ADRs. Many are relatively minor such as nausea, anorexia, headache, and taste alterations and rapidly resolve after cessation of the drug. A skin rash may be the only manifestation of a mild allergic reaction, but anaphylactic reactions can be life-threatening and need to be treated as a medical emergency. An ADR that may be relevant to surgeons is the development of diarrhea. This occurs in approximately 10% of patients and appears to be more common with ampicillin, amoxicillin, and amoxicillin-clavulanate than with other antibiotics. In most of these patients, diarrhea is relatively mild and is thought to be caused by changes to bacterial flora in the small and large bowel.

A particular issue is the development of diarrhea due to *Clostridium difficile* (*C. difficile*). This was first described as pseudomembranous colitis in 1978 and mostly attributed to the use of clindamycin and lincomycin. However, the incidence of the disease has increased in the past decade, and more recent surveys indicate that the antibiotics most frequently associated with *C. difficile* are cephalosporins, penicillins, and macrolides. Presumably, antibiotic-induced changes in the gut microbiome permit the germination of *C. difficile* spores and the subsequent colonization and proliferation of bacteria. The disease is mediated by toxins produced by the organism, largely toxins A and B. Although the overall frequency of *C. difficile* in antibiotic-associated diarrhea is only 10–20%, this infection becomes more likely in the presence of severe diarrhea and accounts for the majority of patients with clinical manifestations of colitis (abdominal cramps, fever, leukocytosis, and a low serum albumin).

Currently, the diagnosis of *C. difficile* infection is mostly based on molecular tests on fecal samples using polymerase chain reaction technology. These tests have high sensitivity and specificity. An alternative test is an enzyme immunoassay for toxins A and B. The "gold standard" is the cytotoxicity assay, but results may not be available for up to 3 days. Flexible sigmoidoscopy or colonoscopy can also be diagnostic when pseudomembranes are present (Fig. 23.1), but this is not universal in milder disease, and pseudomembranes may not be present in the rectum (rectal sparing). Patients with severe disease should have a plain abdominal radiograph to exclude a toxic megacolon.

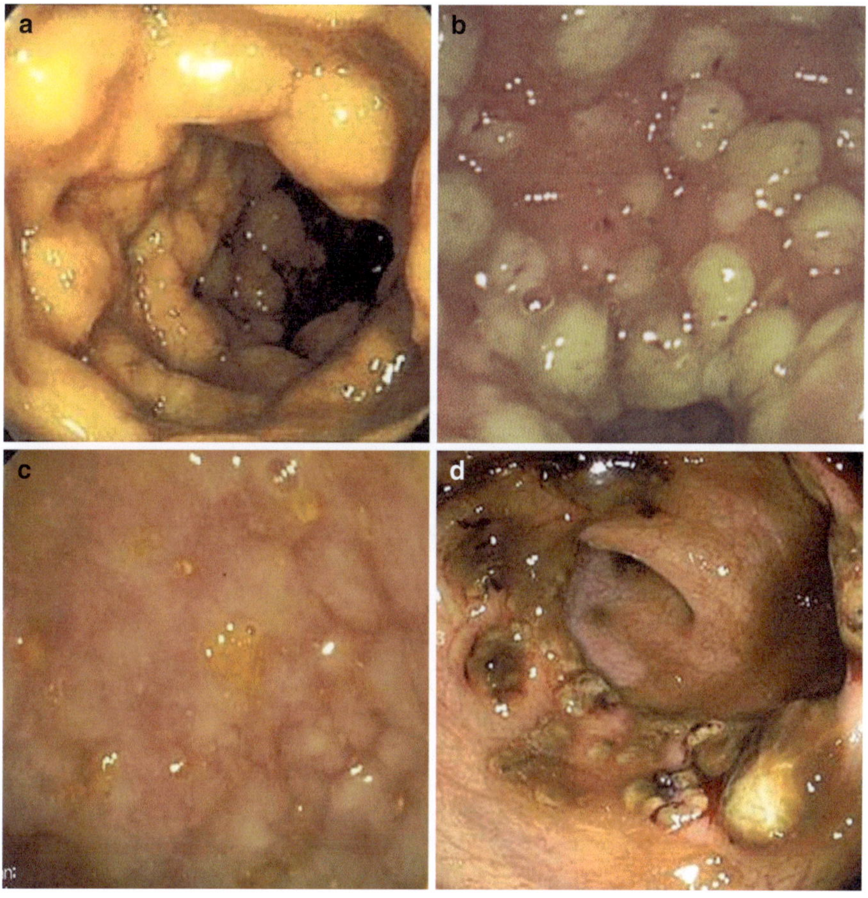

Fig. 23.1 Colonoscopic appearances of colitis caused by *Clostridium difficile*. (**a**) Coalesced pseudomembranes in the rectum in severe colitis. (**b**) Typical pseudomembranes in the rectum. (**c**) Mild colitis with indistinct pseudomembranes in the rectum. (**d**) Occasional pseudomembranes in the cecum

Treatment of *C. difficile* colitis almost always includes cessation of the offending antibiotic. For mild to moderate diarrhea, metronidazole is the drug of choice, while oral vancomycin is usually restricted to patients with more severe disease, those with poor responses to metronidazole and patients with recurrent infections. For very severe disease, oral vancomycin can be given with intravenous metronidazole, and admission to an intensive care unit may be required to monitor fluid and electrolyte balance. Approximately 1% of patients with *C. difficile* infections require surgery because of the development of a toxic megacolon or colonic perforation. This normally involves a colectomy, but an alternative surgical procedure is loop ileostomy with colonic lavage. Operative mortality rates of up 50% have been reported. Fecal transplantation is a newer form of therapy for recurrent disease with cure rates of up to 90% but will usually require transfer to a tertiary center.

Another complication of antibiotic therapy is that of candidiasis. This usually involves the mouth or vagina, but some patients have esophageal candidiasis, particularly in the setting of immunosuppression with anticancer drugs or human immunodeficiency virus (HIV). Symptoms are often minor and include retrosternal discomfort, nausea, and reflux. Most but not all patients have a coexisting oral infection. At endoscopy, the differential diagnosis includes reflux esophagitis and infections with herpes simplex and cytomegalovirus.

23.3 Non-steroidal Anti-inflammatory Drugs

Non-steroidal anti-inflammatory drugs (NSAIDs) are not only the most widely prescribed drugs worldwide but are also available as "over the counter" medication in most countries. In people over 65 years of age, 70% use NSAIDs at least weekly, largely for arthritis and musculoskeletal problems. They act by reducing the production of prostaglandins, chemicals that promote inflammation, pain, and fever. Prostaglandins also have a protective role in the stomach and additional effects on blood coagulation and renal function. The enzymes that produce prostaglandins are called cyclooxygenases (COX) and take two forms, COX-1 and COX-2. Only COX-1 produces prostaglandins that protect the gastric mucosa and activate platelets.

NSAIDs can be categorized as salicylates, non-salicylates, and COX-2 inhibitors. Salicylates such as aspirin and non-salicylates such as ibuprofen, naproxen, and diclofenac inhibit the activity of both COX-1 and COX-2, but there is variation in the degree of inhibition of both enzymes. COX-2 inhibitors provide protection from gastrointestinal side effects, but some of these drugs have been withdrawn from sale because of higher frequencies of vascular disease.

The major adverse events of NSAIDs are focused on the gastrointestinal tract, particularly the stomach. These include gastric erosions, hemorrhagic gastritis, and chronic peptic ulcers. Gastric erosions and hemorrhagic areas (without erosions at endoscopy) are common after a single challenge but become less frequent with longer-term administration. The major mechanism seems likely to be a topical effect of the drug as enteric coating substantially reduces erosive injury.

Overt gastrointestinal bleeding is uncommon with erosions unless NSAIDs are combined with anticoagulants.

It has been estimated that approximately 2–4% of patients treated with NSAIDs for 1 year will develop a chronic peptic ulcer that is either symptomatic or complicated by bleeding or perforation. These ulcers are largely located in the stomach but some are in the duodenal cap. Risk factors include a past history of ulceration, gastric infection with *Helicobacter pylori*, and advanced age. Risks also increase in a parallel fashion with increasing doses of the drugs. For regular use of low-dose aspirin (75–100 mg per day), the risk of an episode of gastrointestinal bleeding is increased by twofold. Erosions and chronic ulcers associated with NSAIDs can largely be prevented by use of a histamine (H2) receptor antagonist drug or a proton pump inhibitor.

A rare adverse effect of NSAIDs is that of diaphragm disease. With this disease, there are one or more strictures in the small bowel caused by the submucosal fibrosis that results from cycles of damage and repair of erosions induced by NSAIDs. The usual mode of presentation is with a partial or complete small bowel obstruction.

23.4 Antithrombotic Agents

Surgeons are likely to encounter an increasing number of patients on antithrombotic medication who are being considered for elective or emergency surgery. These drugs are often categorized as either antiplatelet drugs or anticoagulants. The former inhibit platelet activation and impair the ability of platelets to adhere to one another and to the endothelium of damaged blood vessels. Included in this group are aspirin, clopidogrel, dipyridamole, prasugrel, and ticagrelor, but additional drugs are available in some countries such as the USA. There are also an increasing number of drugs categorized as anticoagulants. These include traditional drugs such as heparins and coumadins (warfarin) and newer drugs such as direct thrombin inhibitors (dabigatran) and direct factor Xa inhibitors (rivaroxaban, apixaban, and edoxaban). The newer drugs are often called non-vitamin K oral anticoagulants or, more simply, direct oral anticoagulants (DOAC).

Common problems for the surgeon include the management of coagulation in patients admitted in an emergency setting and the management of antithrombotic medication in patients booked for elective surgery. Issues to consider include the indication for antithrombotic medication, the risks of cessation of medication, the nature of the emergency or elective setting, the duration of the antithrombotic effect, and the ability or otherwise to reverse the effect of medication. These decisions are sometimes complex and often involve both physicians and anesthetists.

In patients admitted to hospital with significant gastrointestinal bleeding, the site of bleeding is more likely to be the upper gastrointestinal tract than the colon. However, the risks of bleeding from both sites are increased by use of antithrombotic agents. This increase in risk is approximately twofold for antiplatelet drugs and approximately fourfold for use of anticoagulants. When anticoagulants are combined with NSAIDs, there are high additional risks for upper gastrointestinal bleeding but somewhat lower additional risks for colonic bleeding.

The management of gastrointestinal bleeding in patients on anticoagulants needs to be individualized and will depend, at least in part, on the severity of bleeding and type of anticoagulant. For those on warfarin, cessation of the drug will only have a minor initial effect as it may take up to 5 days to normalize the INR. In most settings, patients are given vitamin K intravenously along with prothrombin complex concentrate or fresh frozen plasma (the former is preferred). For DOACs, the risk of major gastrointestinal bleeding seems somewhat lower than warfarin, and, of greater importance, patients have a lower risk of cerebral hemorrhage. An additional benefit is the avoidance of regular blood tests, but the drugs are expensive, and the anticoagulant effect cannot be rapidly reversed. In contrast to warfarin, however, DOACs have a half-life in the range of 5–17 h.

For patients on antiplatelet drugs having elective surgery, the drugs are usually ceased for 2–5 days as the risks of cessation of medication are low. Drugs are also ceased for most patients on anticoagulants apart from very high risk individuals when heparin may be used before and soon after surgery. DOACs are also increasingly used after some operations, particularly orthopedic procedures, to minimize the risk of deep venous thrombosis and pulmonary embolism.

23.5 Opioids

The term opioid refers to a group of substances that produce effects similar to morphine. They act by binding to a variety of opioid receptors, largely located in the central nervous system, the peripheral nervous system, and the gastrointestinal tract. The major receptors in the gastrointestinal tract (μ and γ) are largely located in the submucosal and myenteric plexuses, respectively.

Although opioids are widely used for acute pain, particularly that after surgery, there is increasing use of opioids for both pain associated with advanced cancer and painful, non-cancer disorders such as back pain, musculoskeletal disorders, and fibromyalgia. One estimate suggests that up to 4% of adults in the USA take opioids for at least 3 months for non-cancer indications, while others use the drugs illegally for recreational purposes. This has been associated with an increase in the number of deaths per year for both prescription and illicit drug use. This section will focus on the gastrointestinal effects of opioids, largely excluding issues such as tolerance, physical dependence, and addiction as well as other important public health considerations. In addition, comments largely apply to stronger opioids such as morphine, fentanyl, oxycodone, buprenorphine, hydromorphone, and methadone rather than mild opioids such as codeine and tramadol.

Common adverse effects of opioids include nausea, vomiting, constipation, drowsiness, dry mouth, and itching. Nausea and vomiting occur because of delayed gastric emptying and effects on the vomiting center in the brain. These symptoms often improve after 7–10 days despite continuation of medication because of the development of tolerance. In contrast, constipation is almost universal in people taking opioids long-term but rarely improves with time. Most will need osmotic laxatives, stimulant laxatives, or the intermittent use of enemas. More recently, opioid-induced constipation has been improved by combined treatment with opioid antagonists or the use of the intestinal secretagogue, lubiprostone.

Another adverse effect is the development of abdominal pain syndromes. One of these is biliary-type pain that can develop after single doses of morphine, particularly in patients who have had a previous cholecystectomy (see Chapter 17). This appears to be related to changes in motility in the sphincter of Oddi causing an increase in pressure in the biliary system. This effect is not rapidly reversed by the opioid antagonist, naloxone. The narcotic bowel syndrome describes patients with moderate to severe abdominal pain on most days that continues for at least 3 months. Most take more than 100 mg of morphine equivalents per day, and pain either fails to improve or is aggravated by higher doses of narcotics. Treatment is often difficult but includes either cessation or a reduction in the dose of opioid, use of non-opioid medication, and control of the symptoms of drug withdrawal.

In the postoperative phase, adverse effects from opioids have been a particular problem in children. The most serious adverse events are respiratory depression and prolonged drowsiness. These can be partly reversed by use of opioid antagonists. One issue in adults is a prolonged ileus after abdominal surgery that may be aggravated by continuation of opioid analgesia. The risk of this complication can be minimized by use of non-opioid analgesics as soon as possible, usually with a combination of paracetamol and NSAIDs.

23.6 Chemotherapeutic Drugs

Abdominal symptoms including diarrhea are common in patients with cancer who are being treated with various chemotherapeutic drugs. In the majority of patients, these symptoms seem likely to be related to drug-induced changes in the proliferation of epithelial cells in the small and large bowel. This results in "mucositis" with impaired absorption of fluid and nutrients.

A small minority of patients develop colonic inflammation in the setting of neutropenia, a disorder called neutropenic colitis. The pathogenesis may involve mucosal injury, damage to the myenteric plexus, impaired defense mechanisms, and mucosal ischemia. The disorder has been associated with a variety of drugs including cytosine arabinoside, cisplatin, vincristine, adriamycin, and 5-fluorouracil. The most common presenting symptoms are diarrhea, nausea, vomiting, abdominal pain, and fever. Blood cultures are positive for one or more organisms in 50% of patients. The differential diagnosis of neutropenic colitis needs to include appendicitis as well as *C. difficile* colitis and cytomegalovirus colitis. Initial therapy should involve resuscitation, antibiotics, and correction of neutropenia with granulocyte colony-stimulating factor. A minority of patients develop a toxic megacolon with a risk for colonic perforation, usually at the cecum.

23.7 Glucocorticoids

The hormone, cortisol (or hydrocortisone), is produced in the adrenal cortex and has important homeostatic activities that affect metabolic, immunologic, and cardiovascular functions. Various synthetic glucocorticoids have been produced and are still widely used in the treatment of allergic, inflammatory, and immunologic disorders as well as post-transplantation immunosuppression. Common examples include prednisone, prednisolone, methylprednisolone, and dexamethasone.

For the surgeon, higher doses of glucocorticoids can delay wound healing and are associated with higher risks for postoperative infections such as wound infections and pneumonia. For patients on longer-term glucocorticoids, suppression of corticotropin-releasing hormone and pituitary adrenocorticotropic hormone often results in a degree of atrophy of the adrenal glands. This can cause adrenal insufficiency during times of stress such as operations, particularly when oral medication is overlooked in patients receiving intravenous fluids. Symptoms of drug-induced adrenal insufficiency include malaise, myalgia, disorientation, nausea, and vomiting. The blood pressure is usually low and is accompanied by hypoglycemia and hyponatremia. The emergency treatment of this "adrenal crisis" is intravenous hydrocortisone.

23.8 Biologicals

A newer form of therapy is the use of monoclonal antibodies to target either inflammatory cells or their products or various cancer cells. These medications are called biologicals and have the suffix -mab. Most are formed by fusing myeloma cells with mouse spleen cells that have been immunized with the desired antigen. As murine monoclonal antibodies are rapidly removed from blood by immune mechanisms, the challenge has been to produce part mouse, part human antibodies ("chimeric" antibodies) or "fully" human products. Most monoclonal antibodies are given either by intravenous infusion or subcutaneous injection at intervals of weeks or months. Some are given in combination with immunosuppressive drugs to delay the formation of human anti-mouse antibodies and to augment the therapeutic effect.

In gastroenterology, monoclonal antibodies against tumor necrosis factor alpha are being increasingly used in the management of difficult Crohn's disease and ulcerative colitis. These products include infliximab, adalimumab, golimumab, and certolizumab. Other monoclonal antibodies directed against the integrin receptor (natalizumab and vedolizumab) have also been approved for use in inflammatory bowel disease in several countries. A particular concern was the potential of these drugs to promote serious infections including the reactivation of tuberculosis. In practice, these risks appear to be low. However, monoclonal antibodies against tumor necrosis factor alpha have been associated with a rare form of lymphoma with a poor prognosis. Another interesting adverse effect of monoclonal antibodies is the development of colitis in some melanoma patients treated with ipilimumab and rare cases of colitis with rituximab.

23.9 Laxatives

There is a long list of drugs that have the adverse effect of diarrhea. A short list, however, includes antibiotics as above, metformin, NSAIDs, various anticancer drugs, immunosuppressive drugs such as mycophenolate, proton pump inhibitors, H2-receptor antagonists, and antacids containing magnesium. Laxatives also need to be included in this group but are often overlooked in clinical practice. One area is the regular use of herbal teas, some of which contain senna or other laxatives.

Laxatives are agents that promote a bowel motion or help to loosen stools. Most can be categorized as bulk-forming agents, stool softeners, osmotic agents, stimulant agents, saline laxative agents, or a miscellaneous group that includes serotonin agonists and chloride channel activators. Most of the significant abuse involves stimulant laxatives.

One important area is laxative abuse in individuals with the eating disorders, anorexia and bulimia nervosa. Younger women are most likely to be affected, and up to 60% report abuse of laxatives in order to enhance weight loss. The complications of chronic diarrhea can be life-threatening and include acid-base changes (usually a metabolic alkalosis), hypokalemia, hypotension, and dehydration. Older groups, usually women, often have a history of constipation but continue to use high doses of laxatives because of the fear of recurrent problems. Most of these patients do not have major diarrhea, and significant adverse events are uncommon. A final group has diarrhea as a factitious symptom or induces diarrhea with surreptitious laxatives in order to simulate an illness (Munchausen's syndrome).

At colonoscopy, some patients with laxative abuse have melanosis coli, particularly those who take laxatives containing anthraquinone, a component of senna. This dark brown or black discoloration often involves the entire colon but may be patchy or segmental in some individuals. The appearance is caused by the presence of pigment-laden macrophages in the colonic mucosa. The discoloration slowly resolves after cessation of the drugs.

23.10 Bisphosphonates

Bisphosphonates are used for the treatment of osteoporosis and other disorders causing fragile bones such as Paget's disease. The most popular first-line therapy involves the oral use of either alendronate or risedronate. Adverse gastrointestinal effects include nausea, esophageal reflux, and retrosternal discomfort and pain. At endoscopy, some patients have esophagitis or esophageal erosions caused by retention of tablets in the lower esophagus. The frequency of this adverse effect has been reduced but not eliminated by changes to the medication designed to reduce mucosal adherence and increase solubility. Patients are advised to take the medication in an upright position with a glass of water.

Tetracycline and doxycycline have also been associated with esophageal symptoms including retrosternal pain. Again, esophageal inflammation and erosions have been reported at endoscopy, and symptoms and endoscopic findings have been attributed to the chemical effects of retained tablets in the lower esophagus.

23.11 Cannabinoids

Cannabis is the most widely used drug of abuse in the Western world, perhaps apart from alcohol. The drug is usually delivered by smoking marijuana, the dried leaves and flowers of the cannabis plant. Some individuals also smoke or eat the resinous secretions of the plant known as hashish. The psychoactive effects of the drug are largely mediated by delta-9 tetrahydrocannabinol, widely known as THC.

The effects of cannabinoids include changes in consciousness with feelings of euphoria, relaxation, and sociability. There may also be anxiety symptoms, paranoid thoughts, and disorientation with impaired coordination and concentration. Heavy users of cannabis are at risk of psychosis and the unusual gastrointestinal symptom of repeated episodes of nausea and vomiting. In relation to the latter, a distinctive feature of this syndrome is at least partial relief with long hot baths. Nevertheless, some patients attend the emergency service with dehydration and require treatment with intravenous fluids. This syndrome is often called the cannabinoid hyperemesis syndrome and resolves after withdrawal of the drug.

Recommended Reading

Camilleri M, Lembo A, Katzka DA. Opioids in Gastroenterology: treating adverse effects and creating therapeutic benefits. Clin Gastroenterol Hepatol. 2017;15:1338–49.

Edwards IR, Aronson JK. Adverse drug reactions: definitions, diagnosis and management. Lancet. 2000;356:1255–9.

Einarson TR. Drug-related hospital admissions. Ann Pharmacother. 1993;27:832–40.

Faich GA. National adverse drug reaction reporting: 1984–89. Arch Intern Med. 1991;151:1645–7.

Lanas A, Carrera-Lasfuentes P, Arguedas Y, et al. Risk of upper and lower gastrointestinal bleeding in patients taking non-steroidal anti-inflammatory drugs, antiplatelet agents or anticoagulants. Clin Gastroenterol Hepatol. 2015;13:906–12.

Lazarou J, Pomeranz BH. Incidence of adverse drug reactions in hospitalized patients. A meta-analysis of prospective studies. JAMA. 1998;279:1200–5.

Miller CS, Dorreen A, Martel M, Huynh T, Bankun AN. Risk of gastrointestinal bleeding in patients taking non-vitamin K antagonist oral anticoagulants: a systemic review and meta-analysis. Clin Gastroenterol Hepatol. 2017;15:1674–83.

Ong GKB, Reidy TJ, Huk MD, Lane FR. Clostridium difficile colitis: a clinical review. Am J Surg. 2017;213:565–71.

Roerig JL, Steffen KJ, Mitchell JE, Zunker C. Laxative abuse: epidemiology, diagnosis and management. Drugs. 2010;70:1487–503.

Vieth M, Montgomery E. Medication-associated gastrointestinal tract injury. Virchows Arch. 2017;470:245–66.

Management of Obesity

24

Harsh A. Kanhere and Markus I. Trochsler

24.1 Definition and Magnitude of Current Problem

Introduction: The human race is getting heavier by the day. Until recently, obesity was considered to be a problem of the developed world, but the pandemic is spreading to developing countries and assuming global proportions.

Obesity and its related medical problems, especially the metabolic syndrome (obesity, type 2 diabetes, hypercholesterolemia and hypertension), place a considerable burden on health systems and have significant impact on health-related spending.

According to 2011–2012 data, 63% of Australian adults are above the normal weight range with 35% being overweight and 28% severely obese. There is an almost linear correlation between body mass index (BMI) and health expenditure. Health expenditure increases by 19% for people with BMI between 30 and 35 and skyrockets to 51% higher in people with BMI greater than 35.

In Australia, obesity related diabetes alone had a cost burden of 12 billion dollars to the taxpayers in 2015.

A result of a nationally representative survey showed age adjusted prevalence of obesity to be 35% for men and 40% for women in the United States as of 2013–14.

It is abundantly clear that management of severe obesity is an urgent healthcare issue in western populations and is rapidly becoming a pressing issue all around the world.

H. A. Kanhere (✉) · M. I. Trochsler
Discipline of Surgery, University of Adelaide, Adelaide, SA, Australia
e-mail: Harsh.Kanhere@sa.gov.au; markus.trochsler@sa.gov.au

M. W. Wichmann et al. (eds.), *Gastroenterology For General Surgeons*,
https://doi.org/10.1007/978-3-319-92768-8_24

24.1.1 Classification of Adults According to BMI (Table 24.1)

As a rough guide, the body mass index (BMI) is used to quantify degrees of obesity (Table 24.1). While it is not the most accurate measure, it provides a good starting point for assessments. Another parameter used to classify obesity and related morbidity is waist circumference. The risk of metabolic complications increases with an increasing waist circumference as depicted below (Table 24.2).

The impact of obesity is due to its inherent metabolic consequences and risks associated with being overweight. The following tables chart the problems associated with obesity.

As is evident, obesity affects all organ systems of the body and can have considerable impact on one's quality of life and life expectancy (Table 24.3).

This chapter will concentrate on the principles of secondary prevention and surgical management of severe obesity. A brief framework of non-surgical approaches is provided to start with.

Medical management: General practitioners (GPs) form a major cog in the treatment wheel for morbid obesity. In Australia, the Royal Australian College of General Practitioners (RACGP) has developed a guide for GPs for the management of patients with obesity. It consists of the 5 "As" approach for weight management: "Ask, Assist, Advise, Assess, and Arrange" (Table 24.4).

It is important for GPs, and indeed specialists, to be able to categorise the risks associated with obesity in a simple yet objective manner. The table below is very useful in this regard. Assessment of the risk of disease and effective treatment protocol can be based on these assessments. It is vital to engage patients and caregivers to achieve good outcomes (Table 24.5).

Table 24.1 Risk of comorbidities according to body mass index (BMI)

Classification	BMI kg/m^2	Risk of comorbidities
Underweight	<18.50	Low (but risk of other clinical problems increased)
Normal range	18.50–24.99	Average
Overweight	>25.00	
Preobese	25.00–29.99	Increased
Obese class 1	30.00–34.99	Moderate
Obese class 2	35.00–39.99	Severe
Obese class 3	>40.00	Very severe

Table 24.2 Sex-specific waist circumference and risk of metabolic complications associated with obesity in Caucasians

Risk of metabolic complications	Waist circumference (cm)	
	Men	Women
Increased	≥94	≥80
Substantially increased	≥102	≥88

Table 24.3 Diseases associated with obesity

Relative risk	Associated with metabolic consequences	Associated with weight
Greatly increased	Type 2 diabetes Gall bladder disease Hypertension Dyslipidemia/insulin resistance Atherosclerosis	Sleep apnoea Breathlessness/asthma Social isolation/depression Daytime sleepiness/fatigue
Moderately increased	Coronary heart disease Stroke Gout/hyperuricemia	Osteoarthritis Respiratory disease Hernia Psychological problems
Slightly increased	Cancer (breast, endometrial, colon) Reproductive abnormalities Impaired fertility Polycystic ovaries Skin complications Cataract	Varicose veins Musculoskeletal problems Bad back Stress incontinence Edema/cellulitis

Table 24.4 The "5 As" overweight and obesity management model for adults

	Standard care		Active management		
	BMI < 25	BMI 25–29.5	BMI 30–34.9	BMI 35–39.9	BMI > 40
Ask and assess	Routinely assess and monitor BMI and waist circumference (WC)	Routinely assess and monitor BMI and WC Discuss if BMI and/or WC increasing Screen for and manage comorbidities	Routinely assess and monitor BMI and WC Discuss health issues Screen for and manage comorbidities Assess other factors related to health risk (blood pressure, lipid profile, fasting glucose and liver function tests), and ask about symptoms of sleep apnoea and depression		
Advise	Promote benefits of healthy lifestyle Explain benefits of prevention of weight gain and maintenance of healthy weight		Promote benefits of healthy lifestyle Explain benefits of weight management		
Assist			Assist in setting up weight loss program: • Advise lifestyle interventions • Based on comorbidities, risk factors and weight history, consider adding intensive weight loss interventions (e.g. diets, pharmacotherapy, bariatric surgery) • Tailor the approach to the individual • Refer to multidisciplinary team for specialist treatment recommendations. Suitable patients include those with severe complex obesity, for example, those with a BMI > 40, BMI > 35 with any serious comorbidity and BMI 30–35 with serious comorbidity and a positive weight trajectory		
Arrange			Review and monitoring Long-term weight management Referral to specialist weight management clinic if indicated		

Table 24.5 Classification of disease risks[a] by WHO BMI classification and WC thresholds

BMI (kg/m^2)	Classification	Men WC 94–102 cm Women WC 80–88 cm	Men WC > 102 cm Women WC > 88 cm
18.5–24.9	Normal weight[b]	–	–
25–29.9	Overweight	Increased	High
30–34.9	Obese class I	High	Very high
35–39.9	Obese class II	Very high	Very high
≥40.0	Obese class III	Extremely high	Extremely high

WC waist circumference
Reproduced from the Scottish Intercollegiate Guidelines Network (SIGN).
[a]Disease risk for type 2 diabetes, hypertension and cardiovascular disease
[b]Increased WC can also be a marker for increased risk even in persons of normal weight

24.2 Pharmacotherapy and Diet

24.2.1 Pharmacotherapy

Various pharmacotherapeutic agents have been tried in the management of severe obesity. A few of these agents are approved by the US Food and Drug Administration (FDA) for the management of obesity. These medications are best used together with lifestyle modifications. Some commonly used pharmacotherapeutics are summarised in Box 24.1. Pharmacotherapy is recommended for patients with BMI >30 kg/m^2 for males or BMI >27 kg/m^2 for females with obesity-related medical risk factors. These medications either act centrally to increase levels of satiety or act on the gastrointestinal tract to restrict nutrient absorption. The FDA has recently approved two new medications: lorcaserin and phentermine-topiramate but these medications are not approved worldwide. On average, these medications are associated with a 4 kg weight loss over a 12-month period.

Box 24.1: Commonly Used Pharmacotherapy Agents Used in the Management of Weight Loss

1. Phentermine—This is a dopaminergic agonist. It is approved only for short-term use as an adjunct in a weight reduction program. The average reported weight loss is up to 3.5–3.6 kg. Potential adverse effects limit its use.
2. Orlistat—This is a pancreatic and gastric lipase inhibitor. About 3 kg weight loss is reported over 12 months. It is recommended to follow a low-fat diet while on treatment.
3. Metformin is a biguanide that is used in the treatment of type 2 diabetes. It has moderate effect on weight loss but is not approved as a drug for this indication.
4. Other medications such as exenatide (Byetta) and liraglutide, glucagon-like peptide agonists; lorcaserin, a serotonin 2C agonist; and a combination of phentermine and topiramate have also been tried.

24.2.2 Diet

Numerous commercial diet programs are available on the market, and most utilise diets with a very low-calorie intake.

Readers will be aware of Jenny Craig, Weight Watchers and other well-known weight loss programs. Interestingly over the short-to-medium term, these commercial programs will lead to about a 5% weight loss with strict adherence. A meta-analysis has shown that these programs achieve greater weight loss than self-directed diets or counselling only. This meta-analysis included 45 studies with 39 randomised control trials. Results demonstrated that at 12 months, Weight Watchers participants achieved at least 2.6% greater weight loss than those assigned to control or education. Jenny Craig resulted in at least 4.9% greater weight loss at 12 months than control/education and counselling. Nutrisystem resulted in at least 3.8% greater weight loss at 3 months than control/education and counselling. Very low-calorie programs (Health Management Resources, Medifast and OPTIFAST) resulted in at least 4.0% greater short-term weight loss than counselling, but some attenuation of effect occurred beyond 6 months. Atkins resulted in 0.1–2.9% greater weight loss at 12 months than counselling. Results for SlimFast were mixed. The authors found limited evidence to evaluate adherence or harms for all programs and weight outcomes for other commercial programs.

Adverse effects of medium- to long-term use of very low-calorie diets (VLCDs) are not fully documented. The OPTIFAST® VLCD™ Program is accepted as being a safe form of weight loss with only minor, transient side effects being observed. These side effects are a result of the rapid weight loss and ketosis and may include sensitivity to cold, halitosis (bad breath), headache, hair loss, irritability, postural hypotension, fatigue, muscle cramps and menstrual disturbances. These side effects are generally insufficient in magnitude or duration to warrant cessation of the program. It is advisable that any VLCD program should be medically supervised.

24.3 Interdisciplinary Non-surgical Approach

Severe obesity is a challenging condition and difficult to treat with a single modality. The cornerstone of good outcomes is to incorporate a multidisciplinary approach. A prospective study from Germany has shown that excellent weight loss is achievable by using an interdisciplinary approach using four modules (psychology, medicine, dietetics and exercise), delivered by a team of trained qualified health professionals such as psychologists, medical doctors, dietitians/nutritionists and physical therapists. The program was primarily based around a VLCD diet for 12 weeks. In females, initial body weight was reduced after the 1-year intervention by 19.6 kg (95% confidence intervals 19.2–19.9 kg) and in males by 26.0 kg (25.2–26.8) according to per-protocol analysis of 4850 individuals. Intention-to-treat (ITT) analysis revealed a weight reduction of 15.2 kg (14.9–15.6) in females and 19.4 kg (18.7–20.1) in males. Overall, the intervention resulted in mean reduction in WC of 11 cm; it reduced the prevalence of the metabolic syndrome by 50% and the frequency of hypertension from 47% to 29% of

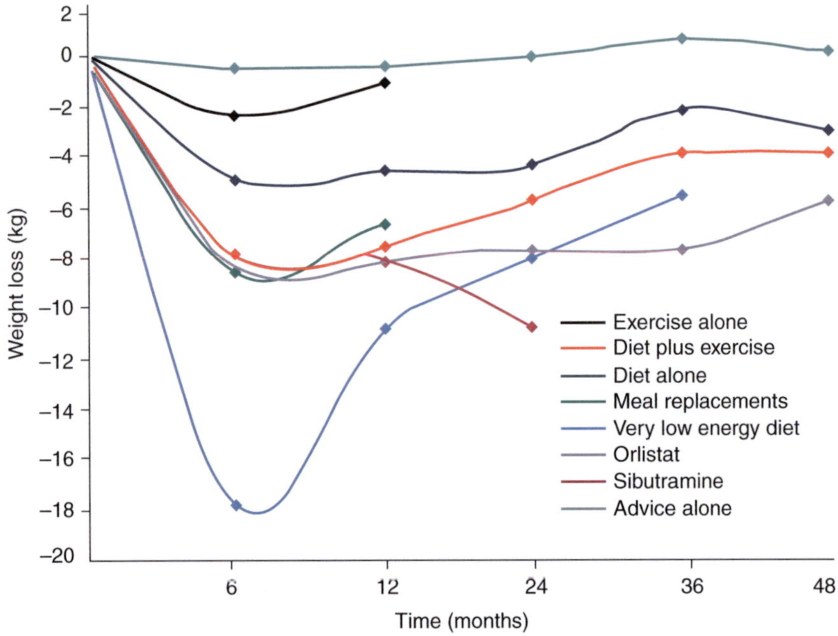

Fig. 24.1 Average weight loss of subjects completing a minimum 1-year weight-management intervention (Franz MJ et. al., Recommended Reading)

all participants (ITT, all $P < 0.001$). The beneficial effects could be documented for up to 3 years and comprised significant improvement in health-related quality of life. The incidence of adverse effects was low; the events repeatedly observed and possibly related to either the intervention or the underlying conditions were biliary disorders.

The population consisted of 20% class 1, 32% class 2 and 47% class 3 obesity. These results are remarkable and difficult to reproduce on such a wide scale. A Swedish Obese Subjects study showed results that were contradictory and provided vital evidence in favour of surgical approach to weight reduction. The average weight change in control subjects was less than ±2% during the period of up to 15 years during which participants' weights were recorded. Maximum weight losses in the surgical subgroups were observed after 1–2 years: gastric bypass, 32%; vertical banded gastroplasty, 25%; and gastric banding, 20%. After 10 years, the weight losses from baseline were stabilised at 25%, 16% and 14%, respectively.

Figure 24.1 demonstrates the typical weight loss curves associated with various non-surgical treatment modalities.

24.4 Surgery

Bariatric surgery is very effective in the management of severe obesity. Surgical interventions have the potential to produce significant and intense weight loss over a short term. Bariatric surgery should only be offered to suitable patients with a multitier approach. Initial attempts with non-surgical therapy using interdisciplinary treatment are essential. Patients need to be educated thoroughly about the pathway to bariatric surgery. A dedicated team of nurses, dieticians, exercise physiologists, clinical psychologists and physicians with a keen interest in weight loss management is essential. Availability of anesthetists with experience in management of such cases is important. Surgeons fully trained in performing open and minimal access bariatric procedures form the core of the team. Surgeons should have full understanding of all procedures, potential complications and physiologic changes occurring with the surgery and weight loss. Experience in both primary and revisional surgeries is essential. Any bariatric surgical program needs to be executed as a part of a multidisciplinary team.

Ideally patients would progress through a pathway of seminars and small education groups, clinical assessment by physicians and endocrinologists, assessment for sleep apnoea, psychological evaluation and consultations with dieticians and exercise physiologists prior to surgical evaluation. Patients generally need to meet the following criteria to be considered suitable for bariatric surgery:

1. BMI >40 kg/m^2 (males) or >35 kg/m^2 (females) with comorbidities correctable by weight loss such as uncontrolled diabetes, obstructive sleep apnoea, hypercholesterolemia and hypertension.
2. Age: Most centres offer bariatric surgery for patients between the age of 18 and 65 years. Adolescent bariatric surgery is a topic in itself with significant ethical considerations and not one for debate in this chapter.
3. Non-smoker.
4. No major psychiatric illness.
5. Efforts to lose weight by other means have been unsuccessful.
6. Fit for general anaesthetic.

In some circumstances patients with BMI of between 30 and 34 may be considered for bariatric surgery if there are severe obesity-related medical comorbidities.

24.4.1 Surgical Options

There is a wide variety of surgical options available. These can be classed as restrictive, malabsorbtive or both.

Restrictive: vertical band gastroplasty, laparoscopic adjustable band and sleeve gastrectomy.

Malabsorbtive: biliopancreatic diversion.

Restrictive and malabsorbtive: Roux-en-Y gastric bypass and omega loop bypass.

Laparoscopic Roux-en-Y bypass, gastric banding, sleeve gastrectomy and recently, the omega or single loop bypass are the procedures routinely performed and will be further detailed.

1. **Restrictive laparoscopic adjustable band**: This procedure consists of applying a band around the proximal stomach to restrict the proximal pouch to about 30–60 mL. The tightness of the band can be adjusted by injecting fluid into a port

positioned subcutaneously and connected to the band by tubing. While good short- to medium-term weight loss results of up to 50–60% of excess weight are reported, the long-term results are less promising. The band has an advantage of being a relatively simple procedure to perform and is fully reversible. However, due to the long-term complications of persistent and worsening reflux, band slippage, proximal gastric dilatation, erosions and failure to achieve sufficient weight loss, laparoscopic band surgery is less popular than previously. A recent study showed an explant rate of 8.74% and maximal weight loss of only 18.7% at 2 years maintained through to 5 years.

2. **Laparoscopic sleeve gastrectomy:** First described as a part of a biliopancreatic diversion, it was observed that the sleeve itself led to significant weight loss. The surgery consists of resection of about 75–80% of the stomach along the greater curvature after detaching the greater omentum. The procedure is technically less challenging than a bypass and is almost always done laparoscopically. The stomach is resected using a laparoscopic stapling device over a bougie. The size of the bougie used depends on surgeon preference, but most prefer between a 32 and 36 F size. About 50–60% excess weight loss has been reported over the short-to-medium term. It is thought that the procedure is mostly restrictive. There is some data to show that ghrelin levels are significantly reduced in people who have a sleeve gastrectomy. Ghrelin is an appetite-stimulating hormone and lower levels may well contribute to weight loss (Fig. 24.2).
3. **Roux-en-Y gastric bypass:** This is a proven gold standard procedure for weight loss. It is now performed laparoscopically in most centres, especially if performed as a primary procedure. This is mainly a restrictive procedure; however some claim that it has a malabsorbtive component. It involves converting the stomach into a small proximal pouch (approx. 30 mL) using a laparoscopic stapling device. A Roux-en-Y gastric pouch-jejunostomy is then constructed.

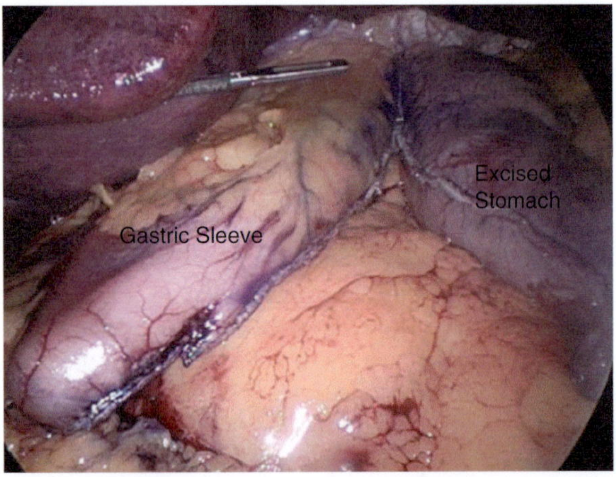

Fig. 24.2 Laparoscopic sleeve gastrectomy

Surgeons have varying opinions as to the length of the Roux limb that is required; however most would agree to a length of around 100 cms. The gastrojejunostomy is performed by varying techniques; our preferred technique is a single-layered handsewn anastomosis. The enteroenterostomy is usually performed as a stapled anastomosis. Some of the steps of the gastric bypass are depicted in Figs. 24.3a–f.

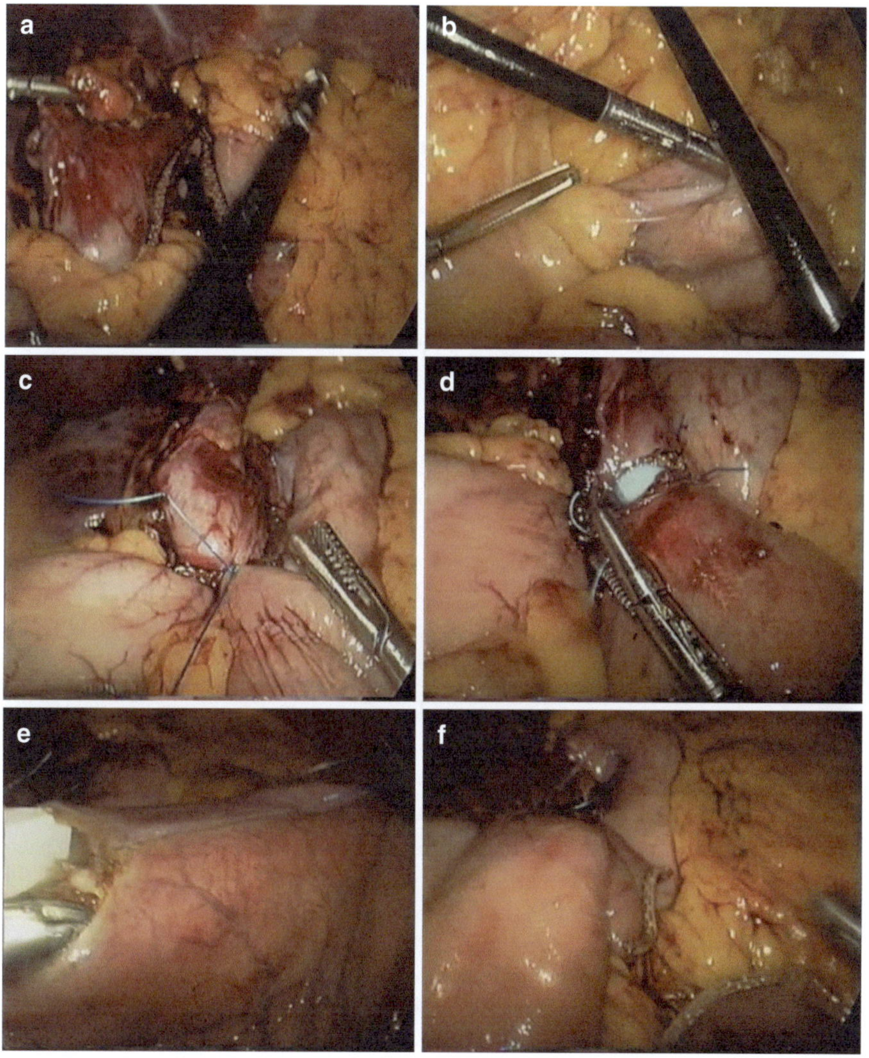

Fig. 24.3 Laparoscopic Roux-en-Y gastric bypass. (**a**) Creating the gastric pouch. (**b**) Identifying the duodenal-jejunal flexure. (**c**) Initiating the Gastric pouch-jejunal anastomosis. (**d**) Anterior layer of the anastomosis being done over a 32 French bougie. (**e**) Stapled enteroenterostomy. (**f**) Formation of the Roux limb by dividing the loop of jejunum

4. **The single loop bypass**: This is the newest addition to the surgical repertoire. It follows essentially the same principles as the Roux-en-Y bypass except a longer pouch and only a loop gastrojejunostomy is constructed. Similar weight loss results to Roux-en-Y bypass have been reported, but long-term results and potential long-term complications are not yet well documented.
5. **Other procedures**: Procedures like the biliopancreatic diversion, vertical band gastroplasty and the duodenal switch are now rarely performed. There are significant side effects and metabolic complications from these procedures.

Recent additions such as the intragastric balloons and endoscopic plications are not routinely performed and should currently be considered experimental.

24.5 Outcomes of Bariatric Surgery

Weight loss: The earliest credible evidence of effectiveness of bariatric surgery over best medical therapy with lifestyle changes and diet came from the Swedish Obese Subjects study (see Recommended Reading). The results showed significant weight loss in the surgical arm as well as a reduction in mortality in the operated patients. The average weight change in control subjects was less than ±2% during the follow-up period of up to 15 years during which weights were recorded. Maximum weight losses in the surgical subgroups were observed after 1–2 years: gastric bypass, 32%; vertical banded gastroplasty, 25%; and banding, 20%. After 10 years, the weight losses from baseline were stabilised at 25%, 16% and 14%, respectively. There were 129 deaths in the control group and 101 deaths in the surgery group. The unadjusted overall hazard ratio was 0.76 in the surgery group ($P = 0.04$), as compared with the control group, and the hazard ratio, adjusted for sex, age and risk factors, was 0.71 ($P = 0.01$). The most common causes of death were myocardial infarction (control group, 25 subjects; surgery group, 13 subjects) and cancer (control group, 47; surgery group, 29). The authors concluded that bariatric surgery for severe obesity is associated with long-term weight loss and decreased overall mortality.

Recent randomised control trials have shown that weight loss with sleeve gastrectomy is comparable to the Roux-en-Y gastric bypass. A prospective randomised trial in 217 patients showed that excessive body mass index loss was similar between laparoscopic sleeve gastrectomy and laparoscopic Roux-en-Y gastric bypass at each analysed time point. At 3-year post-surgery, comorbidities were significantly reduced and comparable for both procedures except gastroesophageal reflux disease and dyslipidemia, which were more successfully treated by laparoscopic Roux-en-Y gastric bypass. Quality of life increased significantly in both groups after 1-, 2- and 3-years post-surgery. There was no statistically significant difference in number of complications treated by reoperation or number of complications treated conservatively.

A systematic review and meta-analysis of 11 randomised trials have been published recently. The results show that Roux-en-Y gastric bypass and sleeve gastrectomy yielded similar weight loss effects and both were superior to laparoscopic adjustable gastric banding. Other factors such as potential complications and patient preference should be considered during surgical consultations.

Overall, evidence suggests that a loss of 50–60% of excess weight is achievable with bariatric surgery over the long term.

Control of comorbidities: Studies have shown that bariatric surgery combined with best medical therapy is superior for the control of diabetes in obese patients compared to best medical therapy alone. The results of the STAMPEDE trial demonstrated that patients who underwent surgical procedures had a greater mean percentage reduction from baseline in glycated haemoglobin level than patients who received medical therapy alone. At 5 years, changes from baseline observed in the gastric bypass and sleeve gastrectomy groups were superior to the changes seen in the medical therapy group with respect to body weight triglyceride levels, high-density lipoprotein cholesterol levels, use of insulin and quality-of-life measures. No major late surgical complications were reported.

This trial showed that, among patients with type 2 diabetes and a BMI of 27–43, bariatric surgery plus intensive medical therapy was more effective than intensive medical therapy alone in decreasing, and in some cases resolving, hyperglycemia over 5 years. A meta-analysis in 2015 provided similar results with comparable outcomes from sleeve gastrectomy and gastric bypass but a lower cardiovascular risk in Roux-en-Y gastric bypass patients.

24.6 Complications

While bariatric surgery has significant benefits, there are a considerable number of potential risks and complications associated with these procedures. The salient surgical risks include intraoperative bleeding, injury to adjacent organs (e.g. spleen), anastomotic/staple line leaks, injury to the bowel as well as internal herniation (especially in gastric bypass).

Patients are also at a risk of complications like deep vein thrombosis and pulmonary embolism, pneumonia and myocardial infarcts. For this reason, it is our practice to commence these patients on a prolonged 28-day course of deep venous thrombosis prophylaxis.

Nutritional deficiencies especially vitamin B12, vitamin D, iron and other micronutrient deficiencies are well known especially after RYGB but can be seen in sleeve gastrectomies and gastric bands as well. Careful monitoring of these elements is required with replacement therapy for those with low blood levels. Hair loss (usually self-limiting) can occur in some patients.

Dumping syndrome and reactive hypoglycemia can occur especially after RYGB. Patients and general practitioners need to remember that if there is hypoglycemia, it should be managed with a complex carbohydrate diet rather than oral glucose (which may complicate matters further).

Anastomotic and staple line leaks are the complications that most surgeons dread. Careful postoperative monitoring, early diagnosis and prompt intervention form the basis of effective treatment. A CT scan with oral contrast is the preferred investigation in a suspected leak. Anastomotic and sleeve gastrectomy leaks are seen in only 1–2% of cases in experienced hands. Sleeve gastrectomy leaks occur in the very proximal part of the sleeve in the majority of cases. While the exact cause is not known, reduced vascularity, increased intragastric pressure and technical issues may play a part. Management of such leaks requires early intervention especially in symptomatic patients. Some of these can be controlled with external drainage, while others need conversion to a bypass and in some instances even a total gastrectomy. A mortality rate between 1 in 200 and 1 in a 1000 has been documented.

Recommended Reading

Agha M, Agha R. The rising prevalence of obesity: part A: impact on public health. Int J Surg Oncol. 2017;2(7):e17.

Bischoff SC, Damms-Machado A, Betz C, Herpertz S, Legenbauer T, Löw T, et al. Multicenter evaluation of an interdisciplinary 52-week weight loss program for obesity with regard to body weight, comorbidities and quality of life—a prospective study. Int J Obes (2005). 2012;36(4):614–24.

Buchmueller TC, Johar M. Obesity and health expenditures: evidence from Australia. Econ Hum Biol. 2015;17:42–58.

Department of Health Website. Prevention and education section. About Overweight and Obesity n.d.

Dixon JB, Eaton LL, Curry T, Lee PC. Health outcomes and explant rates after laparoscopic adjustable gastric banding: a phase 4, multicenter study over 5 years. Obesity (Silver Spring, Md). 2018;26(1):45–52.

Flegal KM, Kruszon-Moran D, Carroll MD, Fryar CD, Ogden CL. Trends in obesity among adults in the United States, 2005 to 2014. JAMA. 2016;315(21):2284–91.

Franz MJ, VanWormer JJ, Crain AL, Boucher JL, Histon T, Caplan W, et al. Weight-loss outcomes: a systematic review and meta-analysis of weight-loss clinical trials with a minimum 1-year follow-up. J Am Diet Assoc. 2007;107(10):1755–67.

Grima M, Dixon JB. Obesity—recommendations for management in general practice and beyond. Aust Fam Physician. 2013;42(8):532–41.

Haddock CK, Poston WS, Dill PL, Foreyt JP, Ericsson M. Pharmacotherapy for obesity: a quantitative analysis of four decades of published randomized clinical trials. Int J Obes Relat Metab Disord. 2002;26(2):262–73.

Holes-Lewis KA, Malcolm R, O'Neil PM. Pharmacotherapy of obesity: clinical treatments and considerations. Am J Med Sci. 2013;345(4):284–8.

Leung F. The Australian bureau of statistics Leung and Fudner 2011–12.

National Health and Medical Research Council. Clinical practice guidelines for the management of overweight and obesity in adults, adolescents and children: draft clinical practice guidelines for primary healthcare professionals. Canberra: NHMRC, 2013. NHMRC. 2013a.

National Health and Medical Research Council. Overweight and obesity in adults: a guide for general practitioners. Canberra: NHMRC, 2003. NHMRC. 2013b.

Schauer PR, Bhatt DL, Kirwan JP, Wolski K, Aminian A, Brethauer SA, et al. Bariatric surgery versus intensive medical therapy for diabetes - 5-year outcomes. N Engl J Med. 2017;376(7):641–51.

SIGN. Management of obesity. A national clinical guideline. Edinburgh: Scottish Intercollegiate Guidelines Network; 2010.

Sjostrom L, Narbro K, Sjostrom CD, Karason K, Larsson B, Wedel H, et al. Effects of bariatric surgery on mortality in Swedish obese subjects. N Engl J Med. 2007;357(8):741–52.

Wang MC, Guo XH, Zhang YW, Zhang YL, Zhang HH, Zhang YC. Laparoscopic Roux-en-Y gastric bypass versus sleeve gastrectomy for obese patients with type 2 diabetes: a meta-analysis of randomized controlled trials. Am Surg. 2015;81(2):166–71.

MIX
Papier aus verantwortungsvollen Quellen
Paper from responsible sources
FSC® C105338

If you have any concerns about our products,
you can contact us on
ProductSafety@springernature.com

In case Publisher is established outside the EU,
the EU authorized representative is:
Springer Nature Customer Service Center GmbH
Europaplatz 3, 69115 Heidelberg, Germany

Printed by Libri Plureos GmbH
in Hamburg, Germany